TEACHING PUBLIC HEALTH

TEACHING PUBLIC HEALTH

Edited by
LISA M. SULLIVAN AND **SANDRO GALEA**

JOHNS HOPKINS UNIVERSITY PRESS | *Baltimore*

© 2019 Johns Hopkins University Press
All rights reserved. Published 2019
Printed in the United States of America on acid-free paper
9 8 7 6 5 4 3 2 1

Johns Hopkins University Press
2715 North Charles Street
Baltimore, Maryland 21218-4363
www.press.jhu.edu

Library of Congress Cataloging-in-Publication Data

Names: Sullivan, Lisa M. (Lisa Marie), 1961–, editor. | Galea, Sandro, editor.
Title: Teaching public health / edited by Lisa M. Sullivan and Sandro Galea.
Description: Baltimore : Johns Hopkins University Press, [2019] | Includes
    bibliographical references and index.
Identifiers: LCCN 2018048634 | ISBN 9781421429809 (hardcover : alk. paper) |
    ISBN 1421429802 (hardcover : alk. paper) | ISBN 9781421429816 (electronic) |
    ISBN 1421429810 (electronic)
Subjects: | MESH: Public Health—education | Education, Public Health
    Professional—methods | Curriculum
Classification: LCC RA440 | NLM WA 18 | DDC 362.1071—dc23
LC record available at https://lccn.loc.gov/2018048634

A catalog record for this book is available from the British Library.

*Special discounts are available for bulk purchases of this book. For more information,
please contact Special Sales at 410-516-6936 or specialsales@press.jhu.edu.*

Johns Hopkins University Press uses environmentally friendly book materials,
including recycled text paper that is composed of at least 30 percent post-consumer
waste, whenever possible.

WE ARE INDEBTED to the editorial assistance of Angelina Casazza, without whom this book would not have been possible. Her attention to detail and care with every aspect of the book elevates the work, and we are forever in her debt. We thank our families always for their support as we took on this book, amid many other ongoing projects. LS in particular thanks her friends, family, and colleagues for their support. SG thanks Isabel Tess Galea, Oliver Luke Galea, and Dr. Margaret Kruk. Both editors would like to thank the amazing faculty, staff, students, and alumni of the Boston University School of Public Health for their commitment to excellence in public health education and learning, which is the inspiration for this book.

CONTRIBUTORS

LINDA ALEXANDER
School of Public Health,
West Virginia University,
Morgantown, WV

SUSAN ALTFELD
School of Public Health, University
of Illinois at Chicago, Chicago, IL

JESSICA S. ANCKER
Mailman School of Public Health,
Columbia University, New York, NY

LAUREN D. ARNOLD
College for Public Health and Social
Justice, Saint Louis University,
St. Louis, MO

MELISSA D. BEGG
Mailman School of Public Health,
Columbia University, New York, NY

ANGELA BRECKENRIDGE
School of Public Health and Tropical
Medicine, Tulane University,
New Orleans, LA

KATHRYN M. CARDARELLI
College of Public Health,
University of Kentucky,
Lexington, KY

ANGELA CARMAN
College of Public Health, University
of Kentucky, Lexington, KY

TREY CONATSER
College of Public Health,
University of Kentucky,
Lexington, KY

LORRAINE M. CONROY
School of Public Health,
University of Illinois at Chicago,
Chicago, IL

YVETTE C. COZIER
School of Public Health, Boston
University, Boston, MA

EUGENE DECLERCQ
School of Public Health, Boston
University, Boston, MA

MARIE DIENER-WEST
Bloomberg School of Public Health,
Johns Hopkins University,
Baltimore, MD

JEN DOLAN
School of Public Health and Health
Sciences, University of Massachusetts
at Amherst, Amherst, MA

GREG EVANS
Jiann-Ping Hsu College of Public
Health, Georgia Southern University,
Savannah, GA

JULIAN FISHER
Hannover Medical School, Germany

ELIZABETH FRENCH
Gillings School of Global Public
Health, University of North Carolina,
Chapel Hill, NC

SANDRO GALEA
School of Public Health, Boston
University, Boston, MA

DANIEL GERBER
School of Public Health and
Health Sciences, University of
Massachusetts at Amherst,
Amherst, MA

SOPHIE GODLEY
School of Public Health, Boston
University, Boston, MA

JACEY A. GREECE
School of Public Health, Boston
University, Boston, MA

PERRY N. HALKITIS
School of Public Health, Rutgers
University, Piscataway, NJ

JENNIFER HEBERT-BEIRNE
School of Public Health, University
of Illinois at Chicago, Chicago, IL

JYOTSNA JAGAI
School of Public Health, University
of Illinois at Chicago, Chicago, IL

KATHERINE JOHNSON
College of Arts and Sciences, Elon
University, Elon, NC

NANCY KANE
T. H. Chan School of Public Health,
Harvard University, Boston, MA

DAVID G. KLEINBAUM
Rollins School of Public Health,
Emory University, Atlanta, GA

WAYNE LAMORTE
School of Public Health, Boston
University, Boston, MA

MEG LANDFRIED
Gillings School of Global Public
Health, University of North Carolina,
Chapel Hill, NC

DELIA L. LANG
Rollins School of Public Health,
Emory University, Atlanta, GA

JOEL LEE
College of Public Health,
University of Georgia,
Athens, GA

LAURA LINNAN
Gillings School of Global Public
Health, University of North Carolina,
Chapel Hill, NC

LAURA MAGAÑA VALLADARES
Association of Schools and
Programs of Public Health,
Washington, DC

UCHECHI MITCHELL
School of Public Health, University
of Illinois at Chicago, Chicago, IL

BETH MORACCO
Gillings School of Global Public
Health, University of North Carolina,
Chapel Hill, NC

ROBERT PACK
College of Public Health, East
Tennessee State University,
Johnson City, TN

DONNA PETERSEN
College of Public Health, University
of South Florida, Tampa, FL

Silvia E. Rabionet
School of Public Health, University
of Puerto Rico, San Juan, PR, and
College of Pharmacy, Nova
Southeastern University, Fort
Lauderdale, FL

Elizabeth Reisinger Walker
Rollins School of Public Health,
Emory University,
Atlanta, GA

Richard Riegelman
Miliken Institute School of Public
Health, George Washington
University, Washington, DC

Kathleen Ryan
School of Public Health, Boston
University, Boston, MA

Nelly Salgado de Snyder
Instituto Nacional de Salud Pública,
Cuernavaca, México

Rachel Schwartz
Jiann-Ping Hsu College of Public
Health, Georgia Southern University,
Savannah, GA

Lisa M. Sullivan
School of Public Health, Boston
University, Boston, MA

Tanya Uden-Holman
College of Public Health, University
of Iowa, Iowa City, IA

Luann White
School of Public Health and Tropical
Medicine, Tulane University,
New Orleans, LA

James Wolff
School of Public Health, Boston
University, Boston, MA

Randy Wykoff, College of Public
Health, East Tennessee State
University, Johnson City, TN

PART I | THE PAST AND THE PRESENT

The Evolution of Public Health Teaching

LISA M. SULLIVAN AND SANDRO GALEA

ACADEMIC PUBLIC HEALTH has been growing steadily over the past seven decades. The first nine schools of public health were accredited in the 1940s, and the first program of public health was accredited in the 1960s (figure 1.1). By the end of the 1990s, there were 31 accredited schools and 32 accredited programs of public health. Ten years later, the counts were 38 and 68, respectively. Those numbers jumped to 50 and 92 over the next decade. As of 2017, there were 64 accredited schools and 115 accredited programs of public health, with more seeking accreditation each year. Nine stand-alone baccalaureate programs secured accreditation by 2017, and many more are currently in the applicant stage.

Interest in public health has also been growing at the undergraduate and graduate levels. Applications to accredited schools and programs have increased nearly eightfold over the past seven decades (figure 1.2). Unfortunately, data for specific degree levels were not available prior to 2010. In 2010, there were 38,588 applications to master's-level programs, which rose to 54,506 in 2017—more than a 40% increase.

Accredited schools and programs are producing more graduates than ever before (figure 1.3), with the sharpest increase seen in baccalaureate degrees. In 2017, nearly 8,000 undergraduates earned baccalaureate degrees in public health or a related discipline, almost 12,000 earned

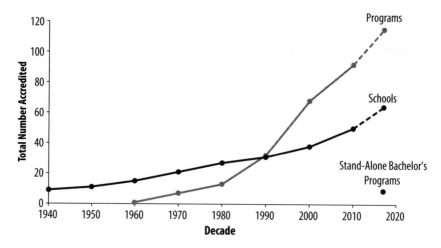

Figure 1.1. Growth in Accredited Schools and Programs of Public Health by Decade, 1940–2017

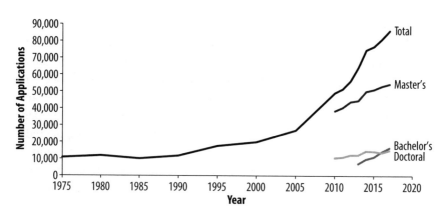

Figure 1.2. Growth in Applications to Schools and Programs of Public Health, 1975–2017

master's degrees, and 1,501 earned doctoral degrees in public health from accredited schools and programs of public health.

There are also more faculty engaged in public health education, research, and practice. In 1975, there were a reported 1,763 faculty at accredited schools and programs of public health. Unfortunately, data reporting was less reliable for faculty head count until about 2005

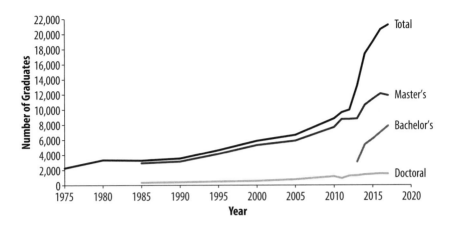

Figure 1.3. Graduates of CEPH-Accredited Schools and Programs of Public Health, 1975–2017

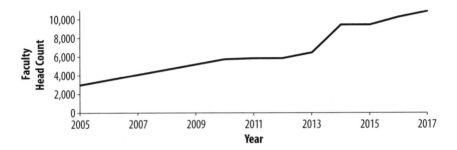

Figure 1.4. Faculty Head Count at Schools and Programs of Public Health

(figure 1.4). From 2005 to 2017, faculty headcounts increased more than threefold, from 2,976 in 2005 to 10,902 in 2017. Approximately half of the current faculty in accredited schools and programs of public health are female, and faculty represent a range of areas of expertise (figure 1.5).

Coincident with this growth, established graduate schools and programs of public health are redesigning curricula to meet the changing needs of incoming students and to ensure that graduates have the knowledge, skills, and attributes to meet the needs of a changing workforce. Rethinking pedagogy is as important as updating curricula. However, there have as yet been no books published that have focused

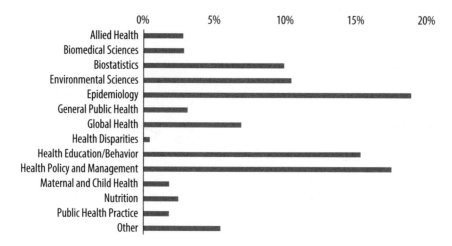

Figure 1.5. Faculty Areas of Expertise, 2017

directly on teaching public health. This book aims to fill that gap, bringing together a state-of-the-field collection of contributions that can serve as a touchstone for the rapid evolution of the field. The book aspires to provide teachers of public health and leaders in academic public health with a cutting-edge primer on the state of teaching public health and with resources that can inform and guide pedagogy in public health programs globally. This book provides academic leaders and experienced faculty with the conceptual underpinning and framing needed to advance curricula, and with the resources to train and support experienced and new faculty in innovative teaching methods. It builds on emerging trends in the field and anticipates where the field is headed, grounded in an appreciation of the importance of interdisciplinary teaching, lifelong learning, and the exigencies of practical skills-based training called for by a pragmatic discipline. The book summarizes the evolution of public health teaching over time, discusses unique challenges of public health teaching, addresses the principles and practice on state of the science for teaching public health at each level of education, highlights innovations in public health education, and looks to the future by anticipating trends in public health education and aiming to offer a resource that has enduring utility.

The Creation of Schools of Public Health

Despite their rapid recent growth, schools of public health are a relatively recent creation in the United States. The oldest schools are just over 100 years old and were developed to meet a specific need in society. In the early 1900s, medical schools and schools of nursing trained medical professionals who were called on to deal with the health issues of the time, mainly infectious diseases such as pneumonia and flu, tuberculosis, and gastrointestinal infections—the top three causes of death in 1900.[1] While the number of medical schools expanded and trained physicians continued to serve as public health officers to address epidemics, these physicians had no distinct training in public health to prepare them for this work.

In 1910, approximately 40% of people living in the South were infected with hookworm.[2] Charles Stiles,[3] a zoologist and parasitologist, convinced the Rockefeller Foundation to donate $1 million over five years to create the Rockefeller Sanitary Commission, whose primary—but not sole—objective was "to bring about a co-operative movement of the medical profession, public health officials, boards of trade, churches, schools, the press, and other agencies for the cure and prevention of hookworm disease."[4] Wyckliffe Rose,[5] a professor of history and philosophy, was named the first executive secretary of the Rockefeller Commission and recruited Abraham Flexner[6] as secretary to the Rockefeller Foundation's General Education Board.

In 1914, the General Education Board convened a meeting of 11 public health representatives, including Wyckliffe Rose, Abraham Flexner, William Welch,[7] Milton Rosenau,[8] and a number of Rockefeller trustees to discuss a separate and distinct curriculum for public health training. Several reports emerged from the meeting, detailing the distinct training needs for public health professionals, including the Welch-Rose report (published in 1915), which articulated a model for schools of public health separate from that of medical schools.[9,10]

The reports produced some differences of opinion regarding, for example, how schools should be organized, whether and to what extent they should connect with other schools within universities as well as with local and state health departments, and what the main focus of public health training should be.[11] Welch leaned toward a research focus and Rose toward public health practice. This tension persists in many schools and programs today, due in part to the need for schools and programs of public health to compete for research funding to support faculty who also teach.

In 1916, the Rockefeller Foundation committed more than $250,000 to establish the Johns Hopkins School of Public Health, and William Welch was named its first dean. The foundation later funded additional schools of public health, both in the United States and abroad. While the first schools of public health were oriented toward training medical professionals in public health, newer schools broadened their focus to address the practical and social needs of their local communities.

Academic Standards for Public Health Education

Accreditation of graduate professional public health programs in the United States began in 1945, when schools of public health were recognized by the American Public Health Association (APHA), the largest professional organization for public health in the country. In 1974, the APHA established the Council on Education for Public Health (CEPH), an independent organization created to handle the accreditation of schools (and, later, programs) of public health, and the Association of Schools of Public Health (ASPH), whose mission is "to strengthen the capacity of members by advancing leadership, excellence, and collaboration for academic public health."[12] In 2016, CEPH revised its accreditation criteria, focusing on more integrated and interdisciplinary competencies that better reflect public health practice of the time. The revised criteria will hold for at least the next five years and represent the most significant change in criteria since the establishment of CEPH.[13] The ASPH became the Association of Schools and Programs of Public Health (ASPPH) in 2013, representing CEPH-accredited schools, programs, and applicants for CEPH accreditation.

Unique Challenges in Public Health Teaching

Public health teaching faces several unique challenges. First, graduate public health is competency based, and these competencies—knowledge, skills, and attributes that graduates can demonstrate in a professional setting—evolve. Second, and related to the first, is the need for innovative and evidence-based pedagogy that meets the needs of a changing student body with varied learning styles. Third, faculty roles are evolving to support diverse students and deeper learning, and fourth, schools are balancing competing priorities to support faculty and educational staff. We briefly discuss each issue.

Since the beginning, public health training focused on preparing professionals to meet the needs of the workforce. As those needs change, so must curricula. Most schools, colleges, and universities have approvals that must be secured before curricular changes go into effect. New curricula need to be advertised to prospective students and appropriately communicated to continuing students well in advance of any implementation. Difficult does not quite describe the logistical challenges of anticipating future needs of public health professionals with sufficient lead time to design, approve, and implement training programs that remain relevant at launch. Adding to the challenge, while these adjustments in pedagogic scope may be right for students and the field, faculty complements may not always be well positioned to effectively execute new curricula, which complicates schools' and programs' ability to respond expeditiously to changing needs.

Innovative pedagogic approaches require that we rethink pedagogy as we update curricula and competencies to ensure that learners truly develop new competencies. Scott suggests a renewed focus on quality education, engaging learners, personalizing learning to meet the needs of different learning styles, and using project-based learning and effective educational technology to motivate and engage learners.[14] Deeper learning occurs when classroom material is applied to real-world, authentic problems. Different educational techniques are also more effective for teaching different content areas, applications, and skills. As curricula evolve, it becomes important to examine all of these factors to ensure that our educational infrastructure, including learning environments, faculty, educational staff, and students, is well positioned for success. In addition, schools and programs must engage in continuous examination of what, how, and why we teach the way we do.

Faculty roles also continue to evolve along with changing curricula and advances in educational technology. Faculty will always teach but are increasingly taking on the role of guide and mentor as well. As public health faculty are asked to teach across disciplinary boundaries—something that is called for more explicitly in current accreditation criteria as well as by potential employers—they must learn new areas and skills. An important element of the latter is in modeling professional confidence and openness to new applications and ideas. Faculty become learners alongside their students, creating more collaborative learning environments and instilling in students critical thinking and resiliency in the face of uncertainties.

While schools and programs of public health aim to recruit and support faculty with the requisite training and practical experiences to effectively teach interdisciplinary and emerging topics, they must face the financial realities of securing research grants and contracts to support faculty work. Sometimes schools and programs have had to invest in research at the expense of public health education and practice. At the same time, research dollars remain focused on medical applications and laboratory sciences and less so on public health and field- or community-based research, creating additional challenges for schools to secure research support, especially for community-based and practice applications.

Overarching Vision for Public Health Education

We recently proposed a vision for graduate public health education based on three principles: "1. Public health education is relevant, authentic and practical, 2. Public health education is inclusive, and 3. Public health education is ongoing," and outlined experiences at our institution in support of these three principles.[15] We suggest that our public health educational programs must prepare graduates to engage with emerging public health issues with knowledge, skills, humility, and personal and professional confidence. We must instill and cultivate a curiosity for ongoing learning that does not end with graduation. Public health curricula will and should evolve. Learning environments must expand beyond our classroom walls, faculty roles must evolve, and pedagogy must adapt. None of this can happen without commitment on the part of schools and administrators, more collaboration among public health faculty and educational staff, and more collaboration around best practices for teaching and learning in public health. This book aims to be a resource toward that end.

This Resource

The book is organized into four parts. In part I, we review the past and frame the present. We recap the distinct educational curricula that were devised for public health professionals and how public health is taught today, with attention to features and challenges that are unique to public health. We highlight the explosion of schools, programs, majors and minors, and partnerships between health departments and academic institutions, along with the coincident demand for qualified faculty. Part I also discusses the new accreditation requirements as a means to innovate in educational programs and approaches for continuous quality improvement.

In part II, we describe in detail the public health teaching continuum and the unique features and challenges at each level. Building a diverse public health workforce starts early. Future undergraduates will select majors based on their interests, aptitudes, and knowledge of careers and opportunities. We begin with techniques to engage high school students in public health, then discuss undergraduate education in public health, which has experienced growth at a staggering rate. We present approaches to undergraduate public health education within a liberal arts framework and as preprofessional training. Next, part II discusses the Master of Public Health (MPH), the most widely recognized public health degree, and its unique challenges as MPH curricula are evolving to include integrated core offerings, interdisciplinary training in an increasing number of specialties, and training in so-called soft skills. We then examine the Doctor of Public Health (DrPH), its growth in popularity, and the variations in DrPH programs across schools and programs. We discuss lifelong learning in public health as a way to ensure that public health graduates have enduring and productive careers. Finally, we address interprofessional education, which is increasingly and critically important for public health and other professionals in health and non-health-related fields.

In part III, we focus on strategies, best practices, and innovations in public health teaching. We begin with strategies for designing public health courses, techniques for developing competencies, devising rubrics to assess competency mastery, linking program competencies and course learning objectives, and developing in-class and out-of-class activities as well as assessments to ensure that students attain appropriate levels of learning. We then discuss techniques for maximizing student engagement, as engaged students make for a better classroom experience for both faculty and students. Next, techniques to develop students' respect for diversity, inclusivity, and cultural competence are discussed. We then focus on techniques that faculty can implement for more effective teaching in diverse classrooms, including acknowledging and appreciating diversity, building relationships, and tailoring teaching strategies to meet the needs of diverse learners.

Next, we discuss practice-based teaching and learning, which is an excellent way to connect education and practice, to build community relationships, and to enhance interdisciplinary teaching and learning. Techniques for faculty to develop learning partnerships and projects that promote deeper levels of learning across public health disciplines are outlined, and we then discuss teaching by the case method, which has proven to be an effective tool to prepare students for decision-making and leadership. We describe techniques for faculty to facilitate engagement with cases, probing for issues and comparisons of alternative solutions. Techniques for selecting appropriate cases and managing student participation are described. Recognizing that public health professionals must always work together, we next discuss group projects focusing on specific techniques to design and evaluate effective group projects across a range of public health disciplines. Related to group projects is team-based learning. The latter can be extremely effective when students are prepared to cooperate and self-manage. Popular models to guide effective teams while recognizing and appreciating diversity among public health students in what they bring to the classroom and respecting various learning styles are described.

No book on public health teaching would be complete without recognition of the difficult topics with which we must engage. Difficult conversations arise in all of our classrooms as we participate in challenging and complex public health issues. We explore techniques to foster, manage, and empower students and faculty to have respectful and constructive discussions within and outside of our classrooms. As our curricula evolve to meet the needs of the workforce, educational technology continues to advance at a rapid pace. Our students are facile with technologies and expect us to use the latest technologies in teaching. We discuss teaching with technology and strategies for incorporating technology in the classroom. We outline strategies to determine when, how, and why technology might be used along with examples of technologies that are particularly effective in public health teaching.

Collaborative teaching teams can make for outstanding classroom experiences. Teaching assistants (TAs) can have a positive influence on students and can assist a faculty member in all aspects of teaching. The TA can also benefit from the experience, as long as there are clearly articulated roles and responsibilities. We outline strategies for defining roles and responsibilities as well as tips for training TAs, including techniques to engage with students, manage difficult situations, use proper email etiquette, and manage difficult conversations.

As we continue to evolve courses and programs to meet the needs of the workforce, we must effectively evaluate courses and programs but also value the hard work of our faculty in teaching public health. Unfortunately, there is no simple system to evaluate teaching. Student course ratings are necessary but insufficient. We discuss the challenges of course ratings and describe multiple methods for evaluating and valuing public health teaching.

In part IV, we discuss the present and the future, with a focus on core issues, challenges, and potential solutions. Interest in public health is expected to continue to grow. Our students will have more choices in schools and programs to earn public health credentials. Accreditors set the floor for what is expected from our educational programs, but we posit that the field must aspire to much more. As curricula evolve and our graduates enter more and more sectors of the workforce, we need to ensure that curricula align with core principles, create more opportunities to connect, and provide outstanding public health education to an increasingly diverse student body. Public health education of the future must be attainable across the life course. Ensuring a healthy public requires an educated citizenry. Schools and programs train public health professionals, but real change will come from communities and from public and private sectors coming together. We describe strategies to communicate public health principles and knowledge to wider audiences as well as techniques to continue to provide lifelong learning opportunities to our graduates as well as other professionals.

REFERENCES

1. Tippett, R. "Mortality and Cause of Death, 1900 v. 2010." Carolina Demography, UNC Carolina Population Center, June 16, 2014, http://demography .cpc.unc.edu/2014/06/16/mortality-and-cause-of-death-1900-v-2010/.

2. The Rockefeller Foundation. "Eradicating Hookworm." https://rockfound .rockarch.org/eradicating-hookworm (accessed November 15, 2017).

3. USDA National Agricultural Library, Special Collections. "Charles W. Stiles." https://www.nal.usda.gov/exhibits/speccoll/exhibits/show/parasitic-diseases-with -econom/item/8206 (accessed November 6, 2017).

4. The Rockefeller Foundation. "By-Laws of the Rockefeller Commission for the Eradication of Hookworm Disease: RG III 2, Series O, Box 52, File 544." https://rockfound.rockarch.org/digital-library-listing/-/asset_publisher/yYxpQ feI4W8N/content/by-laws-of-the-rockefeller-commission-for-the-eradication-of -hookworm-disease (accessed November 15, 2017).

5. The Rockefeller Foundation: A Digital History. "Wickliffe Rose." https:// rockfound.rockarch.org/biographical/-/asset_publisher/6ygcKECNI1nb/content /wickliffe-rose? (accessed November 16, 2017).

6. Encyclopedia Britannica. "Abraham Flexner." https://www.britannica.com /biography/Abraham-Flexner (accessed November 16, 2017).

7. Johns Hopkins Bloomberg School of Public Health. "William Henry Welch, MD." https://www.jhsph.edu/about/history/heroes-of-public-health/william-henry -welch.html (accessed December 11, 2017).

8. Centers for Disease Control. "Milton J. Rosenau, M.D." Morbidity and Mortality Weekly Report. 1999. https://www.cdc.gov/mmwr/preview/mmwrhtml /mm4840b1.htm (accessed December 11, 2017).

9. Rosenau, M. J. "Courses and Degrees in Public Health Work." *Journal of the American Medical Association* 64, no. 10 (1915): 794–796.

10. Welch, W. H., and W. Rose. "Institute of Hygiene: A Report to the General Education Board of Rockefeller Foundation." New York: Rockefeller Foundation, 1915.

11. Hunter, D. J., and J. Frenk. "The Birth of Public Health Education." *Journal of the American Medical Association* 313, no. 11 (2015): 1105–1106.

12. Association of Schools and Programs of Public Health. "About." https:// www.aspph.org/about/ (accessed December 12, 2017).

13. Krisberg, K. "New Criteria for Accreditation to Chart Updated Course for Public Health Education: Bolstering Students." *Nation's Health* (2017): 1–10.

14. Scott, C. L. "The Futures of Learning 3: What Kind of Pedagogies for the 21st Century?" UNESCO Education Research and Foresight. 2015. ERF Working Papers Series, No. 15. http://unesdoc.unesco.org/images/0024/002431/243126E .pdf.

15. Sullivan, L., and S. Galea. "A Vision for Graduate Public Health Education." *Journal of Public Health Management and Practice* 23, no. 6 (2017): 553–555.

[2]

The Current State of Public Health Education

PUBLIC HEALTH is an ever-dynamic field and one notoriously difficult to define. It is also richly interdisciplinary and, in practice, engages multiple sectors, often in systems-level approaches. Public health demands professionals and leaders who are agile and adaptable, excellent communicators, skilled in the methods of public health science and practice, and both competent and confident with a natural inquisitiveness that enables them to continually learn and grow. This creates a significant challenge for those who seek to educate and prepare students and professionals for success in this field, which itself is constantly changing and subject to myriad external forces. Despite opinions to the contrary,[1] most believe public health is a profession, yet employers often decry the lack of professional preparation in the degree programs offered by academic public health programs. Further confounding this situation are the rigid structures imposed within higher education that make it challenging to respond quickly to community needs or student demands. The process of accreditation, designed to ensure and promote quality, is often viewed as a burdensome activity that stifles innovation. Yet, the institutions themselves and sometimes the faculty within them may be slow to adapt, even when the imperative for change is clearly evident and the flexibility to innovate is provided. These and other related issues have been the topic of intense conversation in the United

15

States over the past several years aiming to discover the best means to reshape education in public health for the future. In this chapter, we discuss the current state of education in public health within this context and explore the various factors that can and do create opportunities for transformation.

The 2016 Accreditation Movement

The 1915 Welch-Rose report,[2] supported by the Rockefeller Foundation and following closely on the heels of the Flexner report,[3] outlined the original blueprint for schools of public health and "institutes of hygiene" in the United States. This seminal report outlined a curriculum for a Master of Public Health (MPH) degree and also, presciently, for a Doctor of Public Health (DrPH) degree to assure the ongoing development of the knowledge base to support this growing field. Several schools emerged in response to this report, at such venerable institutions as Johns Hopkins University (where William Welch was dean of the medical school), Harvard University, the Massachusetts Institute of Technology (MIT), and Vanderbilt University. Growth in the number of schools of public health was slow, yet concern for the quality of programs led to calls for an accreditation mechanism in the 1940s, which the American Public Health Association (APHA) agreed to oversee.[4] In the 1970s, the then Association of Schools of Public Health (ASPH) partnered with the APHA to form an independent accrediting organization, the Council on Education for Public Health (CEPH). Accredited by the United States Department of Education, CEPH's purpose has been and continues to be to assure the quality of the educational experience for students as well as the quality of the educational product for the public.

Linked initially to the medical profession and intended to prepare physicians to serve as health officers, the core curricular elements of the Welch-Rose–style MPH were complementary to clinical training: epidemiology and biostatistics to scientifically examine the distribution of disease and the factors contributing to it, environmental sanitation and hygiene to address the control of communicable diseases, and health administration to promote necessary management skills. It would be decades before the social and behavioral scientists effectively lobbied for a focus on chronic disease and, by extension, behavior management and primary prevention. Thus evolved the five core disciplines that served as the backbone for public health education in the United States and the cornerstone of accreditation criteria for decades. These disciplines— biostatistics, epidemiology, environmental health science, health administration, and the social and behavioral sciences—dictated the organization of schools and MPH programs, the recruitment of faculty, the core curriculum, and the MPH concentrations. Concerned that students were not necessarily being afforded opportunities to understand how these disciplines worked in practice nor how they could or would be utilized and applied harmoniously in addressing public health challenges, the accreditors strongly emphasized the need for integrative experiences and field placements as part of master's-level training in public health.

This discipline-constructed model resulted in relative uniformity across schools and programs, from the 1970s to the 2010s. Well into the '90s, many of these MPH programs in schools or programs could be completed in a year if the students came with advanced degrees. Beginning in the 1980s, several schools began offering more comprehensive master's degrees to students without advanced credentials in an effort to prepare professionals for the growing number of jobs at the program or middle management level. These degrees required more credit hours, longer internships, and more in-depth projects, but because of the intended outcome—graduates prepared to contribute to the profession of public health—they were considered professional degrees by the accreditors.

However, faculty members (most of whom, by definition, were discipline trained and discipline focused) did not always embrace the MPH as a professional degree and did not always take seriously the requirement to link classroom learning to real-world experience—experience many faculty members in schools of public health did not themselves have. This disconnect was pointedly brought to light in the 1988 Institute of Medicine report titled *The Future of Public Health*, and although some progress had been made to better connect the field of practice to the institutions that prepared professionals for that field, the basic model of public health education did not substantively change.[5]

It was within this context that the Framing the Future initiative was born in 2011; acknowledging the rapid growth in undergraduate public health programs, the uncomfortable feeling that the MPH had grown stale, and the significant changes occurring in public health practice, higher education, and the world at large, the initiative was intended to reexamine and create a new vision for education in public health to co-incide with the one hundredth anniversary of the Welch-Rose report in 2015. Representing academia, government, employers, and partners, the Framing the Future task force recommended an inclusive process that engaged as many constituents as possible in the conversation.[6,7,8] These conversations and activities included task force meetings, seven expert panels and a Blue Ribbon Employer Advisory Board, presentations at various national conferences, an interactive website, and 50 town halls that engaged hundreds of people in the process of rethinking education in public health. Every draft of every expert panel report was widely disseminated for review, comment, and input. Webinars enabled continuing conversation on each subject, and presentations at ASPH meetings throughout the process ensured the full participation of the member schools and programs. Related efforts by partner organizations (e.g., the Council on Linkages between Academia and Public Health Practice, the Public Health Accreditation Board, the Association of State and Territorial Health Officials, the National Board of Public Health Examiners, and the Interprofessional Education Consortium) were integrated into the task force's work, and representatives of CEPH were active participants to assure alignment with what would ultimately be reflected in accreditation criteria.

The Framing the Future task force conducted its formative work from the fall of 2011 to the spring of 2015. CEPH began an equally rigorous process of reviewing accreditation criteria for schools and programs beginning in 2014, taking full advantage of the work already done by the task force. CEPH mounted an inclusive campaign—unprecedented in its history—utilizing webinars, town halls, ad hoc work groups, and four rounds of public comment. The result, released in October 2016, was the most significant revision of accreditation criteria since the organization's founding.[9]

The 2016 criteria responded both to the recommendations of the Framing the Future expert panels and to persistent concerns of the accredited schools and programs. Beyond the necessary focus on quality assurance, the council addressed the reporting burden expressed by accredited institutions and the desire for more flexibility in curricular design and degree programs offered. The council agreed early in the process to continue to accredit schools (somewhat unique in the accreditation arena, as nearly every other specialty accreditor focuses solely on degree programs) but also clarified that the emphasis of the quality review would be on the public health degree programs—any bachelor's in public health degree offered, the MPH, and the doctoral degree in public health offered by the school. Data reporting was reduced in all areas and limited to those elements required by the US Department of Education and to those needed to determine the requisite level of quality being assured. Wherever possible, schools and programs were given choices of performance metrics to report or were asked to provide examples rather than exhaustive lists.

Of equal if not greater importance were the changes in curricular criteria. For the first time, the new criteria included guidelines for the DrPH degree and clearly distinguished it from the more traditional, disciplinary-focused research PhD, establishing the DrPH as the advanced practice degree in public health. Criteria for undergraduate degrees in public health, wherever offered, were made consistent. Changes in the MPH criteria allowed greater flexibility and were designed explicitly to encourage innovation. Of particular note, in response to the clarion call of Framing the Future to dispense with the five core discipline model, CEPH responded with an entirely new approach to the MPH core curriculum, MPH concentrations, and the calculation of faculty resources needed to assure a quality educational experience.

A New Innovative MPH

It is important to reiterate that the changes formalized in accreditation criteria in 2016 were neither arbitrary nor capricious. They were the result of an intense series of conversations and deliberations on the part of every major organization in the fields of public health, health professions education, and higher education. Still, resistance to change is part of the human condition, and transformation is easier said than done. For decades preceding these efforts, schools of public health followed a relatively simple formula: within each of the five core disciplines, recruit at least five faculty, deliver a core course, and offer an MPH concentration. The new criteria intentionally allow for many approaches to delivering a core curriculum, offer no proscription on concentrations, and, beyond a minimum number (25 full-time faculty), ask only for evidence that the faculty are qualified to teach the concentrations offered. While some faculty inertia is to be expected and makes radical change difficult to achieve, this reticence is further compounded by structural impediments to rapid change in the academy; enforced catalogs, fixed calendars, credit hour strictures, financial aid requirements, and tenure all pose challenges to be overcome. Conversely, early adopters can consider a wide array of innovations such as competency-based assessments for credit, online delivery modalities, just-in-time credentialing, digital badges, community-based experiential learning, flipped classrooms, active learning environments, team-taught courses, and integrated curricula. Any and all of these can be utilized in the design of entirely new concentrations within the MPH, optimizing faculty strengths, community needs, and student interest. If schools no longer have to offer an MPH in environmental health, they can choose to offer an MPH in ecosystem health, climate change, or exposure science. Further, schools can consider entirely new approaches with MPH concentrations in human rights or social justice, in behavioral health or law and policy, in aging or women's health, or in population health science or data analytics. At the same time, across the country, as schools and programs experiment with innovative approaches to a core curriculum, the new criteria assure that regardless of the style or the format of a core curriculum, MPH students will share a common foundational knowledge and competence in a set of skills promoted by a diverse array of organizations committed to elevating the professional practice of public health.

Further advancing these ideals, the new criteria clarify the need for MPH students to have multiple experiences in the world of practice and an opportunity to synthesize and apply foundational and specialization competencies in a culminating project. Acknowledging that for some students in some concentrations, such a project may resemble a research project conducted as part of a larger research study in the community or on campus, the required practice experiences are intended to assure that all students gain exposure to and an appreciation for how evidence is translated into practice and how the public's concerns about their health inform the ongoing study of various approaches to persistent and emerging population health challenges. In effect, the new criteria eschew the age-old arguments that research experiences on topics of public health importance are the real legitimate public health practice experiences, instead opting to simply ask for evidence that students have had practice experiences during their educational journeys, regardless of the nature of their capstone projects.

Public Health Education without Walls

Unlike the education programs of other health professions, students in public health degree programs do not typically rotate through representative practice sites (e.g., teaching hospitals, ambulatory care centers, rehabilitation facilities). Yet, because public health is practiced in the community, students are literally surrounded by natural laboratories in which they can exercise their new skills and experience real-world challenges in myriad settings. Perhaps the abundance of opportunities overwhelms academic systems because the educational journey of public health students has not always provided ready opportunities to engage in practice, either within courses, through extracurricular activities, or through internships. Accreditation criteria have required students in MPH programs to complete formal field experiences for many years, but, as noted previously, without sufficient systems nor structures, such experiences often took the form of data analysis or research assistantships under the supervision of school faculty. While such experiences may well have afforded students important opportunities to hone research-related skills, they failed to provide the intended practical experience in the field. Seeking to rectify this gap in the educational experience, in 2003 ASPH, with funding support from the Centers for Disease Control and Prevention, solicited proposals to build collaboration between state and local health departments and schools of public health.[10] Though streamlining the identification of appropriate practica and the placement of students in them was one objective of the academic health department, joint research, faculty-practitioner collaboration, and more formalized workforce development approaches were also objectives of interest. Resources are available on the website of the Public Health Foundation's Council on Linkages, which has supported, since 2011, the Academic Health Department Learning Community, organized to provide support for the development, maintenance, and growth of these partnerships.

In similar fashion and beyond traditional health departments, many schools and programs have developed partnerships with other community-based organizations to provide ongoing opportunities for students to rotate through, working on projects of local import and contributing to efforts to meet local needs while gaining valuable practical skills. Such organizations can include other governmental entities (e.g., school districts, environmental agencies, human service agencies), nonprofit organizations, or healthcare companies.

Clearly, experiences in the world of practice can be manifold and are not necessarily bound in time or within credit or contact hour requirements. Students are encouraged to select experiences that meet particular competencies they wish to develop, reflecting the principle of greater flexibility that guided the criteria revisions. Opening students to a variety of opportunities to learn and gain experience outside of the classroom should open the entire school or program to greater engagement with the communities they serve and outreach beyond the campus borders. In this way, learning should begin to merge more fully with the service/practice mission of the public health academic institution, further promoting the health of the community while enhancing the education of the students. Giving students the tools to help them learn how to learn, how to think, how to act, and how to be may be the most important curricular enhancement advanced by the Framing the Future initiative and the revised CEPH criteria.

Empowering a New Public Health Faculty

Leadership is clearly necessary and perhaps critical in facilitating the types of transformations intended for public health education. Yet a hallmark of the academy is shared governance, and the role of faculty in curricular matters has long been considered sacrosanct. These cultures have served our institutions well during periods of relative calm, assuring consistency of approach and the integrity of the academic enterprise. In today's world, where our knowledge grows at breakneck speed, information is literally a fingertip (or tap) away, employers are looking for workers who know how to do what they need done at that moment, and students are seeking more meaningful learning experiences, academic institutions need to find ways to be more nimble and more responsive while assuring a solid, quality, academic product. This creates a tension, particularly given the traditional nature of the academy to be deliberative and to subject every proposal to intense scrutiny and robust debate. The revised accreditation criteria were built on the expectation that degree programs would be designed around community needs, student interests, and faculty strengths, understanding that at any given point in time these ideals can and will be in conflict. Community needs can and do change, and student interests are as varied as the incoming class of students each year, but the process by which faculty are recruited, retained, and promoted rewards stability and often an intense focus in a particular area of inquiry. Indeed, the intensity of the effort required to develop a national or international reputation in a clearly defined area of expertise (typically the sine qua non for the granting of tenure) is manifestly contradictory to the need to be responsive to the changing passions of students and emerging challenges in the public health environment. All this exists on top of the persistent discomfort of research-oriented faculty being asked to develop skilled public health professionals.

There are several ways to address these challenges and move toward improving the quality of the educational experience in professional degree programs and encouraging innovation in instruction. Universities themselves and various professional organizations are investing in faculty development programs, particularly around the use of technology. As more and more students demand online options to comport with their work and personal schedules, more and more faculty are being asked to convert learning opportunities to these platforms. This demand has led to the advancement of software packages and new professionals in instructional design and instructional technology. This advanced knowledge and capacity then bleeds into traditional classrooms, as it should, providing new opportunities to promote alternative learning environments in campus-based classrooms. Flipped classes in which content is delivered online prior to class meetings, which can then be used for active learning, are increasing in popularity. These platforms also allow for more creative assignments and assessments beyond quizzes and written papers. Students can develop photo essays, podcasts, or other media-based responses to problems posed, or can design interventions using social media. This speaks to the need for schools and programs to invest in sustainable faculty development programs that enable faculty to competently utilize ever-present and ever-changing sophisticated learning technologies for the advanced education of their students.

Another way to build a more innovative faculty is to recruit faculty who have been trained in more innovative programs and who are comfortable with such approaches as team teaching, technology-enhanced learning, and higher-level assessments. These faculty can serve as important role models or can be given leadership opportunities within the teaching mission of the school or program. Such faculty should also be encouraged to publish in this arena and contribute to the scholarship of learning. The lack of publications by public health educators was a criticism levied at the field in the Lancet Commission report on global public health education,[11] a criticism the field is responding to, albeit rather slowly.

A third way to build a more practice-focused faculty is to engage practitioners in the academic enterprise. Schools and programs often have advisory boards of one sort or another, typically devoted to fundraising or to building community partnerships for research or student career development. Leading practitioners in the community of interest to the school or program should convene to inform and evaluate the curricula for the professional degree programs. Leading practitioners can also be engaged directly in the classroom; many schools and programs feature practitioners as speakers in "grand rounds" or "dean's symposia" series and as guest lecturers, but increasingly, schools and programs are utilizing field-based experts as instructors of record or co-instructors in more intensive ways. Schools and programs are also increasingly developing faculty pathways for leading practitioners with such titles as "professor of the practice" or "practice scholar in residence." Engaging leading practitioners as part of the faculty can change the conversation and ultimately the culture around both the preparation of professionals for public health practice and around the research enterprise, which could, perhaps, be more practice focused. In the words of Dr. Larry Green: "If we want more evidence-based practice, we need more practice-based evidence."[12]

Conclusion

Education in public health should be as dynamic, innovative, and demanding as the field itself. Persistent and emerging challenges to the public's health increasingly call for skilled professionals who are creative and collaborative, nimble and trustworthy, and comfortable with uncertainty and ambiguity. The conversation that began in 1915 continues as academic public health institutions now seek to adapt to a new paradigm, enforced through transformative accreditation criteria. Responding quickly to changing community needs and evolving student interests is challenging in an environment that rewards stability and deliberative processes within the faculty. Scholars and teachers in public health must achieve a balance that promotes a high-quality education within academic norms while assuring professionals are prepared for the work of public health within practice norms. Such educational efforts must also be accompanied by equally vigorous efforts to build the knowledge base for practice, effectively linking education with research with practice and back again. It is incumbent on public health educators to embrace the change that happens in the field and to prepare not only the next generation of professionals but also the next generation of educators to successfully negotiate these different worlds and the challenges found therein. To that end, it is also important that public health educators engage in scholarship around pedagogy and contribute to the evidence base around how best to teach an applied science to a diverse array of students.[13]

REFERENCES

1. Sommer, A. "W(h)ither Public Health?" *Public Health Reports* 110, no. 6 (Nov–Dec 1995): 657–661.

2. Welch, W. H., and W. Rose. "Institute of Hygiene: A Report to the General Education Board of Rockefeller Foundation." New York: Rockefeller Foundation, 1915.

3. Flexner, A. "Medical Education in the United States and Canada: A Report to the Carnegie Foundation for the Advancement of Teaching." New York: Carnegie Foundation, 1910.

4. Council on Education for Public Health. https://ceph.org/about/org-info/ (accessed November 24, 2018).

5. Institute of Medicine. "The Future of Public Health." Washington, DC: National Academy Press, 1988.

6. Association of Schools and Programs of Public Health. "Framing the Future." https://www.aspph.org/teach-research/framing-the-future/ (accessed March 25, 2018).

7. Petersen, D. J., and E. M. Weist. "Framing the Future by Mastering the New Public Health." *Journal of Public Health Management and Practice* 20, no. 4 (2014): 371–374.

8. Council on Education for Public Health. "Accreditation Criteria: Schools and Programs of Public Health." Silver Spring, MD: CEPH, 2016. https://ceph.org/assets/2016.Criteria.pdf (accessed March 25, 2018).

9. Association of Schools and Programs of Public Health. "Blue Ribbon Public Health Employers Advisory Board: Summary of Interviews." 2013. https://www

.aspph.org/ftf-reports/blue-ribbon-employer-advisory-board-report/ (accessed March 25, 2018).

10. Conte, C., C. S. Chang, J. Malcolm, and P. G. Russo. "Academic Health Departments: From Theory to Practice." *Journal of Public Health Management and Practice* 12, no. 1 (2006): 6–14.

11. Frenk, J., L. Chen, Z. A. Bhutta, J. Cohen, N. Crisp, T. Evans, H. Fineberg, et al. "Health Professionals for a New Century: Transforming Education to Strengthen Health Systems in an Interdependent World." *Lancet* 376, no. 9756 (2010): 1923–1958.

12. Green, L. W. "Public Health Asks of Systems Science: To Advance Our Evidence-Based Practice, Can You Help Us Get More Practice-Based Evidence?" *American Journal of Public Health* 96, no. 3 (2006): 406–409.

13. Merzel, C., P. Halkitis, and C. Healton. "Pedagogical Scholarship in Public Health: A Call for Cultivating Learning Communities to Support Evidence-Based Education." *Public Health Reports* 132, no. 6 (2017): 679–683.

[3]

A Conceptual Orientation to Public Health Teaching

ROBERT PACK AND RANDY WYKOFF

WHILE MANY pedagogical principles hold as true for public health training as they do for other academic areas, there are fundamental differences that necessitate alternative approaches to the conceptualization, design, and implementation of an effective education program for a public health practitioner. Effective public health education needs to be different than either a liberal arts or a clinical sciences education. The greatest difference from the liberal arts is that public health education must explicitly provide an educational experience that prepares its graduates with a defined set of practical skills necessary for success in a specific job market. The greatest difference from the clinical sciences is in the wider range of professions and professional settings available to public health graduates. While one might argue that a pediatrician is as different from an orthopedic surgeon as a healthcare administrator is from a biostatistician, the former are both practitioners with a clinical scope of work. The public health practitioner must be trained to work in a wide range of professional areas and professional settings. Graduates of public health programs may work in settings as diverse as hospitals, pharmaceutical companies, institutes of higher learning, environmental protection agencies, state and local public health departments, and nonprofit organizations. Regardless of work setting or industry sector, public health graduates must also have a basic understanding (or mastery, depending on their academic level) of the broad range of essential technical public health skills including epidemiology, biostatistics, environmental health, health administration, health behavior change, and many others. Additionally, to be successful in the workplace, graduates must also possess crosscutting skills that are necessary for professional success, including teamwork, professionalism, problem-solving, communication skills, and innovation, among others.

To assure that its graduates can function effectively across disciplinary areas and in multiple work settings, public health educators must provide a wide range of applied skills and an equally broad knowledge-base for their graduates. It is not enough, for example, for a graduate to simply have an understanding of a theory of adult behavior change—the graduate must also understand how to apply that theory in a range of professional settings and in a wide range of communities. The demonstration of the combination of knowledge, skills, and abilities must also be assessed to assure competency in essential domains.

To this end, a public health education must provide its graduates with the foundational knowledge necessary to understand the breadth and importance of the broad field of public health, the training in specialized skills and techniques required for the specific job market that the graduate will enter, and the crosscutting professional capabilities and competencies necessary in almost all professional settings. Here, we explore how these diverse goals can be achieved through a practice-based conceptual orientation to public health training.

Public Health Teaching: Initial Design

The starting point in designing a public health training program should be an understanding of the specific needs of the public health workforce. While these needs can be approximated by reviewing public health training programs at other institutions and, to a lesser extent, by reviewing the requirements of various accrediting bodies, there is really no substitute for a direct survey of existing public health employers in the region of the training program. Each type of environment—urban, peri-urban, rural—and each state or region of the country offer different employment opportunities for public health graduates. Public health training programs must, therefore, carefully assess the needs of their unique regional employers and assure that their program provides graduates with those skills that employers deem most important. When a significant portion of graduates are employed outside the region, public health training programs should, to the extent possible, assess the needs of those more distant employers. This does not mean, of course, that programs must provide only those skills, but it must assure that, at a minimum, those who are most likely to hire the program's graduates have a level of confidence that their new employees possess the skills they need.

Identification of employers to survey starts with understanding where previous graduates (for existing programs) or potential graduates (for new programs) have been, or are likely to be, employed. Trainees from the Bachelor of Science (BS) in Public Health program at the authors' institution, for example, are more commonly employed in hospital settings (30%) than in governmental public health (14%). Only 22% go on, within two years of graduation, to graduate or professional school. However, trainees from the BS in Environmental Health program at the same institution are much more likely to work in the government sector (38%) or for a for-profit agency such as a laboratory or health service organization (19%). Conversely, trainees from the BS in Health Sciences program, which includes microbiology and human health concentrations, are more likely to immediately pursue further graduate or professional education (47%). In each case, the expectations and requirements of the specific employers or the specific graduate schools must be carefully assessed and, through a systematic process, addressed by curricular revisions. Additional insight can be gathered by interviewing alumni once they are established in the workforce. What skills have been most valuable to them? In what area(s) did they feel underprepared? In what ways do they feel that they are better prepared, or less well prepared, than their counterparts from other degree programs or from other institutions? For programs that require a field experience (which we strongly recommend for all levels of public health training), additional insight about curricula can be provided by the students' preceptors and, importantly, from the students themselves. For example, at the authors' institution, students returning from their field experience are required to include specific recommendations for program improvement in their presentations.

Through this iterative process, program leaders can make significant changes to the curricula, both to meet the existing needs of the workforce and also to assure that programs remain relevant as the workforce evolves.[1]

Public Health Teaching: Academic Level

Because public health is taught at so many levels—from the associate's degree to the doctoral degree—it is important that educational programs teach both skills and content at a level that is appropriate for the learner. Following is a brief overview of Bloom's taxonomy along with an explanation of how the model is used to inform the development of competencies at different levels of public health education.

The educational psychologist Benjamin Bloom and his colleague articulated the hierarchy of cognitive learning (knowledge) by positing that knowledge, comprehension, application, analysis, synthesis, and evaluation represent increasing levels of understanding, and that objectives for educational activities should be commensurate with expectations for the level of the student.[2,3] This intuitive hierarchy is commonly referred to as Bloom's taxonomy. For example, a high school student would not necessarily be asked to evaluate the impact of a social program or synthesize the importance of public health regulations with social needs or norms any more than a doctoral student would be expected to pursue a series of overview courses in the form of a typical general education curriculum for undergraduates.

While the cognitive domain is conceptually distinct from the psychomotor domain wherein skills are taught, the reality is that core, crosscutting, and soft skills must be acquired alongside both knowledge and abilities. Knowledge, skills, and abilities are all component parts of the educational standard model of competency that are understood to define requirements for success in a workplace.

Formal degree program levels such as bachelor's or master's degrees require different levels of training and have different expectations of graduates, and, accordingly, should provide different levels of focus on application. Specifically, learning objectives should be mapped onto the Bloom's taxonomic level associated with the level of the degree. That is not to say that trainees at the bachelor's degree level should not be asked to synthesize concepts. They can and should, to some extent. But a doctoral student should focus on synthesis and evaluation to a much greater extent than a bachelor's degree student. In the following paragraphs, we briefly differentiate the scope of work for different levels of training in the context of applied public health education and workforce readiness. Each level will be elaborated on in subsequent chapters.

The associate's-degree level appears to be emerging as a potential workforce preparatory degree to address several technical and support roles required in the public health workforce. Model curricula have been authored and disseminated by the Association of Schools and Programs of Public Health (ASPPH) and the League for Innovation in the Community College.[4] Though this is an evolving field, degree names appear to be very specific to public health functions, such as healthcare navigator, health information technician, or environmental health specialist. In addition to academic preparation, workforce readiness for graduates at this level should include an introduction to job opportunities, an overview of public health systems, and an introduction to the crosscutting skills necessary for workforce success.

Bachelor's-level degrees have been the fastest growing segment of public health degrees in the past decade. For example, the de Beaumont Foundation and the ASPPH have shown a 750% increase in public health bachelor's degree conferrals between 1992 and 2012.[5] There are a wide variety of conceptual approaches to the bachelor's degree from institutions with a liberal education approach[6] to those with a professional education approach.[7] Bachelor's degree curricula also show great variability in terms of organizational structure and content, but they are increasingly aligned with the accreditation standards from the Council on Education for Public Health and the "Critical Component Elements" defined by the ASPPH.[8] In addition to academic preparation, workforce readiness should include direct exposure to the diversity of the public health workforce, preceptor-guided real-world projects, and direct exposure to the diverse skills needed to succeed in the workforce.

The Master of Public Health (MPH) degree is the traditional graduate-level professional education degree for public health practitioners. The history of the MPH, and related master's degrees, is well documented, but it is worth mentioning that the degree was historically attained by those with previous clinical training. For example, in the mid-twentieth century, more than half of the graduates of MPH programs were physicians, contrasted with a minority today.[9] Today, the market for non-clinically prepared MPH graduates is strong, and the MPH is widely recognized as a professional degree. The accreditation standards for the

MPH have recently been revised to reflect the changing landscape of professional-level public health jobs.

The Doctor of Public Health (DrPH) degree and PhDs in the various disciplines of public health are the terminal degrees in the field. The difference between the two approaches has been addressed extensively elsewhere.[10] The DrPH is often pursued by individuals with previous practice experience and is usually focused on leadership, policy development, intervention evaluation, and systems-level approaches to public health challenges. In addition to being qualified for more senior positions in the same fields that hire those with master's and undergraduate training, those with doctoral degrees in public health are often qualified for academic or research positions in higher education. At the authors' university, about half of DrPH graduates initially accept positions in higher education, with the other half initially taking field-based positions. In addition to academic preparation, DrPH programs should include preparation for major leadership roles with integrative peer- and preceptor-guided projects, exploratory writing assignments on issues of evolving public health importance, mastery of the crosscutting skills necessary for workforce success, and substantive research or evaluation experience. Given that it is the terminal degree in public health and its holders will be tasked with ensuring the quality of the overall federal, state, and local public health systems, including the education of the workforce, DrPH graduates should understand concepts and approaches for public health workforce development, education, and training.

Public Health Teaching: Institutional Alignment

In addition to reflecting the needs of regional employers, degree program priorities should reflect the unique aspects of the mission of the institution. Most readers will recognize the Carnegie Classification of Institutions of Higher Education (http://carnegieclassifications.iu.edu/), which categorizes the more than 4,600 two- and four-year colleges and universities in the United States based on characteristics of degrees offered and the research environment of the host institution. These include such categories of Doctoral Universities (only 335, or 7% of the total in 2015), Master's Colleges and Universities (741, 16%), Baccalaureate (583, 13%), Baccalaureate/Associate's (408, 9%) and Associate's (1,113, 24%). At the time of this writing, 171 different institutions offer degree programs in public health that are accredited by the Council on Education for Public Health. While the majority of these institutions are classified as Doctoral Universities or Master's Colleges or Universities, their degree programs are not the same, in part, because of differences in the missions of the host institutions. Institutional missions are highly variable, often influenced by institutional history, regional needs, proximity to an underserved population, other geographical characteristics, or even long-term aspirations. A public health program at a large doctoral university may focus on research and discovery to a greater extent than one located at a smaller doctoral university or at a master's college or university, which may, in part, focus more specifically on training the workforce to address more regional health needs. Whatever the mission of the institution, however, programmatic educational and research activities should be aligned with that mission. As a concrete example, the authors' parent institution is a regional doctoral university that has a mission statement with an extremely strong focus on regional stewardship—making a real difference in the health, education, and well-being of the people of Central Appalachia. Educational programs, research, and service activities of the college are thus aligned with this mission in that they are applied, community focused, often responsive to local or regional health needs, and typically interprofessional. The college, the other health sciences units, and the university overall are deeply integrated into the local community, creating opportunities for community engagement, community-based research, and community-oriented teaching opportunities for students.

Public Health Teaching: Assuring Practical Skills

As mentioned previously, public health curricula differ from those designed for nonclinical degree programs, to the extent that public health graduates must have a set of practical, applied, and hands-on skills necessary for workforce success. To this end, at least a component of all public health training programs must be experiential and, ideally, field based. The extent to which this can be accomplished is dependent, in part, on the characteristics of the training program, as described earlier in the chapter. Those programs that are more tightly integrated with their surrounding communities may find it easier to initially establish these programs.

There are many models for assuring experiential learning for students, including establishing a variety of relationships and memoranda of understanding with observational field sites, formal internship programs, connection to teams focused on community-based participatory research,[11] or interprofessional healthcare team simulations. For example, although it is a relatively small school of public health, the authors' institution has more than 250 memoranda of understanding with partner organizations across the region and around the world to assure that all public health students can complete a two-to-three-month internship in a real-world setting. These internships, which are mandatory for BS in Public Health, MPH, and DrPH students, require students to complete one or more projects that specifically address the crosscutting competencies required by their academic program.

A model that has been useful for the authors' institution has been the formal establishment of several regional academic health departments (AHDs). The goal of an AHD is to serve as a formalized bridge between the academic program and local or regional health departments. The model at the authors' institution places a graduate student in each regional health department office, where the student gains professional experience with a preceptor while also serving as an agent for faculty and students seeking research or professional collaboration with the practitioners.[12] Dozens of internship placements have been facilitated through this model, which also serves as a recruitment mechanism for the health departments.

Public Health Teaching: Connection to the Workforce

It is essential that public health training programs be based on a careful and ongoing assessment of the needs of the workforce. The creation or modification of curricula based on workforce needs and feedback takes time, and plans should be made accordingly. Most accredited public health programs have developed formal mechanisms to gain insight from alumni, recent graduates, employers, and community stakeholders. These often take the form of surveys or focus groups that provide data for quality improvement and an ongoing assurance that educational programs are meeting the needs of the future workforce. However, other options should also be considered. Formal and informal events such as development galas, dinners, or even sporting events are all opportunities to create links to the workforce. It is our belief that elected officials, the general public, and potential donors are more willing to engage with educational institutions when these programs are striving to make a difference in their home communities. To this end, it is important that programs, activities, and accomplishments be highlighted in the local media and that college faculty be regularly involved as speakers or in other capacities at community, professional, and social events. The more the community sees the college as being active in the community, the more willing they are to both support the college and make training opportunities available to its students. An example of this is the ongoing monthly meetings, co-led by the college, of a large working group of university, faculty, staff and students, community healthcare providers, coalition leaders, and other key workforce stakeholders engaged in the prevention and treatment of opioid use disorder in the region. Multiple trainees have found field internship sites, research projects, and employment through this monthly gathering, and it has led to the development of new educational opportunities focused on treatment of opioid use disorder in rural areas.

It is also important that the community sees that the college is focused on assuring that its graduates have the skills that the workforce wants and expects. This can be accomplished by regular interface with employers, including surveys and meetings, and also by assuring that they are aware of how the college is preparing students with these skills. The authors' institution has created a public health simulation lab on a large rural field site of about 140 acres, where exact replicas of dwellings from urban and rural slums in the developing world have been assembled into a village. At this site, the college offers full semester courses as well as short-term programs of a few hours to a few days that explicitly teach students and others the skills necessary to address public health needs in low-resource and postdisaster settings. At the same time, these programs teach the crosscutting skills, such as teamwork, innovation, problem-solving, and communication skills, that employers have explicitly identified as important for success. Community leaders, even those without a background or particular interest in public health, find the programs appealing and are supportive of the real-world aspect of the training.

A second consideration that may appear antithetical to academic programs funded by tuition dollars is that programs should balance cohort size against workforce opportunities. The public health workforce, while robust and expanding, is still limited in size. It is not in the student's short-term interest, nor in the institution's long-term interest, for the institution to prepare more graduates than the workforce can absorb. Program leaders should stay mindful of the scope and scale of the marketplace by paying close attention to input from their external stakeholders.

Finally, public health training requires constant improvements, and programs should cultivate a deep dedication to a culture of continuous quality improvement. Accreditation standards are just the first level of this culture. Faculty, staff, and students, along with alumni and employers, should be regularly invited to provide ongoing feedback. As with any organization, a public health training program that seeks and values any good idea will provide its graduates with the best educational experience possible.

Conclusion

Public health education is as important today as it has been at any time in the past century and a half. While there will be appropriate variations based on the level of the training program (from associate's to doctoral) and on the regional needs and overarching mission of the host institution, all public health training programs should provide both foundational knowledge and a practical set of skills that are designed, and regularly modified, to prepare graduates for success in the workforce. Programs must have a strong quality improvement ethos and a willingness to rapidly adapt to meet the evolving public health challenges of its regional community and the world.

REFERENCES

1. Stoots, J. M., R. Wykoff, A. Khoury, and R. Pack. "An Undergraduate Curriculum in Public Health Benchmarked to the Needs of the Workforce." *Frontiers in Public Health* 3 (2015): 12.

2. Bloom, B. S., M. D. Englehart, E. J. Furst, W. H. Hill, and D. R. Krathwohl. *The Taxonomy of Educational Objectives, Handbook I: The Cognitive Domain.* New York: David McKay, 1956.

3. Krathwohl, D. R., B. S. Bloom, and B. B. Masia. *The Taxonomy of Educational Objectives, Handbook II: The Affective Domain.* New York: David McKay, 1964.

4. Riegelman, R. K., C. Wilson, J. Dreyzehner, and L. Huffard. "Community Colleges and Public Health Project Final Report." Framing the Future task force, convened by the Association of Schools and Programs of Public Health and the League for Innovation in the Community College. 2014. https://www.league.org /sites/default/files/private_data/imported/league_books/CCPHFinalReport.pdf (accessed March 25, 2018).

5. Leider, J. P., B. C. Castrucci, C. M. Plepys, C. Blakely, E. Burke, and J. B. Sprague. "Characterizing the Growth of the Undergraduate Public Health Major: US, 1992–2012." *Public Health Reports* 130, no. 1 (2015): 104–113.

6. Kiviniemi, M. T., and S. L. Mackenzie. "Framing Undergraduate Public Health Education as Liberal Education: Who Are We Training Our Students to Be and How Do We Do That?" *Frontiers in Public Health* 5 (2017): 9.

7. Stoots et al. "An Undergraduate Curriculum in Public Health Benchmarked to the Needs of the Workforce."

8. Association of Schools and Programs of Public Health. "Undergraduate Baccalaureate Critical Component Elements Report." 2012. https://www.aspph.org /teach-research/models/undergraduate-baccalaureate-cce-report (accessed March 25, 2018).

9. Institute of Medicine. "Who Will Keep the Public Healthy? Educating Public Health Professionals for the 21st Century." K. Gebbie, L. Rosenstock, and L. M. Hernandez, eds. Washington, DC: National Academies Press, 2003. http://www .nap.edu/openbook.php?record_id=10542 (accessed March 25, 2018).

10. Institute of Medicine. "Who Will Keep the Public Healthy?"

11. Viswanathan, M., A. Ammerman, E. Eng, G. Garlehner, K. N. Lohr, D. Griffith, S. Rhodes, et al. "Community-Based Participatory Research: Assessing the Evidence." *Evidence Report/Technology Assessment (Summary)* 99 (2004): 1–8.

12. Brooks, B., D. Blackley, P. Masters, A. S. May, G. Mayes, C. Williams, and R. Pack. "Developing an Academic Health Department in Northeast Tennessee: A Sustainable Approach through Student Leadership." *Journal of Public Health Management and Practice* 20, no. 3 (2014): 315–323.

PART II THE PUBLIC HEALTH TEACHING CONTINUUM

[4]

Activating Public Health Learning for Adolescents and Young Adults

PERRY N. HALKITIS

DEVELOPING AN EFFECTIVE, skilled, and compassionate public health workforce for the twenty-first century that reflects the diverse population of the United States requires that we attract and educate students at earlier educational stages. Engaging potential public health students should begin during their high school years, when they may not be aware of public health as a field, and in the first few years of undergraduate studies, when public health is often conflated with medicine and other health sciences. Successful education of students at these stages of their lives must attend to the realities of being an adolescent, ages 13–17, or an emerging adult, ages 18–25.[1] Thus, curricula must be tailored to the manifestation of cognitive, emotional, and social domains during these developmental periods, and should embrace modern conceptions of intelligence while adhering to the multidisciplinary nature of public health. Strategies for engaging students must involve strategies that activate student learning.

In what follows, consideration is given to theoretical underpinnings and strategies for successful learning in public health for adolescents and emerging adults, in both high school and college. The approaches are as relevant for graduate students as they are for students in any field of study, as excellent pedagogy is universally applicable. The paradigms and strategies addressed here seek to prepare students to develop the requisite applied skills to work effectively in interdisciplinary settings and in interprofessional roles.[2,3]

Educational Approach

The pedagogy for teaching public health to adolescents and emerging adults must be informed by theories of human development and of intelligence as well as from a multidisciplinary perspective. These three elements are described in the following paragraphs as they relate to teaching students in high school and college.

First, teaching adolescents and emerging adults must be undertaken with attention to the complexities of human development that define these periods of life. Students must not be envisioned as mere vessels of learning but as complex organisms whose learning is interrelated with their social and emotional lives, as well as the physical/pubertal manifestations of the time period.[4] Learning during adolescence and emerging adulthood (which may be envisioned as a protracted adolescence) must be shaped by how individuals learn during this stage of life and informed by the biological/physical, psychological/emotional, and social changes that accompany this developmental epoch.[5] This period of life is characterized by the emergence of formal operations whereby adolescents can begin to engage in abstract thinking and reasoning, outgrowing the concrete operations that define childhood.[6] However, this period of life is also characterized by experimentation and development of independence as well as physical changes that occur within the body. As such, teachers must also attend to these components of human development, which may affect learning. Failing to attend to these conditions and engaging students as distinct from these realities result in less successful engagement in the learning process. Teachers must work closely with families, who also may be challenged by the conditions that shape adolescent behavior.[7]

With regard to these cognitive and socio-emotional states, pedagogical techniques—including ones tailored for public health—may take the form of complex group activities, negotiations, simulations, creative expressions, and multidisciplinary activities and projects that bring together public health, art, history, politics, journalism, and the social and natural sciences. Instructors must foster the development of independence and independent thinking as well as shared decision-making,[8] which are key skills of effective public health researchers and practitioners. An example may be the writing of an op-ed in response to a current public health challenge, such as childhood obesity, violence against women, or vaccination for human papillomavirus.

A second and highly critical element is informed by modern conceptions of intelligence. The extant literature is replete with scientific debate on the definition and measurement of intelligence.[9] What is clear is that intelligence is not a unidimensional conception but rather manifests in a variety of different ways. In this view, individuals may possess varying portfolios of intelligence. These ideas are most evident in the writings and research of Howard Gardner. More than three decades ago, in his seminal work, *Frames of Mind*, Gardner challenged traditional conceptions of intelligence[10] rooted in the work of Galton,[11] Spearman,[12] and Binet,[13] where he purported intelligence may be understood as a unitary factor that could be assessed on intelligence tests. In this traditional view of a unitary conception of intelligence, also known as "g" (general intelligence quotient),[14] a student performing well on a verbal test should also perform well on a mathematics test if intelligence truly is a unitary factor. We have ample evidence against this notion.

The final element that must characterize the approach to teaching and learning public health among adolescents and young adults is multidisciplinary education in the health professions.[15] While many public health educators indicate that they espouse such a perspective, the manifestation of this is rarely noted. At the heart of a multidisciplinary approach is the notion that different disciplines must come together to address important topics, issues, or public health challenges. This is also known in the current literature as interprofessional education.[16] A typical learning exercise may ask the students to identify health disparities among a population experiencing HIV. The students can select any global location and identify the manifestation of the disparity as well as challenges of HIV prevention for this population, including racism, homophobia, and other forms of discrimination. Working as a team, students develop a prevention campaign that must take the form of an infographic, a poster to be used in public locations, and a one-minute public service announcement. The three products must be unified in their look and approach, and employ targeted public health communications strategies to address the specific issues and sexual behaviors of the population. This project brings together skill sets from different disciplines, creates opportunities for cooperative learning (discussed later in the chapter), and brings to life a concrete, creative, and engaging application in which to think about a critical public health issue. This authentic exercise illustrates how so many of us work in public health every day.

Strategies for Public Health Teaching and Learning

Teaching public health concepts and skills to high school and college students must incorporate three key strategies. First, teaching must actively engage students in the learning process through discovery, collaboration, and mentorship. Second, teaching must seek to develop higher-level cognitive processes. Finally, effective pedagogy must utilize the power of scaffolding as a means for teaching and learning. The strategies may be effectively used in both classroom and nonclassroom settings, such as research centers where public health concepts can be brought to life. We illustrate how these techniques have been applied in our own courses and at our research site, the Center for Health, Identity, Behavior and Prevention Studies (CHIBPS).

Discovery-Based Learning

Students must learn early in their lives that science is about doing and experimentation, not about recalling facts.[17] This ethos is rooted in an approach to pedagogy that is discovery based, first noted by Bruner,[18] and is as relevant in teaching first graders as it is in teaching adolescents and young adults in programs of public health. It is about activating learning and curiosity. Students learn by doing and actively engaging with concepts and ideas.

Discovery-based learning is rooted in a cognitive constructivist perspective. Underlying this premise is psychologist Jean Piaget's conception of disequilibrium,[19] which posits that learning, in the form of the schemata that humans possess, is enhanced when conceptions are challenged and, in turn, when a learner must accommodate new information. This learning phenomenon occurs within the context of discovery-based learning approaches. For example, a student's conception of health disparity may be that of a low-income person in the United States who has limited access to healthcare. However, when we embed this student in another country or another culture, the schema of health disparity may be disrupted, as the student develops a more expansive view of what a health disparity is and as they consider drivers of heath disparities. Discovery-based learning allows students to actively create cognitive constructions that enhance their understandings of concepts or ideas in public health.

Evidence suggests that discovery-based learning yields the most effective results when the learning is facilitated rather than unstructured,[20] especially when it is coupled with scaffolding (described later in the chapter). An effective approach is student centered, where the instructor functions as a facilitator and the environment is open to ideas and suggestions, creating room for trial and error.

For example, undergraduate students in a biostatistics course might be provided a data set, which includes a variety of variables indicating substance use, demographic states, and psychosocial conditions. In the first session of the course, the students are assigned to work in teams of three, an effective number for group work.[21] The students are briefed on the overriding aims of the study, details on the study design, the protocol, Institutional Review Board approvals, and data collection strategies (a brief intercept street survey using mobile devices), and are shown an animated video illustrating the data collection process. The students are then asked to prepare a brief report of 1,000 words that will be the basis for funding decisions made by lawmakers on what is known about substance use in young adults. They are encouraged to include as many charts and graphs as they deem necessary. Throughout the course, the students learn to generate descriptive statistics as well as produce and interpret bivariable and multivariable statistical analyses. Time is set aside during class for students to work on the report. The instructor acts as a facilitator and guide, navigating the classroom space as students work in their teams, considering which variables to use, how to analyze the variables, and how to best present the results. The students work over the course of the semester and discover, analyze, write, receive guidance and feedback, and revise. At the end of the semester, each team produces a brief report.

It is critical that the instructor is actively involved as a guide, facilitator, and mentor to maximize discovery-based learning. This approach differs radically from traditional biostatistics assignments, where students are given data sets and asked to run certain statistical analyses.

The activity also breaks down the silos across the traditional public health disciplines and aligns with real-world skills, namely "concepts, methods, and tools of public health data collection, analysis and interpretation, and the evidence-based reasoning and informatics approaches that are essential to public health practice."[22]

Cooperative Learning

The second key teaching strategy for high school and college students is cooperative learning, known colloquially as group work.[23] Cooperative learning has been actively studied in primary and secondary schools as well as in higher education environments.[24] Cooperative learning in public health usually involves small teams comprised of students with different interests and levels of ability working together to enhance one another's learning.[25]

For example, students might be asked to create a group to tackle a question posed by the instructor. In each group, one person takes the role of keeping the group on task, one is the record-keeper, and one reports on the work of the group. When roles are clearly defined, struggles for power may be minimized. Another informal mode of cooperative learning may take the form of an activity called "Toss the Ball." The instructor poses a question and then tosses the ball to a student, and that student responds to the question. The student then tosses the ball to another student, and the second student adds their response to the question or comments on the first student's response, and so on. This activity allows students to move around the room, actively engaging with one another, creating active rather than passive learning.

Most of the extant literature on cooperative learning has focused on structured groupings of students, and there is abundant evidence on the effectiveness of cooperative learning in engaging students, enhancing learning, and encouraging the development of student interaction and relationships.[26] One of the key components of cooperative learning is that students are exposed to other ideas and perspectives, other modes of thinking, or skills that others possess. One study found that the use of cooperative learning increased the achievement motivation of female-identified college students.[27] A meta-analysis of empirical studies on cooperative learning detected an increase of 14 percentage points in overall achievement among colleague students who were taught chemistry using cooperative learning techniques.[28]

The composition of groups is key to cooperative learning. Prior to the data analysis learning activity described earlier, students are asked to self-assess their statistical knowledge, skills, and experience. Based on their self-assessments, students are then classified as high, medium, or low knowledge, skills, and experience, and each group is comprised of this triad. Groups of three have advantages over groups of two, including more focus on teamwork.[29]

As is the case with discovery-based learning, cooperative learning is also an effective strategy for enhancing public heath training outside of the classroom as well as a source of mutual beneficence.

Learning through Scaffolding

The final strategy that enhances learning for adolescents and emerging adults in public health is based on the theories of Lev Vygotsky, a Soviet psychologist who wrote extensively about processes for learning in children.[30] The theory that is based on the idea of learning through scaffolding focuses on a concept known as the zone of proximal development[31] and provides a means of conceptualizing teaching and learning thorough a mentor–apprentice model.[32,33,34] The zone of proximal development is defined as the space or the distance between what children can do on their own and what children can do with the assistance of an adult. While originally proposed to understand how children learn, the idea is applicable to any mentor–apprentice relationship and is quite applicable in public health. The mentor works with the apprentice (the learner) to decrease the zone of proximal development, such that through mentoring and support, the learner can eventually undertake a task on their own.

The tenets of the zone of proximal development are highly applicable in higher education with regard to higher-level cognitive skills[35] and in e-learning environments.[36] The techniques of scaffolding and the development of mentor–apprentice relationships also have great potential for engaging adolescents and emerging adults in public health learning.

The principles of scaffolding are also applicable in research centers where students have opportunities to engage with real-world public health issues. For example, scaffolding can be used to teach students to write scholarly public health manuscripts. In our CHIBPS center, we organize paper-writing groups where students work on each section of a manuscript with a mentor. We conceptualize the aims of the paper, develop an outline, strategize the analysis, and then undertake the work side by side on a weekly basis. The discussions are energetic and thoughtful as we push each other to think more strategically and at higher levels. We meet weekly and undertake analyses together so that the student learns how to approach this aspect of the work. We write in between sessions, and feedback is provided when we meet until we are satisfied with the quality of the final product. The instructor is mentor to all, and doctoral students act as mentors to the master's students, undergraduates, and the high school students, creating multiple scaffolds. Over time and after a few iterations, students are able to lead a paper-writing group on their own and serve as first author. Learning through scaffolding occurs at CHIBPS, both formally and informally.

Conclusion

Developmental and intelligence theories, as well as multidisciplinarity, are critical for effective public health teaching and learning among adolescents and emerging adults. Attending to the complexities of these developmental stages and embracing an expansive view of how we understand intelligence and the truly multifaceted nature of public health as a field defined by the perspectives of multiple disciplines must inform how we engage young learners. The elements also complement the pedagogical strategies of discovery-based learning, cooperative learning, and scaffolding, which are all essential elements for developing successful and effective pedagogy for high school and college students.

The pedagogical strategy of discovery-based learning aligns with the key component that must characterize public health education—namely providing in-depth, skills-based education that students are seeking and employers are demanding. Coupled with cooperative learning and scaffolding, discovery-based approaches afford students the opportunity to use hands-on strategies to solve problems individually and as part of a group. Cooperative learning allows students from diverse backgrounds, cultures, and so forth to engage actively with one another. These elements align perfectly with two of the critical content domains for public health—namely, "the cultural context of public health issues and respectful engagement with people of different cultures and socioeconomic strata" as well as "principles of effective functioning within and across organizations and as members of interdisciplinary and interprofessional teams."[37]

Discovery-based and cooperative learning coupled with scaffolding are robust and proven techniques for engaging students and enhancing their learning. There is not anything necessarily unique about teaching public health as compared to biology, music, or writing. What is important to note is that our approaches to pedagogy must engage the student, keep the student at the center of the learning, and enact strategies that interest and stimulate while recognizing that different approaches may be needed for different students.

REFERENCES

1. Arnett, J. J. "Emerging Adulthood: A Theory of Development from the Late Teens through the Twenties." *American Psychologist* 55, no. 5 (2000): 469–480.

2. Association of Schools and Programs of Public Health. "Recommended Critical Component Elements of an Undergraduate Major in Public Health." 2012. https://www.aspph.org/teach-research/models/undergraduate-baccalaureate-cce -report/ (accessed March 25, 2018).

3. Association of Schools and Programs of Public Health. "Master of Public Health Degree for the 21st Century: Key Considerations, Design Features, and Critical Content of the Core." 2014. https://www.aspph.org/teach-research/models /mph-degree-report/ (accessed March 25, 2018).

4. Anderson, L. W., J. Jacobs, S. Schramm, and F. Splittgerber. "School Transitions: Beginning of the End or a New Beginning?" *International Journal of Educational Research* 33, no. 4 (2000): 325–339.

5. Bastable, S. B., P. Gramet, K. Jacobs, and D. Sopczyk. *Health Professional as Educator: Principles of Teaching and Learning.* Sudbury, MA: Jones and Bartlett Learning, 2010.

6. Piaget, J. *The Child's Conception of the World.* Lanham, MD: Rowman and Littlefield, 1951.

7. Hines, A. R., and S. E. Paulson. "Parents' and Teachers' Perceptions of Adolescent Storm and Stress: Relations with Parenting and Teaching Styles." *Adolescence* 41, no. 164 (2006): 597–614.

8. Bastable et al., *Health Professional as Educator.*

9. Neisser, U., G. Boodoo, T. J. Bouchard Jr., A. W. Boykin, N. Brody, S. J. Ceci, D. F. Halpern, J. C. Loehlin, R. Perloff, R. J. Sternberg, and S. Urbina. "Intelligence: Knowns and Unknowns." *American Psychologist* 51, no. 2 (2006): 77–101.

10. Gardner, H. *Frames of Mind: The Theory of Multiple Intelligences.* New York: Basic Books, 2011.

11. Galton, F. "Grades and Deviates: Including a Table of Normal Deviates Corresponding to Each Millesimal Grade in the Length of an Array, and a Figure." *Biometrika* 5, no. 4 (1907): 400–406.

12. Spearman, C. "'General Intelligence,' Objectively Determined and Measured." *American Journal of Psychology* 15, no. 2 (1904): 201–293.

13. Binet, A., and T. Simon. *The Development of Intelligence in Children: The Binet-Simon Scale.* Baltimore: Williams and Wilkins Company, 1916.

14. Kamphaus, R. W. *Clinical Assessment of Child and Adolescent Intelligence.* New York: Springer, 2005.

15. Lary, M. J., S. E. Lavigne, R. D. Muma, S. E. Jones, and H. J. Hoeft. "Breaking Down Barriers: Multidisciplinary Education Model." *Journal of Allied Health* 26, no. 2 (1997): 63–69.

16. Clark, P. G. "What Would a Theory of Interprofessional Education Look Like? Some Suggestions for Developing a Theoretical Framework for Teamwork Training." *Journal of Interprofessional Care* 20, no. 6 (2006): 577–589.

17. Halkitis, P. N. "Grouping of 3 in the Science Classroom." *Gifted Child Today* (July/August 1988): 7.

18. Bruner, J. S. "The Act of Discovery." *Harvard Educational Review* 31 (1961): 21–32.

19. Piaget, J. "The Genetic Approach to the Psychology of Thought." *Understanding Children* 52 (1961): 35–40.

20. Alfieri, L., P. J. Brooks, N. J. Aldrich, and H. R. Tenenbaum. "Does Discovery-Based Instruction Enhance Learning?" *Journal of Educational Psychology* 103, no. 1 (2011): 1–18.

21. Halkitis, "Grouping of 3 in the Science Classroom."

22. Association of Schools and Programs of Public Health, "Master of Public Health Degree for the 21st Century."

23. Gillies, R., and A. Ashman, ed. *Co-operative Learning: The Social and Intellectual Outcomes of Learning in Groups.* New York: Routledge, 2003.

24. Chiu, M. M. "Flowing toward Correct Contributions during Group Problem Solving: A Statistical Discourse Analysis." *Journal of the Learning Sciences* 17, no. 3 (2008): 415–463.

25. Riley, W., and P. Anderson. "Randomized Study on the Impact of Cooperative Learning: Distance Education in Public Health." *Quarterly Review of Distance Education* 7, no. 2 (2006): 129–144.

26. Slavin, R. E. "Cooperative Learning: Applying Contact Theory in Desegregated Schools." *Journal of Social Issues* 41, no. 3 (1985): 45–62.

27. Wang, M. "Effects of Cooperative Learning on Achievement Motivation of Female University Students." *Asian Social Science* 8, no. 15 (2012): 108–114.

28. Bowen, C. W. "A Quantitative Literature Review of Cooperative Learning Effects on High School and College Chemistry Achievement." *Journal of Chemical Education* 77, no. 1 (2000): 116–119.

29. Halkitis, "Grouping of 3 in the Science Classroom."

30. Vygotsky, L. S. *The Collected Works of LS Vygotsky: Problems of the Theory and History of Psychology, Vol. 3*. Berlin: Springer Science and Business Media, 1997.

31. Vygotsky, L. S. *Mind in Society: The Development of Higher Psychological Processes*. Cambridge, MA: Harvard University Press, 1980.

32. Pentimonti, J. M., L. M. Justice, G. Yeomans-Maldonado, A. S. McGinty, L. Slocum, and A. O'Connell. "Teachers' Use of High- and Low-Support Scaffolding Strategies to Differentiate Language Instruction in High-Risk/Economically Disadvantaged Settings." *Journal of Early Intervention* 39, no. 2 (2017): 125–146.

33. Van de Pol, J., M. Volman, and J. Beishuizen. "Scaffolding in Teacher–Student Interaction: A Decade of Research." *Educational Psychology Review* 22, no. 3 (2010): 271–296.

34. Warton, P., and K. Bussey. "Assisted Learning: Levels of Support." *British Journal of Developmental Psychology* 6, no. 2 (1988): 113–123.

35. Harland, T. "Vygotsky's Zone of Proximal Development and Problem-Based Learning: Linking a Theoretical Concept with Practice through Action Research." *Teaching in Higher Education* 8, no. 2 (2003): 263–272.

36. Oliver, R. "Developing E-Learning Environments That Support Knowledge Construction in Higher Education." In *Working for Excellence in the E-conomy*, edited by S. Stoney and J. Burn, 407–416. Churchlands, Australia: We-B Centre, 2001.

37. Association of Schools and Programs of Public Health, "Master of Public Health Degree for the 21st Century."

[5]

Undergraduate Education in Public Health

LAUREN D. ARNOLD

T HE TWENTY-FIRST CENTURY has seen rapid growth in undergraduate public health programs across the United States. In 1992, only 45 colleges and universities offered an undergraduate degree in public health; this number increased to 176 in 2012,[1] with new programs continuing to be developed. This growth may in part reflect Healthy People 2020's goals for public health infrastructure, which specifically cite a target of increasing the number of undergraduate public health degrees earned in the United States by 10% over the 2014–2015 baseline of 10,722 bachelor's degrees awarded.[2] Because programs exist in a number of settings (e.g., schools/colleges of public health, liberal arts institutions without graduate public health degree offerings, research institutions), this growth in undergraduate public health instigated national dialogue about structure and context for the undergraduate degree in public health.

Context for a Liberal Arts Approach

A major shift in the context for public health education occurred in 2003, when the Institute of Medicine's (IOM) Committee on Educating Public Health Professionals for the 21st Century recommended that public health education be available to all undergraduate students, regardless of major course of study.[3] Prior to this, public health education largely focused on graduate professional degrees with some cross-training opportunities for healthcare professionals, such as physicians and nurses; undergraduate programs that did exist were often preprofessional in nature. The IOM's report brought national recognition both to the potential for baccalaureate degrees in public health and to the importance of providing access to public health training to all college students, with the rationale that public health is interdisciplinary and a responsibility of all citizens.[4]

Building on the IOM's recommendation, the Association of American Colleges and Universities (AAC&U) launched the Educated Citizen and Public Health Initiative, a collaborative effort that aimed to integrate public health principles into a liberal arts undergraduate education, support interdisciplinary collaboration, and provide resources for the development of undergraduate public health curricula in all US universities and colleges.[5] They suggested that public health content could be incorporated into the liberal arts in a number of ways, including creating introductory courses in public health and epidemiology that meet general education (or core) requirements and using the liberal arts core as a foundation for the creation of a minor in public health.[6] Additionally, the AAC&U's Liberal Education and America's Promise (LEAP) goals were mapped to public health learning goals to demonstrate the feasibility of viewing undergraduate public health within the lens of a liberal arts education.[7]

In response to the AAC&U's work, the Association of Schools and Programs of Public Health (ASPPH) convened working groups comprised of faculty from across the United States who were tasked with using the LEAP framework to draft a set of undergraduate public health learning outcomes. Working from a list of nearly 400 potential learning outcomes, a Delphi approach was used to develop 34 learning outcomes. These were then mapped to four LEAP domains: (1) Knowledge of Human Cultures and the Physical and Natural World, (2) Intellectual and Practical Skills, (3) Personal and Social Responsibility, and (4) Student-Centered Integrative Learning Methods. The intention was that colleges and universities could draw on this list of learning outcomes to guide integration of public health into the liberal arts curriculum. Because the focus was on suggesting how institutions could integrate public health into existing educational opportunities, specific coursework was not identified. However, perhaps most useful were the concrete examples of in-class and out-of-classroom learning experiences that could be used to expose all undergraduates to public health principles and concepts regardless of major area of study. For instance, examples were related to journalism, public policy, political science, and communications courses.[8] This work helped to solidify the acceptance of viewing undergraduate public health education through a liberal arts lens rather than solely from the perspective of preprofessional training.

Program Structure

A Consensus Conference on Undergraduate Public Health Education was convened with representatives from leaders in public health, health professions, and arts and sciences education to discuss undergraduate public health program structure and focus. The resulting 2007 Consensus Report identified two models for undergraduate public health education: one in which undergraduate degrees are offered in schools/colleges of public health and the other in which degrees are offered in colleges/ universities without schools or (graduate) programs in public health.[9] It is important to note that just because an undergraduate program might be housed in a school/college of public health, it does not mean that the degree is preprofessional in nature; these programs may, in fact, have a liberal arts focus.

Among three of the most well-established undergraduate public health programs in the country, only one—at East Tennessee State University—follows the first model of housing the degree in a school of public health. This distribution reflects findings from a 2008 review of 837 AAC&U four-year institutions, which found that approximately 70% of undergraduate public health degree programs existed outside of schools that offer a graduate public health degree.[10] East Tennessee State University's Bachelor of Science (BS) in Health Education was established in 1955[11] and today exists as a BS in Public Health housed within their College of Public Health. Johns Hopkins University (whose public health studies major was created in the 1970s)[12] and Rutgers University (whose major was established in 1999)[13] offer their under-graduate public health degrees outside of their Schools of Public Health, housed in the Krieger School of Arts and Sciences and Edward J. Bloustein School of Planning and Public Policy, respectively. Rutgers University's program is consistent with a liberal arts approach, preparing students for a range of opportunities after graduation, including medical (or other professional) school, the workforce, and graduate school, both in public health and in related areas. Rutgers was among the first institutions to achieve standalone baccalaureate program accreditation from the Council on Education for Public Health (CEPH), an accreditation that is independent from its School of Public Health's accreditation status.

Curriculum Guidelines: The Undergraduate Degree versus the Master of Public Health

Today, undergraduate public health degrees are offered in a range of departments, including anthropology, health sciences, exercise science, kinesiology, and health education and promotion, as well as in colleges/schools of public health. This variation in program location is important because, as degree programs were developed, the expertise of the faculty in the sponsoring department/unit had the potential to influence the content and structure of the curriculum.

In an effort to bring some consistency to the structure of undergraduate public health education, as well as to distinguish the bachelor's degree from the Master of Public Health (MPH) degree, the ASPPH, with support from the Centers for Disease Control and Prevention (CDC), convened an expert panel in 2012 to develop guidelines for undergraduate public health education. This expert panel was the first in a series of panels that discussed the continuum of bachelor's-master's-doctoral public health education; separate MPH and doctoral degree panels followed. It was critical that the undergraduate expert panel considered this continuum while developing its guidelines, as whatever elements deemed essential to undergraduate education were to be built on and developed further in graduate-level training.

The resulting Recommended Critical Component Elements (CCE) of an Undergraduate Major in Public Health outlined fundamental areas of public health and liberal arts as well as professional development and academic advising that must be addressed at the undergraduate level. The liberal arts nature of undergraduate public health is emphasized in the content guidelines, which include humanities, social science, fine arts, behavioral science, natural science, and quantitative reasoning. Public health domains focus on the need for an introduction to history and philosophy of public health, determinants of health, the role of science in health, the role and importance of data, identification of population health challenges, ethics, and the evidence-based public health framework. The need for both a cumulative (capstone) experience and field experience is articulated, as is the need to expose students to cross-cutting professional skills needed for both the workplace and graduate education.[14] Importantly, the CCE document does not prescribe specific courses to meet the domains/content areas identified. Rather, larger domains are developed that can be used by institutions to create or refine undergraduate public health degrees in a way that respond to the guidelines within the context of general undergraduate education and available resources at each institution. For example, some programs may rely on existing courses in statistics and mathematics to address analytic skills, while others may create specific courses that help students develop these skills while simultaneously emphasizing a public health context.

CEPH used the CCE as a framework to develop criteria for accreditation of undergraduate public health degrees, solidifying the need for programs to emphasize skills development and content in broader areas of public health and the liberal arts.

The 2016 CEPH accreditation criteria require undergraduate programs not only to identify courses and other learning experiences that address the general content areas and public health domains but to articulate how skills are assessed and how students have the opportunity to integrate, synthesize, and apply their knowledge.[15,16] The 2016 criteria apply to all undergraduate public health degrees, regardless of whether or not they are housed within a college/school of public health. This is a significant departure from prior criteria that historically required bachelor's degrees within colleges/schools of public health to provide evidence of competence in five foundational areas of public health: biostatistics, epidemiology, environmental health science, health administration, and the social and behavioral sciences. Existing programs that wish to seek accreditation must update their program structure to respond to the revised criteria. Even if institutions do not plan to seek accreditation for their undergraduate public health degree, these accreditation criteria can be used to guide program development.

It must be acknowledged that despite the guidance from the Association of Schools and Programs of Public Health and CEPH on a framework for undergraduate education, debate still exists as to whether all undergraduate public health programs should follow a liberal arts model or if professional degree training is more (or equally as) appropriate.[17] Other factors must also be considered, including paths that students will pursue after graduation (e.g., medical school, graduate school in public health, graduate school in other areas, the workforce), an institution's capacity for offering required and elective courses in public health, the nature of field experience that can feasibly be supported by the program, and the institution's own strengths.[18] For these reasons, and as is the case with graduate public health programs, no two undergraduate programs will look the same.

Using CEPH Accreditation Requirements to Guide Program Development and Teaching

Regardless of whether or not institutions seek CEPH accreditation, they can use the CEPH criteria to guide program development and revision. Because the criteria require programs to identify how skills and knowledge will be assessed, program administrators and faculty teaching classes can use the accreditation data templates[19] to develop and evaluate courses. Similarly, program administrators can use the data templates as a starting point for examining areas of duplication and to identify gaps across the continuum of required coursework and other learning experiences (e.g., service learning, research rotations, or internships).

Distinction between Undergraduate and Graduate Coursework

It is not uncommon for there to be overlap in bachelor's and MPH degrees with respect to some foundational content, but the distinction between the two is extremely important. Undergraduate public health majors who pursue an MPH must build on their undergraduate coursework and not repeat content in a graduate program. Distinguishing courses with overlap in content is challenging and involves continuous dialogue between undergraduate and graduate programs.[20] For instance, both undergraduate- and graduate-level epidemiology courses include calculating incidence, prevalence, relative risk, and odds ratios. The difference between the classes lies in the depth to which the material is covered. The undergraduate course might focus on computation and basic interpretation and have discussions about whether measures are accurately communicated in a news story. A graduate epidemiology course may go into more depth about who should and should not be included in the numerator and denominator for measures of association, and consider potential threats to validity in specific research applications. When discussing surveillance, an undergraduate epidemiology course might cover the basic definition and approaches and consider examples of how surveillance guides public health practice with flu vaccinations or outbreak investigations. A graduate epidemiology course may have students study surveillance data and discuss what could explain observed trends, as well as how to further investigate possible explanations.

Teaching Undergraduate Public Health beyond the Classroom: Professional Development

In addition to considering curriculum content, undergraduate public health programs must think about teaching and assessing professional development. The CCE specifies that undergraduate public health students "should be exposed to concepts and experiences necessary for success in the workplace, further education, and life-long learning."[21] These include networking, professionalism, teamwork, community dynamics, and advocacy. Moreover, students and parents believe that career development is critical, regardless of whether graduates with bachelor's degrees in public health will enter the workforce or graduate school.[22] A first step to teaching professional skills is to ask employers about skills and characteristics expected of a new hire with a bachelor's degree, such as problem-solving, oral communication, professional writing, ethical behavior, and teamwork.[23] Alumni surveys can provide insight into areas of professional development that should be emphasized and how the undergraduate program can best prepare students.

Professional development can be integrated into the classroom by, for example, having conversations with students about professional dress and networking before a guest speaker comes to class. If a course involves student presentations, faculty can provide an overview of elements of an effective presentation, and then have students critique sample presentations for strengths and weaknesses. To teach students how to manage conflict and delegate responsibilities, group projects can include a requirement that the group develops a contract or memorandum of understanding about each group member's role and responsibilities for the project.

Beyond the classroom, leadership skills can be developed as part of a peer advisor program.[24] Leadership and networking can be fostered by supporting student presentations at conferences and as part of service learning opportunities in the community.[25] While career services staff can discuss career opportunities and provide training in interviewing and resume-writing, alumni and other local public health professionals can also serve to provide real-life examples and mentoring for undergraduates.[26] Requiring students in a specific course to attend job fairs or other career events can help develop networking skills; in preparation, a class session can be devoted to developing 60-second "elevator speeches" for students to introduce themselves to potential employers. Interview skills can be discussed in advising/mentoring sessions and honed through informational interviews supported through faculty introductions of students to professionals.

Field experiences, such as internships and service learning, help undergraduates learn what is expected of them professionally—for example, time management, professional dress, and punctuality. Thus, public health professionals who supervise or otherwise interact with undergraduates in the community serve as teachers and mentors. To bring consistency to professional development training and to build on what is taught in the academic setting, there must be collaboration between the undergraduate public health program and community partners. In instances where students pursue internships independent of academic requirements, undergraduate programs can encourage students to consider professional development goals through conversations with advisors/faculty or through program-sponsored panel/group discussions.

It is important to recognize that not all undergraduate public health students will enter the workforce or continue their education directly in public health. Thus, professional development in undergraduate public health programs should focus on translatable skills, such as oral and written communication, networking, and leadership that can apply to any area a graduate wishes to pursue. Even if some undergraduates do not work directly in public health, they will be an educated citizen and be able to draw on a public health perspective no matter what area they pursue.

Challenges in Undergraduate Public Health Education

As undergraduate public health has gained momentum, individual programs have experienced rapid growth in student numbers,[27] with program size increasing to include several hundred students distributed across all four years of college.[28,29] This growth begets an additional set of challenges related to class size, faculty support, and resources for advising and field experiences.

New undergraduate public health programs may initially support small class sizes (e.g., 20–30 students) and may be able to support individualized field or research experiences. However, as programs rapidly increase in size, challenges arise for course design, support for internships, and academic advising. Resources may not be available to support hiring additional advisors. As such, creative alternatives must be devised in order to effectively interact with students and provide them with the support needed, while also maintaining a reasonable workload for the advisors. For instance, students nearing completion of the major may serve as peer advisors,[30] or group advising through faculty/academic advisors may be done with students in the early stages of the major, when questions are more general.[31] Electronic advising portals may be established with videos messages, forms, and resources to communicate general advising information.

Lastly, program growth results in a greater demand for faculty to teach undergraduates. In institutions that first offered the MPH and later developed the bachelor's degree in public health, faculty may find it challenging to adjust teaching methods to the undergraduate level. Faculty with graduate responsibilities may also have limited availability for teaching additional courses.[32] While public health professionals in the community can be recruited as adjuncts,[33] many may be better suited to and already involved at the graduate level. Alternately, master's and doctoral students may be recruited to teach introductory undergraduate courses with appropriate training and support.

Conclusion

The staggering growth in undergraduate public health programs over the past decade has changed the face of public health education. It has forced the field to reexamine the context for teaching public health and to consider the purpose of bachelor's-level training, including how it fits in with MPH and doctoral education. CEPH accreditation criteria emphasize the liberal arts framework for undergraduate public health and can serve to guide development and refinement of programs regardless of whether they pursue accreditation status.

As undergraduates discover public health, many programs have experienced rapid growth in the number of students interested. This brings challenges for teaching and advising these students. As the field continues to grow, there is a need for undergraduate public health programs to engage in discussion and assessment about best practices for teaching, advising, and supporting professional development in their students and to disseminate this information, not just through conferences but also through peer-reviewed literature. This will build the body of evidence to support effective teaching and strengthen the training of these future professionals.

REFERENCES

1. Leider, J. P., B. C. Castrucci, C. M. Plepys, C. Blakely, E. Burke, and J. B. Sprague. "Characterizing the Growth of the Undergraduate Public Health Major: US, 1992–2012." *Public Health Reports* 130, no. 1 (2015): 104–113.

2. Healthy People 2020. "Public Health Infrastructure: Objectives." US Department of Health and Human Services: Office of Disease Prevention and Health Promotion. https://www.healthypeople.gov/2020/topics-objectives/topic/public-health-infrastructure/objectives (accessed April 7, 2018).

3. Institute of Medicine. "Who Will Keep the Public Healthy? Educating Public Health Professionals for the 21st Century." K. Gebbie, L. Rosenstock, and L. M. Hernandez, eds. Washington, DC: National Academies Press, 2003.

4. Institute of Medicine. "Who Will Keep the Public Healthy?"

5. Association of American Colleges and Universities. "The Educated Citizen and Public Health." https://www.aacu.org/public_health (accessed December 1, 2017).

6. Centers for Disease Control and Prevention. "Notice to Readers: Updated Recommendations of the Advisory Committee on Immunization Practices (ACIP) for the Control and Elimination of Mumps." *Morbidity and Mortality Weekly Report* 55, no. 22 (2006): 629–630.

7. Albertine, S. "Undergraduate Public Health: Preparing Engaged Citizens as Future Health Professionals." *American Journal of Preventative Medicine* 35, no. 3 (2008): 253–257.

8. Petersen D. J., S. Albertine, C. M. Plepys, and J. G. Calhoun. "Developing an Educated Citizenry: The Undergraduate Public Health Learning Outcomes Project." *Public Health Reports* 128, no. 5 (2013): 425–430.

9. Riegelman R., S. Albertine, and N. A. Persily. "The Educated Citizen and Public Health: A Consensus Report on Public Health and Undergraduate Education." Council of Colleges of Arts and Sciences. 2007. http://www.ccas.net/files /public/Publications/Public_Health_and_Undergraduate_Education.pdf (accessed April 7, 2018).

10. Hovland K., B. A. Kirkwood, C. Ward, M. Osterweiss, and G. B. Silver. "Liberal Education and Public Health: Surveying the Landscape." *Peer Review* 11, no. 3 (2009): 5–8.

11. Wykoff, R., A. Khoury, J. M. Stoots, and R. Pack. "Undergraduate Training in Public Health Should Prepare Graduates for the Workforce." *Frontiers in Public Health* 2 (2014): 285.

12. Rienzi, G. "A Major Change." *Johns Hopkins University Arts and Sciences Magazine* (2006): 23–26.

13. Rutgers University. "Rutgers' Undergraduate Public Health Program Receives CEPH Accreditation." https://news.rutgers.edu/news-release/rutgers %E2%80%99-undergraduate-public-health-program-receives-ceph-accreditation /20160803#.WkSNd1WnHIU (accessed December 27, 2017).

14. Wykoff, R., D. Petersen, and E. M. Weist. "The Recommended Critical Component Elements of an Undergraduate Major in Public Health." *Public Health Reports* 128, no. 5 (2013): 421–424.

15. Council on Education for Public Health. "Accreditation Criteria: Schools and Programs of Public Health." Silver Spring, MD: CEPH, 2016. https://ceph.org /assets/2016.Criteria.pdf (accessed March 25, 2018).

16. Council on Education for Public Health. "SBP Data Templates." https://ceph .org/about/org-info/criteria-procedures-documents/templates/ (accessed November 18, 2018).

17. Kiviniemi, M. T., and S. L. Mackenzie. "Framing Undergraduate Public Health Education as Liberal Education: Who Are We Training Our Students To Be and How Do We Do That?" *Frontiers in Public Health* 5 (2017): https://www.ncbi .nlm.nih.gov/pmc/articles/PMC5301016/pdf/fpubh-05-00009.pdf.

18. Friedman, L. H., and J. M. Lee. "Undergraduate Public Health Education: Is There an Ideal Curriculum?" *Frontiers in Public Health* 3 (2015): https://www .frontiersin.org/articles/10.3389/fpubh.2015.00016/full.

19. Council on Education for Public Health. "SBP Data Templates." https://ceph .org/about/org-info/criteria-procedures-documents/templates/ (accessed December 27, 2017).

20. White, L. E. "Success of the Undergraduate Public Health at Tulane University." *Frontiers in Public Health* 3 (2015): https://www.ncbi.nlm.nih.gov /pmc/articles/PMC4403250/pdf/fpubh-03-00060.pdf.

21. Wykoff, Petersen, and Weist, "The Recommended Critical Component Elements of an Undergraduate Major in Public Health."

22. White, "Success of the Undergraduate Public Health at Tulane University."

23. Stoots, J. M., R. Wykoff, A. Khoury, and R. Pack. "An Undergraduate Curriculum in Public Health Benchmarked to the Needs of the Workforce." *Front*

Public Health 3 (2015): https://www.ncbi.nlm.nih.gov/pmc/articles/PMC4330650/pdf/fpubh-03-00012.pdf.

24. Griffin, M., G. T. DiFulvio, and D. S. Gerber. "Developing Leaders: Implementation of a Peer Advising Program for a Public Health Sciences Undergraduate Program." *Frontiers in Public Health* 2 (2014): https://www.ncbi.nlm.nih.gov/pmc/articles/PMC4283432/pdf/fpubh-02-00288.pdf.

25. Nelson-Hurwitz, D. C., L. A. Arakaki, and M. Uemoto. "Insights in Public Health—Training Today's Students to Meet Tomorrow's Challenges: Undergraduate Public Health at the University of Hawai'i at Manoa." *Hawaii Journal of Medicine and Public Health* 76, no. 3 (2017): 89–93.

26. Friedman and Lee, "Undergraduate Public Health Education."

27. White, "Success of the Undergraduate Public Health at Tulane University."

28. Friedman and Lee, "Undergraduate Public Health Education."

29. Perrin K., and L. Merrell. "Undergraduate Public Health Education: Alternative Choices within the BSPH Degree." *Frontiers in Public Health* 2 (2014): https://www.ncbi.nlm.nih.gov/pmc/articles/PMC4144004/pdf/fpubh-02-00127.pdf.

30. Griffin, DiFulvio, and Gerber, "Developing Leaders."

31. Arnold, L. D., E. S. Embry, and C. Fox. "Advising Undergraduate Public Health Students: A Phased Approach." *Public Health Reports* 130, no. 4 (2015): 415–420.

32. White, "Success of the Undergraduate Public Health at Tulane University."

33. Riegelman, R. K., and S. Albertine. "Undergraduate Public Health at 4-Year Institutions: It's Here to Stay." *American Journal of Preventative Medicine* 40, no. 2 (2011): 226–231.

[6]

Community Colleges and Public Health

Building the Continuum of Public Health Education

KATHERINE JOHNSON AND RICHARD RIEGELMAN

C OMMUNITY COLLEGES represent the newest addition to the continuum of public health education. Community colleges have become a central component of higher education in the United States, with more than seven million students taking courses for academic credit. Community colleges in the United States are now majority-minority, with a large number of students coming from underserved communities. Public health education in community colleges therefore presents a unique opportunity for diversifying the public health workforce.

This chapter examines efforts to integrate community colleges into the continuum of public health education, including the Community Colleges and Public Health report of the Association of Schools and Programs of Public Health as well as the League for Innovation in the Community College. It also observes current efforts to develop guided learning pathways for public health. Finally, it studies the unique opportunities and challenges associated with teaching and learning public health in community colleges.

Recent Community College and Public Health Initiatives

Healthy People 2020 included an objective to increase public health education in two-year as well as four-year colleges and universities.[1] As part of this initiative, the American Public Health Association also approved a resolution endorsing the development of public health education for all undergraduates.[2] This was followed by the development of the Community Colleges and Public Health report (referenced hereafter as the Report), issued by the Association of Schools and Programs of Public Health (ASPPH) and the League for Innovation in the Community College (referenced hereafter as the League) in 2014 as part of the ASPPH's Framing the Future initiative.[3]

The League represents more than 800 of the 1,100 community colleges in the United States and is the leading organization in recommending new academic programs. The Report was developed in collaboration with public health–related education and practice organizations, including the Society for Public Health Education, the Association of Environmental Health Academic Programs, the Association of State and Territorial Health Officials, and the National Association of County and City Health Officials. The Report aimed to provide multiple options for the development of public health education within community colleges and their articulation with bachelor's degree programs.

The Report recommended three core and foundational Health Foundation courses that are common to all of the Report's recommended associate's degree and certificate programs. These courses are (1) Personal Health and Wellness with a Population Perspective, (2) Overview of Public Health, and (3) Health Communications.

Health Foundation courses were designed to reach a broad range of community college students and inspire many of them to pursue public health education. In addition, all recommended associate's degree and certificate programs included experiential learning, which was defined as relevant community-based experience as part of a supervised activity with learning outcomes and opportunities for reflection. Electives were recommended, including coursework in public health preparedness.

The Report recommended a series of 30 semester-hour programs as part of associate's degrees or as fulfillment of an academic certificate program in public health or related fields. These were grouped as (1) Public Health Generalist and Specializations and (2) Health Navigation. These degree and certificate programs are described in the following list.

1 Public Health Generalist and Specializations—designed for transfer to bachelor's degree programs in one of the following subjects:
  • General public health
  • Health education (leading to eligibility for the Certified Health Education Specialist examination, a widely used certification administered by the National Commission for Health Education Credentialing, Inc.)
  • Health administration
  • Environmental health
2 Health Navigation
  • Health navigation certificate and associate's degree programs were designed for those working or planning to work as community health workers or health navigators.
  • Health navigation certificate programs are also appropriate for current health and allied health professionals who seek to enhance their skills in health navigation.

Each program included the three Health Foundation courses, required public health courses, experiential learning, and electives. Depending on how community colleges choose to adapt these recommendations, associate's degrees can be modeled on a range of degree types. Associate's of science and associate's of arts degrees are traditionally designed for transfer to four-year programs, whereas associate's of applied science degrees are typically designed for direct entry into the workforce. Similarly, academic certificate programs can vary widely by context and can often be used either as a stand-alone academic credential or as a stackable stepping-stone to continued coursework at the associate's level.

The League has taken a leadership role in encouraging community colleges to develop programs in public health and related fields. Its efforts have included publicizing the Report, developing a webinar series, maintaining a regularly updated website, and presenting annual recognition awards for community colleges developing programs consistent with the Report.[4]

A Community Colleges and Public Health network is being created for faculty and administrators from existing and potential community college public health programs. Linking this emerging network with the rapidly growing ASPPH Undergraduate Public Health and Global Health network of bachelor's degree programs will be an important step in building the continuum of public health education.

Guided Learning Pathways

Guided learning pathways have become a major effort of community colleges designed to provide entering community college students with a discrete number of well-defined options for structuring their education, including academic support, career counseling, and a common foundational curriculum. Successful students are then considered for a range of specific associate's and bachelor's degree programs.

Both the League and the American Association of Community Colleges have encouraged the use of guided learning pathways, and the Gates Foundation has funded their development in 30 community colleges. Additional community colleges are using their own funds to join a network that encourages the use and development of guided learning pathways.[5]

The League is starting to work with ASPPH and the Society for Public Health Education to encourage the development of models for guided learning pathways for public health. These guided learning pathways incorporate the three core Health Foundations courses as well as academic support and career counseling. This Health Foundations curriculum is comprised of foundational coursework common to both the Public Health Generalist and Specializations and the Health Navigation curricular options described earlier, and provides an introduction to public health at the introductory college level.

Students successfully completing the entry-level Health Foundations curriculum should be able to apply to specific associate's degree and bachelor's degree programs in a range of health professions. Transferability of these courses as part of a public health bachelor's degree should help satisfy Council on Education for Public Health criteria D-16, which states: "Bachelor's degree programs have publicly available policies and procedures for review of coursework taken at other institutions, including community colleges."[6]

Challenges and Opportunities in Teaching Public Health in Community Colleges

The diversity of community college students and their communities requires tailored approaches to teaching and learning.

Student Diversity

As open-access institutions, community colleges attract diverse student audiences. In addition to being majority-minority (48% white), they are majority part-time enrolled (62%) and majority female (56%). Additionally, community college students are diverse in age and stage of life, and are likely to have substantial work-life commitments in addition to the requirements of their academic studies. Indeed, 49% of community college students are beyond traditional college age, and 17% are single parents. Close to two-thirds (63%) of community college students are working full time while pursuing their education, and more than one-third (36%) are first-generation students.[7]

While the support of diverse, nontraditional student audiences requires careful and consistent planning on the part of program administrators, this diversity also provides important opportunities, such as the chance to extend academic career ladders to underserved students and ultimately to diversify the public health workforce and better serve the communities in which program graduates often find employment.

Community Characteristics

Community colleges vary widely by setting, and programs must be tailored to fit the local context. For public health programs, two types of partnerships are particularly important—those involving four-year academic institutions (or other specialized higher education partners, as appropriate) and those with local public health organizations. Curricular decision-making regarding the particular focus areas of public health programs is influenced by both types of partnerships.

For academic partnerships, the goal is to ensure that community college programs articulate seamlessly with four-year programs, so that students do not lose time or money by needing to retake similar courses following their transfer to bachelor's degree programs.[8,9] To this end, community colleges should involve four-year partners in the program planning process. By seeking input on the partner institution's needs, community college programs can better articulate to public health programs at the bachelor's level and match learning objectives across courses.

For partnerships with public health organizations, the goal is to ensure that community college programs successfully train program graduates in the skills and abilities prioritized by local employers and that colleges calibrate program size to the local market. Even for transfer programs where the intended goal for program graduates is matriculation into bachelor's degree programs, it is important to recognize that not all students will immediately or ultimately transfer. Close collaboration with local public health organizations can help to facilitate job readiness for students who do not immediately continue their studies.

Additionally, local professional partnerships are important in establishing robust experiential learning opportunities. The value of promoting such opportunities for applied learning in community college settings has been demonstrated.[10] A variety of local organizations can serve as valuable partners, from local health departments and community health centers to hospital networks to insurance companies.[11]

Teaching Strategies

As with other settings for public health education, community college programs have the primary goal of providing sound training for the public health workforce of the twenty-first century. However, given the diverse student characteristics highlighted previously, community colleges have an added mandate to focus on the unique needs of their students.

Past research has articulated high-impact practices, specifically for community college settings. For example, the Center for Community College Student Engagement has closely examined 13 promising practices, while others have emphasized five to six core strategies or "game-changers" for the full range of program offerings provided by community colleges, such as corequisite remediation, incentivizing 15-credit full-time enrollment, and simplifying and structuring student learning through an emphasis on guided learning pathways.[12,13,14,15]

While it is beyond the scope of this chapter to delve deeply into high-impact practice research as it concerns public health, it is worth describing a few examples that highlight the ways in which programs have applied some of these core principles. Key strategies described in this section include designing flexible class schedules to meet student needs, considering the strengths and drawbacks of online learning for specific student populations, and recognizing the necessity of educating community college audiences about the nature of public health and the ways in which it can be integrated into diverse academic formats.

First, community college programs pay special attention to scheduling classes around student needs. In addition to structuring schedules to consolidate time spent on campus,[16] programs regularly report other special programming efforts, such as electing to host classes at off-campus sites or working around student schedules for internship placements.

An additional strategy sometimes used to promote program flexibility is online learning. The perceived benefit of online learning at community colleges is somewhat mixed, and research findings vary as to whether online or blended learning opportunities raise or lower student learning outcomes.[17,18] If online learning is used, programs must prioritize current best practice on course format, recognizing that not all students may benefit equally.[19,20,21,22]

Another key lesson is the need to raise awareness about the nature of public health. This theme has been highlighted by current teaching faculty as well as by executive administrators in community college settings. As a relatively new program offering, public health is still often poorly understood by broader audiences. Thus an important function of successful public health programs is persistent marketing and education.

In community colleges, the need to contextualize and personalize student learning is clear. By focusing on the specific needs of students and understanding how student learning fits within the broader community context, community colleges are helping to prepare the next generation of public health professionals.

Conclusion

Community colleges and public health share a commitment to communities, diversity, and career advancement for students. Yet until recently, there has been little attention paid to public health education in community colleges.[23] Therefore, it is not surprising that misinformation and lack of information exist in both public health and in community colleges.

The Community Colleges and Public Health report and the subsequent efforts by the League for Innovation in the Community College to champion public health education have gone a long way in educating community college faculty about the role and importance of public health.

The development of a true continuum of public health education that articulates community college public health education and public health bachelor's degree programs is still a work in progress. The efforts to create guided learning pathways provide an opportunity to build on an important initiative of the community colleges to support and guide students into well-defined career directions.

It is important that public health becomes one of these career directions that provides new opportunities for students and helps to diversify the public health workforce. The initial success of efforts by community colleges and public health educational organizations to work together holds great promise for progress in the years to come.

REFERENCES

1. Healthy People 2020. "Public Health Infrastructure." US Department of Health and Human Services: Office of Disease Prevention and Health Promotion. https://www.healthypeople.gov/2020/topics-objectives/topic/public-health-infra structure (accessed April 7, 2018).

2. American Public Health Association. "The Integration of Core Public Health Education into Undergraduate Curricula." 2009. https://www.apha.org/policies -and-advocacy/public-health-policy-statements/policy-database/2014/07/22/09/58 /the-integration-of-core-public-health-education-into-undergraduate-curricula (accessed April 7, 2018).

3. Riegelman, R. K., C. Wilson, J. Dreyzehner, and L. Huffard. "Community Colleges and Public Health Project Final Report." Framing the Future Task Force, convened by the Association of Schools and Programs of Public Health and the League for Innovation in the Community College. 2014. https://www.aspph.org/ftf -reports/community-colleges/.

4. League for Innovation in the Community College. "Community Colleges and Public Health." https://www.league.org/ccph (accessed April 7, 2018).

5. American Association of Community Colleges. "The Movement toward Pathways." https://www.aacc.nche.edu/wp-content/uploads/2017/10/TheMovement TowardPathways112.pdf (accessed April 7, 2018).

6. Council on Education for Public Health. "Accreditation Criteria: Schools and Programs of Public Health." Silver Spring, MD: CEPH, 2016. https://ceph.org/assets/2016.Criteria.pdf (accessed March 25, 2018).

7. American Association of Community Colleges. "Fast Facts 2017." https://www.aacc.nche.edu/ (accessed April 7, 2018).

8. US Government Accountability Office. "Higher Education: Students Need More Information to Help Reduce Challenges in Transferring College Credits." 2017. http://www.gao.gov/products/GAO-17-574 (accessed April 7, 2018).

9. Lederman, D. "The Bermuda Triangle of Credit Transfer." *Inside Higher Ed.* September 14, 2017. https://www.insidehighered.com/news/2017/09/14/reports -highlight-woes-faced-one-third-all-college-students-who-transfer.

10. Center for Community College Student Engagement. "A Matter of Degrees: Engaging Practices, Engaging Students (High-Impact Practices for Community College Student Engagement)." Austin: University of Texas at Austin, Community College Leadership Program, 2013.

11. Johnson, K. J. "Health Professions Education: A National Survey of Community College Leaders." *Pedagogy in Health Promotion* 2, no. 1 (2016): 20–33.

12. Center for Community College Student Engagement, "A Matter of Degrees."

13. Center for Community College Student Engagement. "A Matter of Degrees: Practices to Pathways (High-Impact Practices for Community College Student Success)." Austin: University of Texas at Austin, Program in Higher Education Leadership, 2014.

14. Pescarmona, D., and A. Green. "Implementing High-Impact Practices for First-Year Student Success." Association of American Colleges and Universities— Developing a Community College Student Roadmap. Fall 2014. https://www.aacu .org/sites/default/files/files/Roadmap/RoadmapFall2014Newsletter.pdf.

15. Complete College America. "New Rules: Policies to Strengthen and Scale the Game Changers." 2016. http://completecollege.org/wp-content/uploads/2016 /11/NEW-RULES.pdf (accessed April 7, 2018).

16. Complete College America. "New Rules."

17. Jaggars, S. S. "Online Learning in Community Colleges." In *Handbook of Distance Education 3rd Edition*, edited by M. G. Moore, 594–608. New York: Routledge, 2013.

18. Means, B., Y. Toyama, R. Murphy, M. Bakia, and K. Jones. "Evaluation of Evidence-Based Practices in Online Learning: A Meta-Analysis and Review of Online Learning Studies." US Department of Education. May 2009. https://eric.ed .gov/?id=ED505824.

19. Jaggars, S. S., and D. Xu. "How Do Online Course Design Features Influence Student Performance?" *Computers and Education* 95 (2016): 270–284.

20. Kauffman, H. "A Review of Predictive Factors of Student Success in and Satisfaction with Online Learning." *Research in Learning Technology* 23 (2015): https://doi.org/10.3402/rlt.v23.26507.

21. Xu, D., and S. S. Jaggars. "The Impact of Online Learning on Students' Course Outcomes: Evidence from a Large Community and Technical College System." *Economics of Education Review* 37 (2013): 46–57.

22. Goldrick-Rab, S. "Challenges and Opportunities for Improving Community College Student Success." *Review of Educational Research* 80, no. 3 (2010): 437–469.

23. Honoré, P. A., G. N. Graham, J. Garcia, and W. Morris. "A Call to Action: Public Health and Community College Partnerships to Educate the Workforce and Promote Health Equity." *Journal of Public Health Management and Practice* 14, no. 6 (2008): S82-S84.

[7]

Master of Public Health Education

MARIE DIENER-WEST

T HE MASTER OF PUBLIC HEALTH (MPH) is the most widely recognized public health degree, and graduates are highly sought after by a wide range of employers. MPH curricula are evolving to include integrated core offerings, interdisciplinary training in an increasing number of specialties, and training in skills and values that have not been historically emphasized. These changes place an increasing demand on faculty to stay current in their disciplines and to employ techniques that are relevant to students' learning and to their preparation for careers as public health practitioners. In this chapter, we outline educational changes, challenges for faculty, and strategies to address them.

For almost a century, the MPH degree has been the desired degree in public health training for health professionals—predominantly physicians at first—working in health departments and other governmental and nongovernmental agencies. The appreciation that schools of public health are obligated to provide "relevant, efficient, and effective" education to advance the cause of public health has been emphasized,[1] as well as the urgency for appropriate and high-quality educational preparation and training of public health professionals to meet the public health challenges of the twenty-first century.[2,3] The Commission on the Education of Health Professionals for the 21st Century concluded that a new transdisciplinary approach and health systems outlook was needed for professional public health education.[4]

This need is also reflected in the proliferation of public health degrees over time. In 1936, a public health degree or certificate requiring at least one year of residence was offered by only 10 schools.[5] Monitoring of the standards of public health education was instituted in the 1940s; by 1960, there were 12 accredited schools of public health in the United States, and 8 more schools were added between 1965 and 1975.[6] In 2003, there were 32 schools of public health and an additional 45 MPH programs accredited by the Council on Education for Public Health (CEPH).[7] By 2017, this number had increased to 64 schools and 122 programs, including 3 schools (Canada, Mexico, and Taiwan) and 3 programs outside of the United States (Canada, Lebanon, and the West Indies).[8] In 2017, there were 40,840 MPH applications (including dual degrees) and 8,990 MPH graduates across schools and programs.[9]

Educational Challenges

Over time, the reach of public health has expanded in many ways, making it difficult to define a public health professional by previous education or training, professional category, or organizational setting.[10] In addition, the value of the broad-based MPH curriculum has been recognized as a complement not only to medical and nursing degrees but also to training in law, social work, business, dentistry, and international affairs. As the role of public health practice expanded to address evolving knowledge and skills in diverse fields across science, communication, and technology, it was recognized that public health competencies would also need change.[11] Today, with increasing focus on public health at the undergraduate level, the MPH degree may be pursued by students directly out of college, or, conversely, by midcareer professionals seeking additional training. The need to appropriately train this more heterogeneous MPH student body in the foundations of public health and to meet its diverse needs for knowledge and skills in the twenty-first century has challenged the public health educational community to reexamine the required components and competencies of MPH education and to innovate in novel and creative ways.

Traditional MPH Core Competency Model

In 2004, the Association of Schools of Public Health (then ASPH) initiated the development of an MPH Core Competency Model to address the changing needs of public health, to incorporate recommendations from national organizations and the added emphasis on competency-based training, to include competencies within accreditation criteria, and to consider the possible development of a certification exam. Using work groups consisting of members from public health programs and practitioner organizations, and employing a modified Delphi process and expert panel discussion, the final project included 119 competencies for the five core areas of public health (biostatistics, environmental health sciences, epidemiology, health policy and management, and social and behavioral sciences) as well as seven cross-cutting areas (communication, diversity and culture, leadership, professionalism and ethics, program planning and assessment, public health biology, and systems thinking).[12,13]

Emphasis on Interdisciplinary Learning and Foundational Knowledge and Skills

However, as the number of schools and programs offering MPH degrees proliferated, the Association of Schools and Programs of Public Health (now ASPPH) constituted the Framing the Future task force.[14] To broaden the work of the task force, expert panels were created for specific areas, including the undergraduate public health major, the MPH degree, and the Doctor of Public Health (DrPH) degree. The work of the MPH expert panel was finalized in November 2014. It concluded that key considerations of the twenty-first-century MPH degree should distinguish the MPH from the bachelor's and doctoral public health degrees, increasing the attention paid to population health and healthcare, responding to the needs of employers, being connected to applied public health practice, and emphasizing global health issues. Necessary design features would include a rigorous interdisciplinary and interprofessional curriculum for core components but also an in-depth concentration area. It was recommended that an in-depth concentration be a distinguishing element of a twenty-first-century MPH degree, but the panel emphasized that this feature still allowed for a generalist or customized approach.[15,16]

Building on the work of these groups and task forces, and after a lengthy process of seeking feedback from multiple stakeholders through many different forums, CEPH released their new accreditation criteria for all schools and programs of public health in October 2016.[17] The criteria now call for six foundational knowledge learning objectives related to "Profession and Science of Public Health" and six related to "Factors Related to Public Health" as well as 22 MPH foundational competencies, ranging from evidence-based approaches to systems thinking. The foundational competencies are no longer tied directly to the five traditional core areas in the silos of their own disciplines, thus providing schools and programs the opportunity to design and teach MPH curricula in creative and novel ways that are informed by the strengths of their faculty.

MPH Professional/Practical Training

The 1988 Future of Public Health report by the Institute of Medicine (IOM) made several recommendations for strengthening the link between professional education and professional practice, and tasked schools of public health with developing "a greater emphasis on public health practice and to equip them to train personnel with the breadth of knowledge that matches the scope of public health."[18] In particular, the IOM report recommended new linkages between schools and state and local health departments as well as the practice community, the development of new training and practice opportunities, and expanded relationships between schools of public health and other professional schools. All MPH students are now required to demonstrate the application of public health concepts through an applied practice experience focusing on foundational competencies and competencies relevant to their areas of specialization.[19]

Students' applied practice experiences may vary across governmental, nongovernmental, nonprofit, and for-profit settings or university-affiliated settings with external partners. Achieving practice competencies in an organizational setting is typically supervised and evaluated by an organizational partner. However, a faculty member may be a preceptor if the work is with an external agency or community-based organization. Numerous schools have developed a practicum office or office for field practice that serves to centralize the support for selecting, supervising, and evaluating applied experiences. Novel ways of offering applied practice experiences include developing academic-community partnerships,[20] academic courses that have practice-based additions, and pathways for students to seek out independent projects at local, national, and international organizations.

MPH Interdisciplinary Training

The IOM report also recommended that schools of public health expand their relationships with other professional schools to encompass the full scope of public health practice.[21] The attention to public health problems through interdisciplinary solutions and interprofessional work is apparent through the newly required foundational competency on interprofessional practice and the growth and interest in joint graduate degrees combined with the MPH degree. The emerging need to prepare the next generation of public health leaders in integrated approaches to solving these evolving problems has guided the development of numerous dual and combined degree programs.

MD/MPH, MSN/MPH, DDS/MPH

The introduction of combined MD/MPH programs serves to meet the changing needs of physicians, their patients, and the healthcare system while also promoting the health of the public. Public health training has been of interest even before the advent of changes in the graduate medical curriculum that have taken place over the past decade. It ranges from integrated training within a four-year medical program[22] to stand-alone MPH training between the third and fourth years of medical school. Some evidence suggests that dual training results in educational experiences that pique student interest in careers as primary care physicians (family medicine, pediatrics, or general internal medicine).[23] Such combined MD/MPH programs have expanded to developing areas outside of the United States, where the need for such training in their health systems is even more critical.[24] Similarly, combined MSN/MPH and DDS/MPH training prepares nurses and dentists for public health positions outside of conventional practice settings.

DVM/MPH

The One Health approach has stimulated the recognition that the health of humans is related to that of animals and the environment. This established need has initiated novel educational programs for public health veterinarians working in private practice, industry, and government, such as the Centers for Disease Control and Prevention.[25]

PharmD/MPH

With pharmacists' increasing roles in the community, as well as in hospitals and health systems, their function in public health has evolved from providing medications and immunizations to taking an active role in prevention (e.g., health screenings) and intervention (e.g., that may be required for the opioid epidemic). Dual PharmD/MPH programs will prepare pharmacists to play a larger role as the need for public health workers increases in the future.[26]

MBA/MPH

Multiple schools have designed dual MBA/MPH programs to train healthcare managers and consultants. Changes in the nature and complexity of the healthcare system have increased the demand for managers having skills in both population health and business.[27] It is projected that employment in the United States will increase by 11.5 million over the next decade, and that healthcare industries will account for a large share of this increase due to the aging of society and other factors.[28] MBA/MPH graduates obtain leadership roles at for-profit and nonprofit hospitals, healthcare organizations, nongovernmental organizations, and consulting companies.

MSW/MPH

With evolving changes in the healthcare system and the emphasis on the importance of the social determinants of health, dual MSW/MPH degree programs prepare social workers with the broader lens of population-based health.[29]

The addition of these dual degree programs has broadened the interdisciplinary scope of MPH students at public health schools and allows for tailored applied practice experiences and integrative learning experiences that advance their combined knowledge for future professional endeavors.

Creative Educational Strategies in the MPH Curriculum

Integrated Core Curriculum or Multidisciplinary Experiences

Teaching the foundational knowledge and core competencies is no longer solely the responsibility of the faculty of traditional departments. An integrated approach to teaching the core areas, employing case studies, and using shared cross-cutting examples across cores has been developed, implemented, and evaluated at a number of schools.

In 2001, the University of Alabama at Birmingham School of Public Health introduced an integrated MPH core curriculum that is team-taught and structured around a series of modules on topics lending themselves to interdisciplinary discussion and skills.[30]

The Columbia University Mailman School of Public Health completed a curriculum renewal in which faculty revised the core curriculum to be taught by interdisciplinary teams to integrate knowledge and skills across disciplines. They also introduced two new courses, a case-based course titled Integration of Science and Practice and a leadership skills course. Lastly, in addition to departmental (disciplinary) course requirements, all MPH students are required to elect a certificate for specialization, although the generalized approach was also available.[31]

A slightly different approach has been taken by the Loma Linda University School of Public Health, which created three integrated and interdisciplinary public health core courses—Public Health for Community Resilience, Public Health for a Healthy Lifestyle, and Public Health and Health Systems.[32]

Most recently, Boston University redesigned their MPH curriculum to consist of four integrated courses—Health Systems, Law, and Policy; Individual, Community, and Population Health; Quantitative Methods for Public Health; and Leadership and Management.[33] Similarly, other schools are in the process of developing or implementing changes in their curricula. The Harvard T. H. Chan School of Public Health has designed a new integrated MPH core course titled Critical Thinking and Action for Public Health Professionals, which will be required for all MPH students in 2018.[34]

Alternatively, the School of Public Health at University at Albany, State University of New York designed an integrated first-year MPH experience in which a common cross-cutting current public health issue such as diabetes was discussed in each core course and related across core courses. This enables students to explore the issue from multiple disciplines and perspectives.[35]

Other multidisciplinary approaches to facilitating students' comprehension and appreciation of MPH competencies and interdisciplinary skills have included the case study approach that is used by the Harvard T. H. Chan School, the flipped classroom model, and teaching with technology method that is employed by the Johns Hopkins Bloomberg School of Public Health and others for both online and on-site instruction.

Global MPH Training: Meeting International Challenges

Advances in technology and global access to the internet have increased the opportunities for public health education beyond the conventional walls of on-site instructional programs. Education through multiple modalities and increasing innovation is required and may range from intensive institute courses and online course offerings to tailored global education and open education initiatives. There is a continued need for broadly rethinking and evaluating the future needs and delivery of global public health education beyond the conventional walls of full-time on-site programs.

Intensive Institute Programs

The offering of short on-site courses in a concentrated learning format has been utilized by a number of schools of public health. In these institutes, didactic courses are offered in compressed one-to-three-week sessions and, more recently, in an online format. Course readings may be required prior to the on-site instruction, and course papers or projects may be completed after the session ends. Attendees may take the courses for academic credit or not. This institute model also has expanded internationally.

Online Degrees

The first online public health courses were developed in 1997, with funding from the Centers for Disease Control and Prevention (CDC), for a Graduate Certificate Program for CDC employees and were offered at four schools: Emory, Johns Hopkins, Tulane, and the University of Washington.[36] Today, numerous schools of public health offer part-time graduate certificates and online MPH programs, which allow public health professionals to augment their education and skills for immediate application to the workplace.

Tailored Global Education

There is a growing need for versatile and available public health education and training. New multimedia resources and technology provide a viable and inexpensive format for addressing changing needs in both global health and global MPH education. Tools and platforms for viewing course content and for communication via computers, tablets, and mobile phones make access possible for more people in more locations than ever before. Increased access to technology, even in remote locations, provides opportunities for specialized and tailored education that were not previously possible.

The Johns Hopkins Bloomberg School of Public Health has initiated several unique part-time degree programs in targeted geographic areas, including Taiwan, Abu Dhabi, and China. A more recent cooperative MPH program was developed with the Indian Institute of Health Management Research University in Jaipur, India.

Open Education Initiatives

Since 2005, public health course content has been widely available on OpenCourseWare (OCW).[37] Funded by a grant from the Hewlett Foundation, the Johns Hopkins Bloomberg School of Public Health originally published materials from ten courses on OCW, thereby joining the

Massachusetts Institute of Technology (MIT) and other institutions in the growing open educational resources movement. The content of more than 110 public health courses is now available for free under the Creative Commons license. In addition to course content, OCW also includes some student-generated work and symposia as well as the OCW Image Library of graphs and illustrations, making it a valuable resource for both faculty and students.[38]

Many schools of public health have partnered with either Coursera or edX in the offering of massive open online courses on their online platforms.[39]

Opportunities for Enhancing the Impact of the MPH Degree

Certification in Public Health

With the increase in numbers of schools and programs in public health, the role of credentialing or certifying in public health has been under discussion as a means for validating the knowledge, skills, and principles mastered by public health graduates in preparation for the workplace, similar to the certification acquired by those trained in other health professions.[40] The National Board of Public Health Examiners was established in September 2005 to recognize public health as a certified profession and to "ensure that public health professionals have mastered the foundational knowledge and skills relevant to contemporary public health."[41] This is done through the administration of a voluntary certification exam, the Certified in Public Health (CPH) exam, which can be taken by students and graduates from schools and programs of public health accredited by CEPH or by other public health professionals. The exam is a mandatory graduation requirement for some schools of public health. The first offering of the exam was in 2008, but the effects of the CPH exam and credential on subsequent hiring, jobs, and quality of work by the public health workforce are still unknown and must be evaluated.[42]

Job Task Analysis and Meeting Employer Needs

As part of the necessary evaluation of the CPH exam, the National Board of Public Health Examiners conducted a survey in 2014 to determine the extent to which the education and experiences of MPH graduates matched the knowledge, attitudes, and skills needed in the workplace. An advisory committee reviewed all available documents highlighting public health competencies and activities and identified 200 common job tasks in each of 10 content domains: critical and strategic analysis; biological and environmental applications in public health; leadership and systems thinking; management, finance, and policy; program planning; collaborating and partnering; communication; advocacy; ethics; and diversity and cultural proficiency. More than 4,800 responses were collected and analyzed to assess the relative rankings of the domains as well as tasks within domains. The three most highly rated job tasks were: collecting valid and reliable data, using information technology for data collection, and employing ethical principles in the collection, use, and dissemination of data.[43] This suggested that the majority of respondents feel that working with public health data is a critical component of their workplace. Future plans include conducting a more systematic survey of employers and using the results from the job task analysis as a tool for refining the CPH exam in the future. The goal of the exam should be to capture the necessary knowledge and skills that are mapped to success in the workplace.

Conclusion

The CEPH accreditation criteria of 2016 provide an opportunity for all schools and programs of public health to critically evaluate their MPH curriculum, learning objectives, and competencies. Optimizing the approaches to creatively teach in different ways, with different strategies and modalities, and sharing these approaches, will be the hallmark of the second 100 years of public health education. Assuring success through the valid assessment of competencies and measurements of outcomes will be a focus of faculty, institutions, and accrediting agencies. Improving public health education using some of the multiple methods outlined here will translate to better public health for all when meeting the challenges of the twenty-first century.

REFERENCES

1. Sommer, A. "Toward a Better Educated Public Health Workforce." *American Journal of Public Health* 90, no. 8 (2000): 1194–1195.

2. Institute of Medicine. "Who Will Keep the Public Healthy? Educating Public Health Professionals for the 21st Century." K. Gebbie, L. Rosenstock, and L. M. Hernandez, eds. Washington, DC: National Academies Press, 2003.

3. Koh, H. K., J. M. Nowinski, and J. J. Piotrowski. "A 2020 Vision for Educating the Next Generation of Public Health Leaders." *American Journal of Preventative Medicine* 40, no. 2 (2011): 199–202.

4. Frenk, J., L. Chen, Z. A. Bhutta, J. Cohen, N. Crisp, T. Evans, H. Fineberg, et al. "Health Professionals for a New Century: Transforming Education to Strengthen Health Systems in an Interdependent World." *Lancet* 376, no. 9756 (2010): 1923–1958.

5. Institute of Medicine, "Who Will Keep the Public Healthy?," 43.

6. Institute of Medicine, "Who Will Keep the Public Healthy?," 48.

7. Institute of Medicine, "Who Will Keep the Public Healthy?," 50.

8. Council on Education for Public Health. "List of Accredited Schools and Programs." https://ceph.org/about/org-info/who-we-accredit/accredited/ (accessed November 17, 2018).

9. Association for Schools and Programs in Public Health. "Data Center." https://data.aspph.org (accessed November 16, 2018).

10. Institute of Medicine, "Who Will Keep the Public Healthy?," 29.

11. Clark, N. M., and E. Weist. "Mastering the New Public Health." *American Journal of Public Health* 90, no. 8 (2000): 1208–1211.

12. Association of Schools of Public Health. "Master's Degree in Public Health Core Competency Development Project—Version 2.3." ASPH Education Committee. 2006. https://s3.amazonaws.com/aspph-wp-production/app/uploads/2014/04/Version2.31_FINAL.pdf (accessed April 7, 2018).

13. Calhoun, J. G., K. Ramiah, E. M. Weist, and S. M. Shortell. "Development of a Core Competency Model for the Master of Public Health Degree." *American Journal of Public Health* 98, no. 9 (2008): 1598–1607.

14. Petersen, D. J., and E. M. Weist. "Framing the Future by Mastering the New Public Health." *Journal of Public Health Management and Practice* 20, no. 4 (2014): 371–374.

15. Association of Schools and Programs of Public Health. "Master of Public Health Degree for the 21st Century: Key Considerations, Design Features, and Critical Content of the Core." 2014. https://www.aspph.org/teach-research/models/mph-degree-report/ (accessed March 25, 2018).

16. Petersen, D. J., J. R. Finnegan Jr., and H. C. Spencer. "Anticipating Change, Sparking Innovation: Framing the Future." *American Journal of Public Health* 105, Suppl. 1 (2015): S46-S49.

17. Council on Education for Public Health. "Accreditation Criteria: Schools and Programs of Public Health." Silver Spring, MD: CEPH, 2016. https://ceph.org/assets/2016.Criteria.pdf (accessed March 25, 2018).

18. Institute of Medicine. *The Future of Public Health*. Washington, DC: National Academy Press, 1988, 157. https://www.nap.edu/catalog/1091/the-future-of-public-health.

19. Council for Education in Public Health, "Accreditation Criteria."

20. Rutkow L., M. B. Levin, and T. A. Burke. "Meeting Local Needs While Developing Public Health Practice Skills: A Model Community-Academic Partnership." *Public Health Management and Practice* 15, no. 5 (2009): 425–341.

21. Institute of Medicine, "Who Will Keep the Public Healthy?"

22. Boyer, M. H. "A Decade's Experience at Tufts with a Four-Year Combined Curriculum in Medicine and Public Health." *Academic Medicine* 72, no. 4 (1997): 269–275.

23. Wei McIntosh, E., and C. P. Morley. "Family Medicine or Primary Care Residency Selection: Effects of Family Medicine Interest Groups, MD/MPH Dual Degrees, and Rural Medical Education." *Family Medicine* 48, no. 5 (2016): 385–388.

24. Salehi, A., N. Hashemi, M. Saber, and M. H. Imanieh. "Designing and Conducting MD/MPH Dual Degree Program in the Medical School of Shiraz University of Medical Sciences." *Journal of Advances in Medical Education and Professionalism* 3, no. 3 (2015): 105–110.

25. Minucci L. A., K. A. Hanson, D. K. Olson, et al. "A Flexible Approach to Training Veterinarians in Public Health: An Overview and Early Assessment of the DVM/MPH Dual-Degree Program at the University of Minnesota." *Journal of Veterinary Medical Education* 35, no. 2 (2008): 166–172.

26. Gortney, J. S., S. Seed, N. Borja-Hart, et al. "The Prevalence and Characteristics of Dual PharmD/MPH Programs Offered at US Colleges and Schools of Pharmacy." *American Journal of Pharmacy Education* 77, no. 6 (2013): 1–7.

27. Pettigrew, M. M., H. P. Forman, and A. F. Pistell. "Innovating in Health Care Management Education: Development of an Accelerated MBA and MPH Degree Program at Yale." *American Journal of Public Health* 105 (2015): S68-S72.

28. Bureau of Labor Statistics. "Employment Projections: 2016–26 Summary." 2017. https://www.bls.gov/news.release/ecopro.nro.htm (accessed December 19, 2017).

29. Ziperstein, D., B. J. Ruth, A. Clement, J. W. Marshall, M. Wachman, and E. E. Velasquez. "Mapping Dual-Degree Programs in Social Work and Public Health: Results from a National Survey." *Advances in Social Work* 16, no. 2 (2015): 406–421.

30. Peterson D. J., M. E. Hovinga, M. A. Pass, et al. "Assuring Public Health Professionals Are Prepared for the Future: The UAB Public Health Integrated Core Curriculum." *Public Health Reports* 120 (2005): 496–503.

31. Begg, M. D., S. Galea, R. Bayer, J. R. Walker, and L. P. Fried. "MPH Education for the 21st Century: Design of Columbia University's New Public Health Curriculum." *American Journal of Public Health* 104, no. 1 (2014): 30–36.

32. Loma Linda University School of Public Health. "MPH Program." https://publichealth.llu.edu/academics/mph (accessed December 19, 2017).

33. Sullivan, L. M., A. Velez, V. B. Edouard, and S. Galea. "Realigning the Master of Public Health (MPH) to Meet the Evolving Needs of the Workforce." *Pedagogy in Health Promotion* (2017): 1–11.

34. Harvard T. H. Chan School of Public Health. "MPH Program." https://www.hsph.harvard.edu/office-of-education/master-of-public-health/for-students/mph-program-competencies (accessed December 19, 2017).

35. Dewar, D. M., M. S. Bloom, H. Choi, L. Gensburg, and A. Hosler. "The Integrated First Year Experience in the Master of Public Health Program." *American Journal of Public Health* 105, Suppl. 1 (2015): S97-S98.

36. Institute of Medicine, "Who Will Keep the Public Healthy?," 55–56.

37. OpenCourseWare, http://ocw.jhsph.edu (accessed December 19, 2017).

38. Kanchanaraksa S., I. Gooding, B. Klaas, and J. D. Yager. "Johns Hopkins Bloomberg School of Public Health OpenCourseWare. *Open Learning* 24 (2009): 39–46.

39. Gooding I., B. Klaas, Y. D. Yager, and S. Kanchanaraksa. "Massive Open Online Courses in Public Health." *Frontiers in Public Health* (2013): 1–8.

40. Gebbie, K., B. D. Goldstein, D. I. Gregorio, W. Tsou, P. Buffler, D. Petersen, C. Mahan, and G. B. Silver. "The National Board of Public Health Examiners: Credentialing Public Health Graduates." *Public Health Reports* 122, no. 4 (2007): 435–440.

41. The National Board of Public Health Examiners. "Credentialing Public Health Graduates." www.nbphe.org (accessed December 19, 2017).

42. Institute of Medicine, "Who Will Keep the Public Healthy?," 44.

43. Kurz, R. S., C. Yager, J. D. Yager, et al. "Advancing the Certified in Public Health Exam: A Job Task Analysis." *Public Health Reports* 132, no. 4 (2017): 518–623.

[8]

The DrPH Degree in Contemporary Public Health Education

EUGENE DECLERCQ

IN ITS 1912 BULLETIN, the Massachusetts Institute of Technology (MIT) noted that it had changed the name of its biology department to the Department of Biology and Public Health

> in recognition of the readiness and the ability of the institute to prepare
> men and women technically trained for this new and important branch
> of the government service. Experience has shown that the sanitary
> biologist and the sanitary engineer are sometimes even more successful
> than the medical man in such positions and that a medical training is no
> longer regarded as necessary is shown by the fact that some of our
> leading Universities are now awarding the degree of Doctor of Public
> Health [DrPH] after courses of work and study quite different from
> those required for the degree of Doctor of Medicine.[1]

In that same year, a joint Harvard-MIT program awarded their first two DrPHs, including one to the redoubtable Arthur Isaac Kendall, who also had a PhD and a ScD.[2]

By 1918, an article in the *American Journal of Public Health* cataloging the state of DrPH education in North America noted that 20 schools were offering the DrPH degree, although most were new and had not yet actually awarded a DrPH degree. They generally required a medical degree for admission, and though only Harvard formally limited their admissions to men, the requirement for a medical degree may have sufficed to prevent female enrollments. The curricula, where listed, focused on sanitary engineering, bacteriology, and water supply, though courses in statistics and public health administration were noted.[3] This was a time of great hope for public health as C. E. A. Winslow wrote in 1920: "The public health movement has been expanding so rapidly that what was 'the New Public Health' fifteen years ago includes only the more conventional interests of the present day."[4]

From this enthusiastic beginning, the DrPH degree grew rapidly, in just a few years, in popularity, with 37 graduates by 1925. Growth, however, slowed to a trickle soon thereafter. The degree languished as medical doctors increasingly focused on the Master of Public Health (MPH), with its shorter training period, as the degree of choice. The 1925 total of DrPH graduates would not be matched for almost half a century.[5] As public health education grew in popularity, the PhD became the doctoral degree of choice, as faculty in schools of public health were expected to become specialized researchers capable of successfully competing for major research grants. The DrPH, as a degree preparing generalists to lead public health departments, was becoming increasingly rare as fewer schools even offered the degree, and among those that did, many were legacy programs in departments that barely distinguished the DrPH from the corresponding departmental PhD.[6]

The Revival of the DrPH

While the number of doctoral students in public health has been growing steadily over the past 30 years, to more than 8,000 in 2016, the growth has been primarily in PhD students.[7] The rise in DrPH students is a more recent phenomenon. The growth in PhD students continued a long-term trend as the number of schools of public health increased and schools needed to staff their faculty with PhD-trained researchers. In turn, faculty were drawn to schools with large numbers of PhD students, who could serve as their research and lab assistants as they pursued ever-more competitive grant funding.

The more recent surge in DrPH students (figure 8.1) is likely the result of several factors. First is the growth in the number of individuals with an MPH degree who have an interest in pursuing the "next degree." Between 2010 and 2016, more than 43,000 students graduated from ac-

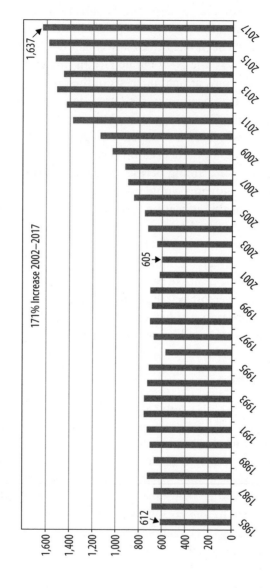

Figure 8.1. DrPH Student Trends, 1985–2017

credited schools of public health with an MPH.[8] The proliferation of MPH graduates created a large pool of those interested in advancing to higher-level training in public health. Second, the demands of the field are calling for individuals with higher-level skills to address increasingly complex problems that require training beyond the MPH. PhD training, with its emphasis on developing exceptional research skills in a specialized area, may not prepare individuals for such leadership positions. A third factor may have been the desire for new schools of public health to achieve accreditation, which required them to offer at least three doctoral degrees in core areas of public health.[9] Because establishing a DrPH at a school of public health typically did not require approval from a university graduate school, it was more efficient for some schools to offer DrPH degrees. As the number of schools of public health increased rapidly from 28 in 2000 to 59 in 2016, the number of DrPH programs increased from 18 to 33 and the number of DrPH students increased by 161% to almost 1,600 (figure 8.1). The increases have slowed in recent years, which is likely a reflection of students completing their programs as the number of DrPH graduates has begun to increase rapidly from 72 in 2003 to 249 in 2016.[10]

Distinguishing DrPH and PhD Public Health Students

The available data for 2010–2016 identifies some distinctions between PhD and DrPH students. While approximately 70% of both DrPH and PhD students are female, there are differences by nativity and race. PhD students are more likely to be foreign born (25% vs. 16%). Almost half of DrPH students are nonwhite (49%), as compared to about one-third (34%) of PhD students. DrPH students are twice as likely to self-identify as black (20%) as compared to PhD public health students (9.7%).[11]

Differences in areas of study can be identified from Association of Schools and Programs of Public Health (ASPPH) data, which reports on program areas by type of doctoral degree (e.g., biostatistics, epidemiology, environmental sciences). DrPH students focus to a far greater degree on health policy and management (25%), behavioral science (21%), generalist public health (12%), and public health practice (10%). Notably, one in five DrPH students (22%) are in areas that ASPPH did not even include in its 1995 survey: general public health and public health practice. Conversely, PhD students tend to concentrate in epidemiology (25%), biostatistics (16%), behavioral science (14%), and health policy and management (13%).[12]

Curriculum Development for DrPH Programs

The evolution of the DrPH degree has been reflected in the changing accreditation expectations concerning the DrPH curriculum. The 2011 accreditation requirements from the Council on Education for Public Health (CEPH) make no mention of DrPH curriculum, and schools often maintained small legacy DrPH programs as minor offshoots of departmentally based PhD programs. The slight program variation for the DrPH candidates was typically seen in a more practice-relevant dissertation. The lack of clear precedents and the fact that almost half of existing DrPH programs have come into existence since 2000 created considerable opportunity for innovation.

For example, at the time of the development of the DrPH program at our institution, in 2002–2003, we reviewed the curricula of other DrPH programs and found very little variation across programs. In our case, we already had four PhD degree programs—in biostatistics, environmental health, epidemiology, and health services—and we set out to design a DrPH for early and midcareer professionals who sought advanced training in management, policy, and leadership. With no consensus in the field on how best to implement such a curriculum in schools of public health, we opted to work with practitioners and faculty to identify the skills necessary for public health leadership. In doing so, we found that our curriculum, which was rich and diverse in research courses, did not have all the practice-oriented courses necessary to provide the scope or level of training we sought. Therefore, we developed a number of new courses to address those needs. This had the advantage of allowing us to create an integrated curriculum in which core courses were sequenced and targeted the desired competencies. However, it raised the administrative challenge of finding faculty willing and able to teach practice-oriented courses when the program began in fall 2004.

In 2005, an informal meeting of DrPH directors was held in Philadelphia at the American Public Health Association conference to discuss mutual interests and the challenges of running DrPH programs. The informal discussions led to a formal committee of the Association of

Schools of Public Health, which in turn led to a project to formalize competencies for DrPH graduates. Committees cochaired by academics and practitioners met and initially agreed that the competencies for DrPH graduates did not need to conform to the MPH competencies, which were strongly linked to the five core areas of public health. Instead, the emphasis was on cross-cutting skills; the resulting 2009 document titled "Doctor of Public Health (DrPH) Core Competency Model" described 7 domains of skills, with 6 to 9 specific competencies identified in each area, for a total of 54 competencies.[13] The competencies were advocacy, communication, community/cultural orientation, critical analysis, leadership, management, and professionalism and ethics.

Of note was how much these competencies represented a commitment to the practice-oriented model of DrPH education. Schools that had used their DrPH as a way to facilitate accreditation through the development of three doctoral degrees that were indistinguishable from PhDs (i.e., a DrPH in biostatistics or epidemiology) needed substantial restructuring of their programs to ensure that their students addressed domains involving topics such as developing financial and business plans, organizing teams for implementation, engaging communities in implementation plans, guiding an organization in setting communication goals, or presenting positions on health issues, law, and policy. Of note, schools were not required to incorporate these competencies into the curriculum planning; they were at the time only advised to do so. As expected, however, accreditation requirements soon followed, and when CEPH issued new accreditation criteria for the DrPH in 2016, many of these principles were reflected in an explicit commitment to practice-oriented education.[14]

After establishing the need for foundational public health knowledge for both the MPH and the DrPH, the opening statement of the accreditation section on DrPH competencies reads: "The DrPH is the professional doctoral degree in public health, designed to produce transformative academic and practice leaders with expertise in evidence-based public health practice and research. These individuals are able to convene diverse partners; communicate to effect change across a range of sectors and settings; synthesize and translate findings; and generate practice-based evidence that advances programs, policies, services and/or systems addressing population health."[15] The 2016 criteria identified 20 DrPH competencies in four specific areas: (1) data and analysis;

(2) leadership, management, and governance; (3) policy and programs; and (4) education and workforce development. By far, the greatest attention was devoted to management and leadership, with 10 specific competencies. The new accreditation requirements also spell out the need for a practicum so that "DrPH programs ensure that graduates have significant advanced-level practical experiences collaborating with practitioners, allowing opportunities to develop leadership competencies and contribute to the field."[16]

Current Challenges for DrPH Education

The new accreditation criteria should have a profound impact on DrPH programs going forward. Schools will have to either commit to implementing practice-oriented programs or simply close their programs. Given the increasing demand for DrPH education among the growing cohort of MPH graduates, schools may be reluctant to forgo such a growing market. Having succeeded in more clearly defining the distinction between a public health PhD and a DrPH, schools now face an array of challenges as they move into an area of education that they have not traditionally emphasized at the doctoral level.

Practice-Based Education in a Research Institution

The financing model for many large schools of public health has rested on three elements—an active National Institutes of Health–based research program; a large MPH program; and, for a handful of more established schools, an endowment. Faculty have been traditionally hired largely based on their ability to bring in research funding. PhD and postdoctoral programs fuel the research engine by providing a steady stream of research assistants and colleagues.

Schools wanting to support a practice-based DrPH program under the new accreditation requirements need faculty to teach those students and supervise their dissertations and practicums—little of which will assist the National Institutes of Health grant-writing process. The goal of DrPH education—producing generalists who are comfortable working on a variety of problems in a wide range of contexts—is the antithesis of the targeted specialist education at the core of PhD training.

Sustaining Faculty Enthusiasm

Schools that have opted to develop a DrPH program must continue to support faculty involvement in the program. For faculty hired for their research specialization in a well-funded area, working with DrPH students whose interests are not closely associated with their own may be seen as counterproductive. For the many faculty who are more practice oriented, their promotion and tenure opportunities are not typically determined by the quality of practice-based teaching. Therefore, while these faculty may support the concept of a DrPH program in practice, they may have little incentive to get heavily involved. Thus, schools need to value and recognize faculty contributions in DrPH programs in promotion and tenure decisions.

Admitting the Right DrPH Candidates

Admissions committees have a variety of tools—grades, graduate record examinations (GREs), writing samples—to help them determine the most academically promising applicants; however, judging leadership potential is not clearly identified by a GRE percentile. Even if someone demonstrates a strong potential for leadership through their early career accomplishments, how do you weigh that against less-than-stellar academic performance that may be more than a decade old? Faculty and staff must therefore devise new systems for evaluating potential of DrPH applicants that will best fit their programs and have the greatest potential for success.

Assessing Field-Based Competency

For a PhD student, the assessment of the quality of their work generally falls into the comfort zone for faculty—demonstrated performance of methodological skills and writing of research papers and grants. For DrPH students, faculty must assess such things as leadership performance, policy savvy, ability to work in diverse communities, and strategic thinking. Metrics can be developed and applied to all these areas, but faculty may need additional support and training to develop course offerings and student work products that allow for assessment of desired competencies.

The DrPH Comprehensive Examination

If DrPH candidates are expected to display the ability to work on myriad public health problems, one possible means of assessment is a comprehensive examination. At our institution, we wrestled with the best approach to assessment and determined that a case analysis was a reasonable solution. Students are given a case that is explicitly not in their area of expertise, but they do choose the geographic setting. Students therefore develop the ability to quickly learn about a new problem, as well as become immersed in the data and resources of their chosen area. This approximates a challenge they would face in the field, and their preparation allows them to develop critical skills. They have four days to develop a written solution, and then orally defend it. The grounded nature of the examination has proven attractive to both students and faculty.

Flexibility of Programs

In the most recent data available (2010–2011), DrPH students more often attended part time (52%) than did PhD students (21%).[17] A 2014 survey of DrPH directors found most all DrPH programs involved both part-time and full-time students. The same survey found only 5 of the 27 responding programs reporting an online-only or hybrid format.[18] The midcareer status of many DrPH students suggests the need for more flexible forms of class offerings in terms of online, weekend, and evening classes.

Practice-Based Culminating Product (Dissertation)

Only 4 of 28 responding DrPH directors identified an option other than a dissertation as a student's final product in their program.[19] If dissertations are the norm, what should a DrPH consist of? The "three-paper" model of public health research programs is sound preparation for an academic career, but does it prepare students for field leadership? DrPH programs are often better served with field-oriented dissertations given the desired competencies. At our institution, we added a step to our dissertation process in which a school-wide committee reviews dissertation topics to assess their practice relevance before approving them for development. Our criteria for judging the practice nature of the dissertation are rigor, relevance to a current entity in the field (either a governmental or nongovernmental organization), and consideration of transferability of findings to other settings.

Global Focus

There is considerable interest among students in global public health. In training individuals to work in major leadership positions, there is an obligation to take global issues into account, even for those working domestically. This implementation is a matter of balance and specialization in trying to blend global content into the overall curriculum because only four schools with DrPH programs in 2016 listed any global health concentrators. For students committed to working locally, how much of the world should be introduced into their curriculum?

DrPH as Faculty

There are clear benefits associated with having faculty with the kind of field experience and high-level training offered in DrPH programs. Given the need for faculty to acquire external research funding, DrPH programs, particularly under the new competencies, may not adequately be preparing students for that career. DrPH-trained faculty can often identify outside funding sources through contracts and foundations. The challenge is for schools of public health to identify funding models that respect the considerable benefits that DrPH-trained faculty can bring with reasonable expectations for promotion and tenure.

Financing of DrPH Programs

Many schools offer PhD students full tuition remission with a stipend. The benefits of PhD students as research assistants is an attractive inducement for faculty recruitment and retention, as is the prestige associated with a notable PhD program. For DrPH programs that emphasize practice-based education of midcareer professionals, the financing model shifts. Most DrPH students are not interested in serving as research assistants given their leadership focus. DrPH graduates are not as likely to go on to academic careers, rising to become deans and thereby able to support their alma maters in reputation-based school rankings. They often return to where they came from—to become leaders in the seldom-lucrative world of public health practice. Unfortunately, entering from public health practice means that DrPH students are no more able to self-finance than PhD students. Thus, schools need to consider ways to ease the financial burden in order to support the education of these future leaders and ensure the continued growth of DrPH programs.

Conclusion

Several trends are converging to increase demand for DrPH education. The growing complexity of the field requiring better-trained generalists who can lead efforts to combat problems arising from diverse sources, combined with the apparently endless flow of students seeking training to improve the human condition, will keep demand high.

The challenges described in this chapter are real. Training high-level leaders requires resources that many schools have not expended before and a culture change in how we structure our doctoral programs to include an emphasis on practice. The benefits are considerable as we will not only prepare professionals to lead the response to challenges we have not conceived of yet, but the emphasis on practice education will also facilitate the strengthening of practice-level education at the master's and undergraduate levels.

The ultimate test of the success of these changes will be seen in the work of the core of leaders who represent the highest levels of public health practice. Almost a century ago, C. E. A. Winslow, commenting on the importance of the growth of the DrPH, remarked: "It will be long, however, before the supply of doctors of public health is nearly adequate to the demand."[20] His plea remains unfulfilled, but the potential for change to rectify that problem in schools of public health has never been greater.

REFERENCES

1. Massachusetts Institute of Technology. "President's Report." *Bulletin of the Massachusetts Institute of Technology* 47, no. 2 (1912): 1–152.

2. Doyle, L. "Arthur Isaac Kendall: An Artisan of Living." *Northwestern University Medical School Quarterly Bulletin* 20 (1946): 342–360.

3. Howe, E. "Professional Instruction in Public Health in the United States and Canada." *American Journal of Public Health* 8, no. 8 (1918): 600–607.

4. Winslow, C. E. A. "The Untilled Fields of Public Health." *Science* 51, no. 1306 (1920): 23–33.

5. Venezia, R. A. "An Analysis of DrPH Degree Programs in the United States." Washington, DC: Association of Schools of Public Health, 1993.

6. Lee, J. M., S. E. Furner, J. Yager, and D. Hoffman. "A Review of the Status of the Doctor of Public Health Degree and Identification of Future Issues." *Public Health Reports* 124, no. 1 (2009): 177–183.

7. Association for Schools and Programs in Public Health. "Data Center." https://data.aspph.org (accessed December 19, 2017).

8. Association for Schools and Programs in Public Health. "Data Center."

9. Council on Education in Public Health. "Accreditation Criteria Schools of Public Health and Public Health Programs." Silver Spring, MD: CEPH, 2011. https://ceph.org/assets/PHP-Criteria-2011.pdf (accessed April 8, 2018).

10. Association for Schools and Programs in Public Health. "Data Center."

11. Association for Schools and Programs in Public Health. "Data Center."

12. Association for Schools and Programs in Public Health. "Data Center."

13. Association of Schools of Public Health. "Doctor of Public Health (DrPH) Core Competency Model. Version 1.3." ASPH Education Committee. November 2009. https://s3.amazonaws.com/aspph-wp-production/app/uploads/2014/04/DrPHVersion1-3.pdf.

14. Council on Education for Public Health. "Accreditation Criteria: Schools and Programs of Public Health." Silver Spring, MD: CEPH, 2016. https://ceph.org/assets/2016.Criteria.pdf (accessed March 25, 2018).

15. Council on Education for Public Health. "Accreditation Criteria."

16. Council on Education for Public Health. "Accreditation Criteria."

17. Association for Schools and Programs in Public Health. "Data Center."

18. Sherman, B., R. Hoen, J. M. Lee, and E. R. Declercq. "Doctor of Public Health Education and Training: Where Are We Now?" *Public Health Reports* 132, no. 1 (2017): 115–120.

19. Sherman, Hoen, Lee, and Declercq, "Doctor of Public Health Education and Training."

20. Winslow, "The Untilled Fields of Public Health."

[9]

Lifelong Learning

JOEL LEE

THE CHARGE TO the Committee on Educating Public Health Professionals for the 21st Century was to "develop a framework for how, over the next five to ten years, education, training, and research in schools of public health could be strengthened to meet the needs of future public health professionals to improve population-level health." In their consensus report, the committee noted that there is an existing public health workforce that requires education and training to address their lack of previous training and/or needs to update existing skills due to change. In recognition, the committee stated that access to lifelong learning for the public health workforce is one of the six responsibilities of schools of public health.[1] It is now well past the suggested five-to-ten-year timeline, and many changes have occurred in both public health and in educational technology. In this chapter, we present an overview of issues related to and strategies for lifelong learning for public health professionals.

What Is Lifelong Learning?

The First Global Conference on Lifelong Learning defines lifelong learning as the "acquisition of knowledge, values, skills, and understanding that we will require throughout our lifetimes whereby we apply them with confidence, creativity, and enjoyment in all roles, circumstances, and environments." The conference defined the characteristics of life-long learning as: (1) continuous, in that it never ceases; (2) supportive, in that it is not achieved independently; (3) stimulating and empowering, in that it is self-directed and active rather than passive; (4) incorporating knowledge, values, skills, and understanding, in that it is more than what we know; (5) applied, in that the knowledge is not just for knowledge's sake; (6) incorporating confidence, creativity, and enjoyment, in that it is a positive and fulfilling experience; and (7) inclusive of all roles, circumstances, and environments, in that it applies not only to our chosen profession but also to our entire lives.[2,3]

While these findings apply to lifelong learning in its broadest terms, here we focus specifically on lifelong learning in public health. The breadth of career paths linked to public health and the lack of either a required formal educational program for employment or a credential for eligibility to practice make the need for lifelong learning in public health very different than other health professions. Limited preemployment education in public health along with a rapidly changing external environment emphasize the critical importance of lifelong learning for public health professionals.

The 2010 Institute of Medicine (IOM) report titled *Redesigning Continuing Education in the Health Professions* discusses moving traditional continuing education (CE) to continuing professional development (CPD), stating: "CE often is associated with didactic learning methods, such as lectures and seminars, which take place in auditoriums and classrooms." Most health professionals engage in CE to maintain licensure and certification, while CPD applies multiple formats that are learner driven. The IOM report notes that CPD focuses on individual performance improvement and better aligns with lifelong learning more appropriate for the health professions.[4]

Microlearning

In 1959, the American Public Health Association (APHA) established the Continuing Education Program in Public Health. Courses were offered to serve the 13 states in the APHA's Western Region using the innovative (for the time) technologies of videotape, closed-circuit television, programed instruction, and telephone conferences.[5] These tools have now been replaced by newer technologies, including the internet, personal computers, and smartphones. With a generation fluent in their use, these technologies facilitate a transition to a new approach to lifelong learning and the development of microcredentials for lifelong learning in public health.

Lifelong learning opportunities may be categorized on a learning continuum from macrolearning to microlearning. Definitions of these terms vary in the literature; however, there appears to be consensus in several areas. Macrolearning is cognitive and reflects broad concepts, principles, and practices. It is offered in longer sessions, working with others—including an instructor or coach—and typically over a period of hours. Examples include courses, workshops, conferences, and certificate programs offered over days or weeks. In contrast, microlearning typically is topical or problem based; may be private; is offered in a shorter time frame, perhaps even minutes; and is frequently delivered using the internet and digital media.[6,7,8,9]

Public health professionals and educators commonly understand the framework of macrolearning, while microlearning may be less familiar. While microlearning may have been available in the past, the tools to offer microlearning have evolved, thus increasing options and accessibility.[10] Bersin notes that the type of learning is linked to the individual's career stage.[11] Macrolearning is aligned with beginning a career and microlearning is more aligned with maintenance of skills until someone who is proficient moves on to a new role, which could potentially require additional macrolearning.

Learning Management Systems

While large private organizations may offer lifelong learning on their own learning management systems, the limited resources of local public health agencies make this a challenge. The Public Health Foundation maintains the TRAIN Learning Network (https://www.train.org) as a free service and operates through collaborative partnerships with state and federal agencies, local and national organizations, and educational institutions. TRAIN enables lifelong learners to find and enroll in more than 34,000 courses available to any interested user as well as an additional 13,000 courses with limited access to certain groups based on employment site. Three federal agencies—the Centers for Disease Control and Prevention (CDC), Medical Reserve Corps, and Veterans Health

Administration—along with 27 state health and preparedness agencies, academic institutions, professional associations, Public Health Training Centers, nonprofits, and other institutions post content to TRAIN. In addition, the Public Health Agency of Canada offers 13 fee-based and four free courses. TRAIN reports more than 97% of offerings are free and have a completion rate of more than 80 percent. More than 820,000 courses were completed in 2015. Users may track their coursework, print transcripts, and apply work for CE credit in some professions.

The National Network of Public Health Institutes is developing a second learning management system (the Public Health Learning Navigator), which launched in 2018. The Public Health Learning Navigator is described as a "curated, guided, and individualized experience to help public health learners navigate to high-quality training, tools, and resources."[12]

Digital Badges

Digital badges are described as online visual representations demonstrating achievements that serve as a substitute for traditional physical recognitions such as certificates, physical badges, or transcripts. Ostashewski and Reid describe digital badges developing from a history of game culture, visuals on the internet, and traditional use of badges.[13] Digital badges can serve as a valid indicator of specific achievements, knowledge, skills, and competencies that can be earned in formal or informal learning environments.[14] In addition, multiple badges can be stacked to demonstrate greater achievement or specialization in a particular area. Advantages over traditional coursework may include low or no cost, flexible access to online resources, a focus on specific competencies rather than overall course goals, translation of achievement of specific skills to employers, and the potential to motivate lifelong learning.

Each badge, based on its function, is validated differently. Foster describes badges as "in their infancy," "gaining traction," and "no longer considered a technology of the future."[15] However, in public health there is not a well-established model for the development or use of digital badges. Validation could involve many people, such as knowledge experts (instructors), applications specialists (real-world knowledge practitioners), curriculum designers, career services professionals, trainers, and assessment specialists.[16]

Massive Open Online Courses (MOOCs) are open educational resources that aim to facilitate efficient creation, distribution, and use of knowledge and information for learning serving "massive" audiences, "open" to users, offered "online," providing a defined activity or "course."[17] Siemens describes MOOCs as offering "a middle ground for teaching and learning between the highly organized and structured classroom environment and the chaotic open web of fragmented information."[18] De Waard et al. expand this description, describing MOOCs as using social media to build a community for discussion and learning to take place.[19] MOOCs are at an early stage of development still addressing a series of issues including high dropout rates, the lack of an economic or sustainable model, challenges of plagiarism, and risk of de-skilling the professoriate.[20]

Presently, there is wide variation in popular MOOC offerings. Searches based on the terms "public health" and related subjects such as "epidemiology" and "environment" identify relevant courses for public health professionals offered on the following platforms: www.edx.org, www.udacity.com, www.lynda.com (operated by LinkedIn), and www.udemy.com. However, sites are highly variable in their definition of public health content. Costs vary widely, ranging from free to fee-based, although some financial aid opportunities exist. Offerings vary from open, around-the-clock to scheduled courses with set start and finish dates. Assessment of performance ranges from documented completion of watching a video to formal assignments and testing of competencies. Each MOOC operates its own independent learning management system, with variation in reporting via digital and printable badges and certificates with some online availability to employers. Presently, there are few multicourse pathways or formal degrees in public health; however, growth is anticipated. As an example, in March 2018, Coursera (www.coursera.org) announced two public health graduate degrees.

Types of Lifelong Learning

Candy describes four types of learning after graduation as follows: (1) workplace-based learning, (2) continuing professional education, (3) further formal study, and (4) self-directed learning.[21] Each of Candy's four types of lifelong learning are available in public health, as well as a unique fifth hybrid category spanning multiple categories. Each is described in detail in the following sections.

Workplace-Based Learning

Ilyas notes that many organizations are adopting a corporate university model (described later) to meet their training requirements and to add value to their business, including improved employee productivity and retention.[22] His research addresses change and evolution in training and development, defining the corporate university and its value to the culture of knowledge and learning acquisition. As an example of the corporate university model, the Human Resources Office of the CDC operates CDC University (CDCU), a series of online and face-to-face courses developed exclusively for CDC employees and available 24 hours a day, seven days a week through its intranet portal. CDCU offers courses within seven schools: (1) career development, (2) business management, (3) information resources management, (4) leadership and management development, (5) preparedness and emergency response, (6) public health, and (7) public health science, research, and medicine.

CDCU is accredited by seven organizations to provide CE, at no cost, for US health professionals and the global public health community. The CDC is accredited to award CE to physicians (AMA PRA Category 1), the International Association for Continuing Education and Training; Certified Health Education Specialists (CHES) by the National Commission for Health Education Credentialing, Inc.; Certified in Public Health (CPH) recertification credits by the National Board of Public Health Examiners; continuing nursing education by the American Nurses Credentialing Center's Commission on Accreditation; the Accreditation Council for Pharmacy Education, as a provider of continuing pharmacy education; and the American Association of Veterinary State Boards' (AAVSB) Registry of Approved Continuing Education (RACE), to provide AAVSB/RACE contact hours.

While an organization of the scale of the CDC is capable of mounting a broad workplace-based program, smaller state and local departments may have difficulty gathering the necessary resources to do the same.

The National Association of County and City Health Officials reported that in 2005, many local health departments (LHDs) lacked the basic workforce development infrastructure needed to ensure competent staff, and that 38% of all LHDs (and 43% of LHDs serving populations of fewer than 50,000) did not have specific line items in their budgets for staff training.[23] A recent driver promoting workplace-based learning is the Public Health Accreditation Board, which provides voluntary accreditation of state, local, tribal, and territorial public health departments on quality and performance. In its Accreditation Standards Domain 8, the Public Health Accreditation Board requires "the provision of individual training and professional development and the provision of a supportive work environment."[24] Reaccreditation calls for examples of implementation of workforce development plans and the impact of these plans.

Continuing Professional Education

While continuing professional education can conceivably incorporate any lifelong learning activity, it typically refers to the maintenance of professional credentials. The IOM appointed a Committee on Planning a Continuing Health Care Professional Education Institute, which reported that "a vision will be key in guiding efforts to address flaws in current CE efforts and to ensure that all health professionals engage effectively in a process of lifelong learning aimed squarely at improving patient care and population health."[25]

The APHA conducts a Learning Institute at its annual meeting, offering CE courses compliant with the accreditation criteria of four accrediting bodies: Certified Health Education Specialists (CHES) and Master Certified Health Education Specialists (MCHES), Continuing Medical Education, Continuing Nursing Education, and CPH. While these fee-based courses are open to all attendees, offerings address the needs of members seeking to maintain their professional credentials.[26] In addition, there are public health practitioners with other professional licenses, certifications, and registrations, including law, engineering, and the allied health professions, with their own requirements taking advantage of these offerings. Some state public associations also offer their attendees similar continuing professional education credits at regular meetings.

Professionals working in public health hold a wide variety of clinical, legal, and social work credentials; however, there are two voluntary public health–specific credentials requiring additional education for recertification. The National Board of Public Health Examiners (NBPHE) awards the Certified in Public Health (CPH) credential based on education or work experience and a passing score on a standardized examination. To maintain certification, CPH professionals are required to complete a minimum of 50 educational credits every two years for recertification. Maintenance of certification may be achieved through a variety of micro- and macrolearning experiences in the following categories: attending public health professional events, attending public health college or university courses, attending Coursera courses, instruction, writing or professional contribution, residencies and dissertations, public health fellowships, experiential activities, earning other certifications, service as an item writer for CPH exam or CPH study guide, and service activities. NBPHE's website functions as a modest learning management system providing both letters confirming current certification and digital certificates. NBPHE maintains a web-based learning management system for the reporting of educational credits. Digital badges are displayed for each certified professional as they complete and report CE in each category of learning, with three levels of competency (https://www.nbphe.org). NBPHE is currently exploring linkages with TRAIN.

The National Commission for Health Education Credentialing offers two levels of certification for the health education workforce. Eligibility for the CHES credential requires academic preparation and passing a competency-based examination. The MCHES certification requires academic preparation with courses in health education, experience requirements in the health education field, and passing a comprehensive written examination. Professionals seeking recertification must demonstrate continued competence throughout their professional careers. Both CHES and MCHES recertification is conducted on a five-year renewal cycle requiring 75 hours of CE. In addition, MCHES recertification requires that 30 hours be directly related to advanced-level competencies. Presently, the National Commission for Health Education Credentialing, Inc. is not linked to TRAIN and does not offer digital badges as part of its recertification process.

Further Formal Study

The 2015 Public Health Workforce Interests and Needs Survey reports that only 17% of the public health workforce have a formal public health degree.[27] While academic degrees may be required for some public health positions, they may be viewed as part of lifelong learning (career ladders or stacked credentials) for others. Undergraduate and graduate public health degrees, including the BSPH, MPH, MS, DrPH, and PhD, as well as academic certificates in public health awarded by university programs and schools of public health accredited by the Council on Education for Public Health (CEPH), clearly fit the definition of formal study as lifelong learning. Public health degrees that are not accredited by CEPH are a less clear fit, as they may vary in content and quality. Academic certificates may offer a more abbreviated experience, concentrating in a specific practice area. While academic degrees may be required for some public health positions, they may be viewed as part of lifelong learning for others. For working professionals, the growing availability of online and executive degrees provides new opportunities for formal degree completion. Practitioners in nursing, medicine, social work, law, or other areas may seek a complementary degree in public health to advance professionally.

Self-Directed Learning

With many public health organizations lacking the capacity to offer workplace-based learning, self-directed lifelong learning serves an important role in public health. Candy describes six personal attributes and qualities of lifelong learners: (1) an inquiring mind, (2) "helicopter vision," (3) information literacy, (4) a sense of personal agency, (5) a repertoire of learning skills, and (6) interpersonal skills and group membership.[28] Professionals possessing these characteristics are likely to have greater decision-making autonomy in the pursuit of their lifelong learning. To date, there has been limited study of why public health professionals voluntarily pursue lifelong learning; however, based on the TRAIN Learning Network experience, public health professionals are engaging actively.

There are options for the workplace-based learning offered by both public and private organizations for the self-directed learner. For example, in addition to its internal CDCU, the CDC also offers free CE through the CDC Learning Connection (https://www.cdc.gov/learning /index.html), a source for information about public health training developed by the CDC, CDC partners, and other federal agencies. Their website encourages learners to connect through social media and to stay informed through an e-newsletter.

Hybrid Resources

In addition to the traditional four types of lifelong learning identified by Candy,[29] additional resources exist in public health. Various learning opportunities are offered by the National Association of County and City Health Officials and the Association of State and Territorial Health Officials, as well as by a variety of discipline-specific public health–related associations. Two examples of these category-spanning resources are the federally funded US Public Health Training Centers and the private nonprofit Institute for Healthcare Improvement Open School, described later in the chapter. While not offering further formal study, these organizations do have the potential to provide workplace-based learning to large audiences, as well as individual continuing professional education and self-directed lifelong learning.

US Public Health Training Centers

Beginning in 1999, the US Department of Health and Human Services, Bureau of Health Workforce, began designation and funding of Public Health Training Centers with the purpose of "increas[ing] the number of individuals in the public health workforce; strengthen[ing] and expand[ing] the education, training, and capacity of the current and future public health workforce."[30] The program seeks to achieve the following: (1) develop tailored training and technical assistance; (2) create or enhance training curricula to provide skill-based, interactive instruction using multiple modalities; (3) establish and enhance collaborative partnerships among state and LHDs, primary care providers, and related organizations; 4) involve faculty members and students in collaborative projects; and (5) establish or strengthen field placements for students. These activities are being currently implemented by 10 regional training centers, with 40 local sites with technical assistance.

Institute for Healthcare Improvement Open School

The Institute for Healthcare Improvement (IHI, www.ihi.org) describes its Open School as a global learning community offering online courses, short videos, case studies, games and other online activities, and project-based learning opportunities addressing healthcare improvement. In 2017, Andrew Jacaruso, project manager at IHI, reported 611,459 registrants completing 486,441 courses and 115,609 basic certificates in quality, safety, and leadership over the institute's history. While many of its offerings are clinically oriented, others address a variety of healthcare quality and leadership issues relevant to public health. Courses vary in price, but many are free, and others include scholarship opportunities. Completion of a course generates a certificate in PDF format; digital badges are not currently available. IHI maintains its own learning management system that is not currently linked to TRAIN.

Conclusion

The consensus report *Who Will Keep the Public Healthy?* states that assuring access to lifelong learning for the public health workforce is a responsibility of schools of public health. In some schools, this may be a new endeavor.[31] While there are practical, logistical, and financial challenges, there are also opportunities for alumni engagement, enhanced connections with community partners, and faculty research identifying factors that motivate practitioners to pursue lifelong learning as well as assessing the learning efficacy of different methods to generate best practices for lifelong learning. The needs of the workforce, along with the availability of new technologies, provide an opportunity for public health educators to explore and contribute to lifelong learning.

REFERENCES

1. Institute of Medicine. "Who Will Keep the Public Healthy? Educating Public Health Professionals for the 21st Century." K. Gebbie, L. Rosenstock, and L. M. Hernandez, eds. Washington, DC: National Academies Press, 2003.

2. Carlson, E. R. "Lifelong Learning and Professional Development." *Journal of Oral and Maxillofacial Surgery* 74, no. 5 (2016): 56–79.

3. Duyff, R. L. "The Value of Lifelong Learning: Key Element in Professional Career Development." *Journal of the American Dietetic Association* 99, no. 5 (1999): 538–543.

4. Institute of Medicine Committee on Planning a Continuing Health Professional Education. "Redesigning Continuing Education in the Health Professions." Washington, DC: National Academies Press, 2010.

5. Parlette, G. N., and A. R. Leonard. "Continuing Education in Public Health: The Experience of the Western States 1959–1966." *American Journal of Public Health* 58, no. 3 (1968): 558–568.

6. Bersin, Josh. "The Disruption of Digital Learning: Ten Things We Have Learned." 2017. http://joshbersin.com/2017/03/the-disruption-of-digital-learning -ten-things-we-have-learned/ (accessed April 8, 2018).

7. Buchem, I., and H. Hamelman. "Microlearning: A Strategy for Ongoing Professional Development." *eLearning Papers* 1, no. 21 (2010): 1–15.

8. Curry, M., and J. Killon. "Slicing the Layers of Learning." *Journal of Staff Development* 30, no. 1 (2009): 56–79.

9. Neelen, M., and P. A. Kirschner. "Microlearning—A New Old Concept to Put out to Pasture." 3-Star Learning Experiences. 2017. https:// 3starlearningexperiences.wordpress.com/2017/06/13/microlearning-a-new-old -concept-to-put-out-to-pasture/ (accessed April 8, 2018).

10. Neelen and Kirschner, "Microlearning."

11. Bersin, "The Disruption of Digital Learning."

12. McKeever, Jennifer. "The Public Health Learning Navigator: Preparing the Public Health Workforce of Today and Tomorrow." *National Network of Public Health Institutes.* 2017. https://nnphi.org/public-health-learning-navigator -preparing-public-health-workforce-today-tomorrow/ (accessed April 8, 2018).

13. Ostashewski, N., and D. Reid. *A History and Frameworks of Digital Badges in Education.* Edited by T. Reiners and L. C. Wood. Switzerland: Springer International Publishing, 2015.

14. Ifenthaler, D., N. Bellin-Mularski, and D. Mah, eds. *Foundation of Digital Badges and Micro-Credentials: Demonstrating and Recognizing Knowledge and Competencies.* Switzerland: Springer International Publishing, 2016.

15. Foster, J. C. "The Promise of Digital Badges." *Techniques: Connecting Education and Careers* 88, no. 8 (2013): 30–34.

16. Ahn, J., A. Pellicone, and B. S. Butler. "Open Badges for Education: What Are the Implications at the Intersection of Open Systems and Badging?" *Research in Learning Technology* 22 (2014): 1–13.

17. McGreal R., W. Kinuthia, and S. Marshall, eds. *Open Educational Resources: Innovation, Research and Practice.* Vancouver, BC: Commonwealth of Learning and Athabasca University, 2013.

18. Siemens, G. "Massive Open Online Courses: Innovation in Education?" in *Open Educational Resources: Innovation, Research and Practice,* edited by R. McGreal, W. Kinuthia, and S. Marshall, 5–16. Vancouver, BC: Commonwealth of Learning and Athabasca University, 2013.

19. de Waard, I., A. Koutropoulos, R. J. Hogue, S. C. Abajian, N. O. Keskin, C. O. Rodriguez, and M. S. Gallagher. "Merging MOOC and mLearning for Increased Learner Interactions." *International Journal of Mobile and Blended Learning* 4, no. 4 (2012): 13–25.

20. Siemens, "Massive Open Online Courses."

21. Candy, P. C. "Reaffirming a Proud Tradition Universities and Lifelong Learning." *Active Learning in Higher Education* 1, no. 2 (2000): 101–125.

22. Ilyas, M. "Making of a Corporate University Model: Transition from Traditional Training to Learning Management System." *Journal of Education and Practice* 8, no. 15 (2017): 85–90.

23. National Association of County and City Health Officials. "The Local Health Department Workforce: Findings from the 2005 National Profile of Local Health Departments Study." archived.naccho.org/topics/infrastructure/profile /upload/LHD_Workforce-Final.pdf (accessed April 8, 2018).

24. Public Health Accreditation Board. "Public Health Accreditation Board, Standards and Measures, Version 1.5." http://www.phaboard.org/accreditation -process/public-health-department-standards-and-measures/ (accessed April 8, 2018).

25. Institute of Medicine, "Redesigning Continuing Education in the Health Professions."

26. American Public Health Association. "Continuing Education at the APHA Annual Meeting." 2017. https://www.apha.org/professional-development /continuing-education/continuing-education-at-the-annual-meeting (accessed April 8, 2018).

27. Association of State and Territorial Health Officials and the de Beaumont Foundation. "Information to Action: The Workforce Data of Public Health WINS: Summary Report." Arlington, VA: Association of State and Territorial Health Officials and Bethesda, Maryland: The de Beaumont Foundation, 2015. http://www.debeaumont .org/phwins/ (accessed April 8, 2018).

28. Candy, "Reaffirming a Proud Tradition Universities and Lifelong Learning."

29. Candy, "Reaffirming a Proud Tradition Universities and Lifelong Learning."

30. US Department of Health and Human Services, Health Resources and Services Administration. "Public Health Workforce Development." https://bhw.hrsa .gov/grants/publichealth (accessed April 8, 2018).

31. Institute of Medicine, "Who Will Keep the Public Healthy?"

[10]
Interprofessional Education

TANYA UDEN-HOLMAN

PUBLIC HEALTH EDUCATION is critically important for professionals in health fields as well as for professionals trained in a variety of
nonhealth fields. In this chapter, we discuss ways to create and support
opportunities for public health students and students from other disciplines to engage in interactive interprofessional learning so that they can
work effectively together toward common goals.

The importance of interprofessional education (IPE) and practice has
been recognized for more than 30 years by respected national and international health organizations. In 1972, the Institute of Medicine
(IOM) report titled *Educating for the Health Team* discussed the need
to redeploy the functions of health professions in new ways in order to
provide effective, efficient, and comprehensive healthcare.[1] Other reports made similar recommendations.[2,3]

In 2010, the World Health Organization (WHO) defined IPE as occurring when "two or more professions learn about, from and with each
other to enable effective collaboration and improve health outcomes"
and interprofessional collaborative practice in healthcare as occurring
"when multiple health workers from different professional backgrounds
provide comprehensive services by working with patients, their families, carers [*sic*] and communities to deliver the highest quality of care
across settings."[4] Integral to the WHO's definition and efforts by the

Interprofessional Education Collaborative (IPEC), IOM, and others is the view that academic institutions and their faculty must realign their institutional culture, teaching approaches, and environments in order to successfully integrate IPE into their curricula and learning opportunities. Facilitating this transformational change requires institution-wide recognition and resolve tied to a realistic time frame, institutional self-assessment of IPE challenges and opportunities, adequate resources, and flexible implementation strategies. The importance of working together in our practice settings is well known. Today, there is also a growing recognition that we need to start early in the educational process to move away from professional silos and toward IPE.

The need for IPE and collaborative practice is reaching a critical juncture as we look for strategies to address the challenges of the changing healthcare landscape, including provider shortages, rising healthcare costs, an aging population, increases in comorbidity and chronic disease, patient safety (including medical errors), and addressing the Institute for Healthcare Improvement's Triple Aim: (1) improving the patient experience of care, (2) improving the health of populations, and (3) reducing the per capita cost of healthcare. Given the vital role of public health in addressing these challenges, it is important that public health students are engaged in interactive learning with other health professionals. Although in the past IPE was often limited to health sciences students taking a class in common, today the focus has shifted to an emphasis on the importance of interprofessional competencies related to real-world interdisciplinary practice.

Finally, the importance of IPE is also reflected in accreditation criteria. In late 2014, the Health Professions Accreditors Collaborative (HPAC) was created. As noted on its website, HPAC was formed to "enhance accreditors' ability to ensure graduates of health profession education programs are prepared for interprofessional collaborative practice."[5] In less than three years, HPAC has grown in size from 6 to 23 members who are all committed to working together to advance IPE and collaborative practice. The Council on Education for Public Health (CEPH), the accrediting body for schools and programs of public health, was one of the six initial members. Signaling the increased importance of interprofessional collaborative practice for public health professionals, the 2016 CEPH criteria includes the following as one of the required Master of Public Health (MPH) Foundational Competencies: "Perform effectively on interprofessional teams."[6]

Interprofessional Education Collaborative Core Competencies: The Foundation of IPE Efforts

Recognizing the importance of IPE and collaborative practice, in 2009 the six national health professions' education associations (American Association of Colleges of Nursing, American Association of Colleges of Osteopathic Medicine, American Association of Colleges of Pharmacy, American Dental Education Association, Association of American Medical Colleges, and Association of Schools of Public Health) formed the IPEC with the goal of advancing IPE learning experiences to better prepare students for collaborative and team-based care. In May 2011, an expert panel appointed by the IPEC published *Core Competencies for Interprofessional Collaborative Practice*. The goal was to ensure that students have the knowledge, skills, and values they need to perform interprofessional teamwork and to function as part of a team to provide effective patient-centered collaborative care. The four competency domains identified were (1) values/ethics for interprofessional practice, (2) roles/responsibilities, (3) interprofessional communication, and (4) teams and teamwork.[7]

In 2016, IPEC grew to include nine new institutional members and expanded the professional representation from six to fifteen. In their 2016 report, the IPEC board broadened the interprofessional competencies to better address the Triple Aim, with a greater emphasis on the health of populations. Additionally, they organized the competencies within an overarching competency domain of interprofessional collaboration, which now includes the four topical areas from the 2011 report.[8] Below is a brief description of the core competencies and examples of subcompetencies from the 2016 IPEC report.

Values/Ethics for Interprofessional Practice

The first competency is to work with individuals from other professions to maintain a climate of mutual respect and shared values. Examples of subcompetencies include embracing the cultural diversity and individual differences that characterize patients, populations, and the health team; managing ethical dilemmas specific to interprofessional patient/population-centered care situations; and placing the interests of patients and populations at the center of interprofessional healthcare delivery and population health programs and policies, with the goal of promoting health and health equity across the life span.

Roles/Responsibilities

The second competency is to use the knowledge of one's own role and those of other professions to appropriately assess and address the healthcare needs of patients and to promote and advance the health of populations. Examples of subcompetencies include engaging diverse professionals who complement one's own professional expertise, as well as associated resources, to develop strategies to meet specific health and healthcare needs of patients and populations; communicating with team members to clarify each member's responsibility in executing components of a treatment plan or public health intervention; and describing how professionals in health and other fields can collaborate and integrate clinical care and public health interventions to optimize population health.

Interprofessional Communication

The third competency is to communicate with patients, families, communities, and professionals in health and other fields in a responsive and responsible manner that supports a team approach to the promotion and maintenance of health and the prevention and treatment of disease. Examples of subcompetencies include choosing effective communication tools and techniques, including information and communication technologies, to facilitate discussions and interactions that enhance team function; listening actively and encouraging ideas and opinions of other team members; giving timely, sensitive, constructive feedback to others about their performance on the team and responding respectfully as a team member to feedback from others; and communicating the importance of teamwork in patient-centered care and population health programs and policies.

Teams and Teamwork

The fourth competency is to apply relationship-building values and the principles of team dynamics to perform effectively in different team roles to plan, deliver, and evaluate patient- and population-centered care and population health programs and policies that are safe, timely, efficient, effective, and equitable. Examples of subcompetencies include describing the process of team development and the roles and practices of effective teams; engaging health and other professionals in shared patient-centered and population-focused problem-solving; engaging self and others to constructively manage disagreements about values, roles, goals, and actions that arise among health and other professionals and with patients, families, and community members; and using process improvement to increase effectiveness of interprofessional teamwork and team-based services, programs, and policies.

The core competencies and subcompetencies are important as they provide the foundation for curriculum development. Additionally, the increased emphasis on population health as well as on the promotion of health and the prevention of disease—the hallmarks of public health—provide additional opportunities for public health students to be involved in IPE initiatives on their campuses.

Critical Elements for a Successful IPE Initiative

In reflecting on the experiences of institutions with successful IPE programs, several common themes can be identified.

- An explicit, observable, and measurable philosophy of IPE that permeates the institution must be in place for an institution to successfully implement IPE.
- Faculty champions from all disciplines involved are critical for long-term success.
- The implementation process must be flexible and tailored to the institution's unique features so that interprofessional relationships and collaborations can emerge naturally.
- Communication, trust, honest reflection, and openness to team development are essential at both the organizational level and the individual professional level.

- Organizational infrastructure should foster IPE by providing support for faculty time to participate in faculty development opportunities, integrate IPE into learning activities, and cocreate learning opportunities with faculty from different professions.
- Organizational infrastructure is critical to support educational programming for students.
- Comprehensive and ongoing faculty development is imperative.
- Incentives for and recognition of faculty efforts in IPE must be created or incorporated into existing formal and informal reward programs, including the promotion and tenure process.
- Developing an IPE initiative with a centralized coordinating function that promotes IPE integration across academic units is a long-term and incremental process.
- Sustained funding is critical to long-term success—although program grants from external agencies are helpful in catalyzing programming, the institution must identify sustainable funding sources for IPE to thrive long term.

In reviewing the aforementioned elements, some might argue that sustained funding is the most important component in ensuring a successful IPE initiative. Although funding is necessary, it is not sufficient. Additionally, much emphasis is given to developing educational programming for students. However, once again, although IPE programming for students is important, students are not the only group on campus that needs education and training. Without faculty onboard and trained in the content of the IPE competency domains and the importance of interprofessional collaborative practice in the current and future delivery of healthcare and preventive services, an IPE initiative will not have long-term impact or success. In fact, the Professional Affairs Committee of the American Association of Colleges of Pharmacy noted that IPE faculty development should be initiated before the educational process begins and that as faculty members learn to work together to implement IPE curriculum, they can serve as important role models to students.[9] Faculty development is even more critical as IPE brings in additional professions beyond the more traditional clinical professions. Current faculty and practitioners must understand the role that other professions, including public health, play in meeting today's healthcare challenges, including achieving the Triple Aim.

Challenges for Implementing IPE and Integrating Public Health Students into IPE Curricular Activities

Some of the more general challenges in implementing IPE are reflected in the previous discussion, including faculty development and the recognition of faculty contributions to IPE in promotion and tenure. Logistical issues such as development of courses that span multiple colleges, harmonization of schedules and calendars, coordinated communication, and shared learning venues present challenges but can also provide tangible evidence of intent to implement IPE. Acquiring adequate resources to effectively implement and sustain a comprehensive IPE center is another significant challenge. Leveraging the growing interest in IPE by health systems, healthcare professionals, and philanthropic organizations may offer additional new sources of support. Most important for changing the institutional culture, leadership and faculty must be role models for the behaviors taught and expected of students, and implement policies that reinforce these precepts.

There are additional challenges as we look to incorporate public health students into IPE educational activities. Many of the educational programs utilized by health sciences colleges still have a heavy clinical focus. For example, scenarios may be used with simulated patients in inpatient settings. Information is provided about the patient's symptoms, diagnosis, vital signs, prescriptions, and lab results during their hospitalization. The IPE student team is then charged with reviewing this information, interviewing the patient to obtain additional information, and presenting a discharge plan to the patient. For public health graduate students without clinical training, it can be hard to determine how they can contribute to the discussion and ultimate discharge plan. And yet with the increased emphasis on population health and the importance of promotion of health and the prevention of disease, public health clearly has important contributions to add to the discussion. However, the successful incorporation of public health students into IPE activities takes careful and deliberate consideration and planning.

Engaging Public Health Students in IPE Learning Activities

As schools and programs continue to develop opportunities for public health students to engage in interprofessional learning opportunities, there is no singular right approach. An important starting point is the definition of IPE and the IPEC Core Competencies. In reviewing the definition of IPE, it is clear that learning opportunities do not always have to involve students from a wide variety of professions. Sometimes IPE involves students from public health and one other discipline. The key aspect is the authenticity of the learning opportunity, where students have the chance to interact and share through the lens of their profession. They need to be able to learn about, from, and with one another. Students cannot be sitting next to one another in a lecture hall or watching an online video with no chance for meaningful interaction or learning. Additionally, the IPEC Core Competencies should be the foundation for the curricula. Although an individual training does not have to address all four competencies (values/ethics for interprofessional practice, roles/responsibilities, interprofessional communication, teams and teamwork) by the end of their program, students should have learning opportunities in all four competencies and be able to meet the required MPH Foundational Competency of "perform effectively on interprofessional teams."

IPE learning opportunities should not be "one and done." Schools and programs need to provide students with multiple opportunities across their time in the program. And although some of these opportunities will likely need to be required to ensure that students meet the competencies, electives, such as service learning, and cocurricular activities, such as student organizations, provide additional ways for students to interact and learn about, from, and with students in other disciplines. Finally, IPE content can be delivered through multiple modalities. While we might argue that in an ideal world IPE learning opportunities would all be delivered face-to-face, this is often not realistic due to some of the barriers previously mentioned, such as curricular requirements, academic calendars, room availability, or distance-based students. In practice, IPE is delivered in a range of formats, including in person, online, or in a blended format of in person and online. For example, online formats may include interactive learning modules, online discussions among students, asynchronous discussion boards, and video conferencing. In-person sessions might utilize simulations and standardized patients, where students have the opportunity to practice in a safe environment.

Examples from Public Health Schools and Programs

Sibbald et al. discuss three pedagogical approaches that they argue better support interprofessional teaching and learning: case-based pedagogy, team-based learning, and competency-focused curriculum.[10] Common to these approaches is that they allow for higher levels of student engagement and learning. A specific example of how team-based learning is being used for IPE programming that includes public health students is provided by the University of Florida.[11] Students apply knowledge on topics including patient safety, professional ethics, and health systems and disparities. The authors note that a positive of the team-based learning approach is that it does not require a faculty facilitator for each small group, and that a few faculty with appropriate training can facilitate multiple groups simultaneously. Finally, and as previously mentioned, due to logistical and curricular constraints, IPE programming is often delivered in a blended format. Once again, the key is that no matter the format, students need to have the opportunity for meaningful interaction and exchange of ideas through the lens of their profession.

Again, one of the challenges of incorporating public health students into IPE educational activities is that many trainings have a clinical focus. However, given the increased focus on population health and the importance of promotion of health and the prevention of disease, in both the IPEC competencies and healthcare in general, there are no shortage of topics that can be utilized for IPE, where public health students have key content knowledge to share and help inform discussions in important ways. Examples of topics include the role of the determinants of health, including the social determinants of health, in informing how teams might develop an interdisciplinary care plan for a patient. For example, in developing a patient discharge plan, lack of transportation; limited availability of healthy, affordable foods; and limited access to health services for routine follow-up tests because of where one lives can adversely impact patient compliance and outcomes. In an example from a public health program, faculty at Des Moines University created an asynchronous, six-week online learning activity that integrated the social determinants of health.[12] Public health students participated on the IPE teams along with students from several other clinical programs. The authors noted that without the participation of public health students, the social determinants of health might have been over-looked in the team's development of an interdisciplinary care plan.

Another frequent topic of IPE offerings is patient safety, which is a key component of the Triple Aim. Public health students within health management departments typically have training in quality improvement methods that can improve patient safety. Their knowledge can benefit teams as they review cases where errors occurred and how they might best be prevented through clearer interprofessional communication and teamwork. For example, the University of South Carolina provided IPE for public health and social work students with a focus on patient safety. Specifically, students conducted a root cause analysis involving a complex stroke patient living in a rural community with multiple barriers to care outcomes.[13]

Emergency preparedness and response is another topic that brings together a wide range of professions, and where public health has a critical role to play. Simulations and table-top exercises can be developed for health profession students, including public health, that address a number of natural and humanmade disasters, such as infectious disease outbreaks, hurricanes, and chemical spills. For example, the University of Minnesota utilizes simulations as part of their IPE programming. After completing online programming as well as several hands-on workshops led by first responders, students participate in two immersive simulations involving a bomb blast and structural collapse, respectively.[14]

Topics related to social justice, health disparities, and health equity are also appropriate for IPE trainings, and is another area where public health can inform the discussion. For example, if an IPE training were focusing on the competency of values and ethics, students could engage in a discussion of the book *The Immortal Life of Henrietta Lacks,* by Rebecca Skloot, which brings issues of health disparities, health equity, and social justice into a larger discussion of values and ethics.

In addition to formal coursework, cocurricular activities provide important opportunities for public health students to learn about, from, and with students from other disciplines. Examples include volunteer activities such as student-run mobile clinics, which provide care to underserved populations and involve students from across the health sciences, including public health. Student organizations are another mechanism for IPE. And reflecting the growing interest in IPE and collaborative practice, a number of schools and programs have student organizations specifically focused on IPE opportunities. These organizations undertake a variety of activities, from promoting programming on campus, to developing their own educational offerings, and to submitting and presenting posters and oral presentations at regional and national conferences. A specific example of a well-known student organization dedicated to improving healthcare through interprofessional collaboration is CLARION at the University of Minnesota. CLARION has been hosting the University of Minnesota's student case competition since 2002. Teams, which must include at least two professions, are given a case and are charged with creating a root cause analysis.[15] Other schools have developed their own case competitions with a more specific focus on public health–related issues. For example, the School of Public Health at the University of Memphis developed an interdisciplinary case competition to allow public health and health administration students to work with students from other disciplines to address a community health concern.[16]

Conclusion

It is important to note that the examples provided in this chapter are by no means an exhaustive list of all the IPE activities currently happening in schools and programs of public health. However, they clearly illustrate that public health students can be successfully incorporated into a range of IPE activities. Furthermore, given the importance of public health in addressing today's healthcare challenges, it is imperative that the IPE taking place on health sciences campuses include public health so that other professions better understand the knowledge, skills, and abilities that public health professionals can contribute toward improving the health of populations.

REFERENCES

1. Institute of Medicine. "Educating for the Health Team." Washington, DC: National Academy of Sciences, 1972.

2. O'Neill, E. H., and the Pew Health Professions Commission. "Recreating Health Professional Practice for a New Century: The Fourth Report of the Pew Health Professions Commission." San Francisco: Pew Health Professions Commission, 1998.

3. Institute of Medicine. "Health Professions Education: A Bridge to Quality." Washington, DC: National Academies Press, 2003.

4. World Health Organization. "Framework for Action on Interprofessional Education and Collaborative Practice." Geneva: World Health Organization, 2010.

5. Health Professions Accreditors Collaborative. "Home." http://healthprofes sionsaccreditors.org (accessed October 29, 2017).

6. Council on Education for Public Health. "Accreditation Criteria: Schools and Programs of Public Health." Silver Spring, MD: CEPH, 2016. https://ceph.org /assets/2016.Criteria.pdf (accessed March 25, 2018).

7. Interprofessional Education Collaborative Expert Panel. "Core Competencies for Interprofessional Collaborative Practice: Report of an Expert Panel." Washington, DC: Interprofessional Education Collaborative, 2011.

8. Interprofessional Education Collaborative. "Core Competencies for Interprofessional Collaborative Practice: 2016 Update." Washington, DC: Interprofessional Education Collaborative, 2016.

9. Buring, S., A. Bhushan, G. Brazeau, S. Conway, L. Hansen, and S. Westberg. "Keys to Successful Implementation of Interprofessional Education: Learning Location, Faculty Development, and Curricular Themes." *American Journal of Pharmaceutical Education* 73 (2009): Article 60.

10. Sibbald, S. L., M. Speechley, and A. Thind. "Adapting to the Needs of the Public Health Workforce: An Integrated Case-Based Training Program." *Frontiers in Public Health* 4 (2016): https://www.ncbi.nlm.nih.gov/pmc/articles/PMC506 3848/.

11. Black, E. W., A. V. Blue, R. Davidson, and W. T. McCormack. "Using Team-Based Learning in a Large Interprofessional Health Science Education Experience." *Journal of Interprofessional Education and Practice* 5 (2016): 19–22.

12. Duffy, P. A., J. A. Ronnebaum, T. A. Stumbo, K. N. Smith, and R. A. Reimer. "Does Including Public Health Students on Interprofessional Teams Increase Attainment of Interprofessional Practice Competencies?" *Journal of the American Osteopathic Association* 117 (2017): 244–252.

13. Addy, C. L., T. Browne, E. W. Blake, and J. Bailey. "Enhancing Interprofessional Education: Integrating Public Health and Social Work Perspectives." *American Journal of Public Health* 105 (2015): S106-S108.

14. Miller, J. L., J. H. Rambeck, and A. Snyder. "Improving Emergency Preparedness System Readiness through Simulation and Interprofessional Education." *Public Health Reports* 129 (2014): 129–135.

15. CLARION. "Case Competition." https://www.chip.umn.edu/clarion/case -competition (accessed October 29, 2017).

16. Carlton, E. L., M. P. Powell, S. E. Dismuke, and M. C. Levy. "Our Future's Brightest: Developing Interprofessional Competencies through an Interdisciplinary Graduate Student Case Competition." *Journal of Health Administration Education* 32 (2015): 47–57.

PART III INNOVATION IN PUBLIC HEALTH TEACHING

[11]

Public Health Course Design

MELISSA D. BEGG AND JESSICA S. ANCKER

WHILE THE DESIGN of the overall curriculum for a degree program is paramount in public health education, the next most important consideration is the design of the building blocks of that curriculum—the individual courses. The goal of this chapter is to outline the process of designing a public health course—from the very beginning steps in conceptualizing the course through the ultimate delivery, evaluation, and revision of that course. This chapter provides guidance on course design for adult learners in general, in addition to advice on courses in the public health domain specifically. There are many excellent resources available on course design, both in general and in public health, and although this chapter draws on those resources, it is not meant to serve as a comprehensive summary, nor does it present novel methods. Rather, it represents the authors' experiences in course planning and implementation and points to existing research, resources, and references that they have found especially helpful in their teaching public health at the graduate level.

General Principles of Course Design for Adult Learners

Conceptualizing the Course

Effective course design might be best undertaken in the same way that a good journalist approaches a news story—by articulating the "who, what, where, why, when, and how" behind the course. Careful consideration of these questions, outlined in the following list, can help the instructor craft the goals, content, requirements, and delivery methods for the course most successfully.

- Who: Who will take the course? Are they graduate students or undergraduates? Are they primarily majors in this discipline or students studying in a broad range of departments? What do they already know? What do they need to know?
- What: What are the goals of the course? What are the learning objectives? What knowledge, skills, and attitudes will students attain by the end of the course? What types of assignments and activities would be best suited for achieving these learning goals and objectives?
- Where: Where do the students in this course come from, and where will they end up? What are the backgrounds of the students who will enroll? Where will their careers take them, and how will the skills and knowledge gained in this course be useful to them?
- Why: Why should students be excited to take this course? How will it relate to their academic and career goals? Why is this content relevant to public health research and practice?
- When: When is this course offered relative to the students' progress in the degree program? Which courses have they already taken? Which courses will they take next?
- How: How will you achieve the goals of the course and ensure that students meet the learning objectives that have been set? How will you know students have gained the knowledge and skills that you set out to impart? How will students be assessed and graded? How will you evaluate the overall success of the course? How will you revise the content and implementation of the course in the future, based on feedback received?

The initial result from addressing the aforementioned questions is the course description—a brief summary of the scope of the course. A good course description is more than a laundry list of topics; ideally, it provides some indication of the course's context within the field of public health (or a subfield), rationale, key skills and topics, intended audience, and fit within the overall program.[1] A particularly helpful course description should include the overarching questions or challenges in public health that the course is designed to address, so that prospective students can evaluate whether it will be a good fit for their career goals and aspirations. A really well-written course description can, in fact, generate excitement among potential participants.

It might be tempting to write a very long course description. However, course descriptions should be as brief as possible. Many colleges and universities set a maximum length for a course description. For example, Stanford University characterizes the course description as a "short, pithy statement" with information on "the subject matter, approach, breadth, and applicability of the course," with a target length of no more than 80 words.[2] (For comparison, note that this paragraph contains nearly 100 words, excluding this parenthetical.) The course description should be written to provide students (and perhaps prospective employers) with a concise summary of the course content and context within a curriculum or discipline.

Setting Course Goals, Competencies, and Learning Objectives

Having completed the initial conceptualization of the course and drafted its description, the next step is to carefully articulate the overall course goals and learning objectives. To begin, it is helpful to enumerate the competencies that students will gain from the course. Competency-based education is centered on the acquisition of specific knowledge and skills rather than time spent in a particular course of study. The concept of competency-based education originated in the 1960s and 1970s, primarily in the areas of teacher and vocational training.[3] While it is not very common in general undergraduate education, it has gained traction in public health and other professional education settings.[4,5] In 2005, the Council on Education for Public Health revised its accreditation criteria to specify competencies for programs, rather than learning objectives.[6] This then led to the development of required competencies in public health, promoted by the Association of Schools and Programs of Public Health, which are necessary for accreditation of new programs.[7,8]

The strategic decision to embrace competency-based education in public health was likely motivated in part by the desire to encourage schools and programs to adopt a learner-centered rather than content-centered approach to teaching, which eschews structuring courses around a list of topics in favor of structuring courses around what students need to learn and how to help them learn it.[9]

The competencies should be derived from an understanding of the needs of the public health professional, with each competency representing a collection of knowledge and skills that will serve the learner well on entering the workforce.[10] Thus, a competency defines at a high level what the student is able to do at the end of the course (or program), while learning objectives can be viewed as more discrete, highly specific steps that map to a competency. As Hooper et al. describe this process, learning objectives represent an "unbundling" of competencies, achieved by addressing the question, "What would a student need to know to perform this competency at a given level?"[11] Another important step in this process is to relate the competencies for an individual course back to the competencies set for the overall program. Instructors should set course competencies in context, taking note of which courses have been completed previously, and which courses students will take subsequently, so that knowledge and skills accumulate in logical fashion as a student progresses through a curriculum.

The development of the broad course description, followed by the competencies, then by the learning objectives, might best be described as an exercise in reverse engineering. This builds on the Understanding by Design (or UbD) framework, which proposes a three-stage, backward-design process for curriculum planning.[12] The first stage in UbD course design is to identify the desired results—specifically, the competencies. The process of moving from competency to learning objectives involves breaking down the competency into its component parts in an iterative fashion until each learning objective is articulated as a specific, measurable statement and written in behavioral terms. Each learning objective is comprised of two parts—an action verb and a content area, following Bloom's taxonomy.[13,14] Bloom suggests appropriate verbs that represent observable characteristics rather than internal states that are not visible to an external evaluator, echoed by the UbD framework, which focuses on students' abilities at the end of a course. Bloom's taxonomy covers six levels of learning outcomes, from lowest to highest level of functioning, moving from knowledge, to comprehension, to application, to analysis, to synthesis, and ultimately to evaluation. Core courses in public health will likely fall into the first three or four categories of Bloom's taxonomy, from knowledge through analysis; advanced courses will likely target learning objectives in the highest taxonomic levels, such as synthesis and evaluation.[15]

Student Assessments

Once measurable learning objectives are finalized, this leads nicely into the second stage of the UbD: determining assessment evidence. In this stage, the instructor must stipulate how they will know when a student has achieved the desired results. Backward design supports this approach very naturally, as it begins by requiring a statement of what students are able to do; the next step is to determine the types of evidence that could be used to demonstrate students' abilities. In this stage, both performance tasks and other evidence may be used to establish that a student can understand and apply the knowledge and skills acquired through the course. Performance tasks can be selected that mimic the activities that public health students will be required to pursue in the workplace. For example, this might include analyzing a public health data set and summarizing its findings, or writing a grant proposal for external funding, or drafting a manuscript for a peer-reviewed publication. Other evidence might include more typical academic requirements, such as homework assignments, term papers, quizzes, and exams. Various methods of assessment are discussed later in this chapter.

Course Content

The third and final stage in UbD course design is to plan learning experiences and instruction. The goal here is for the instructor to map out how she or he will actually teach the course; the beauty of the UbD framework is that this process should be much more direct since the learning goals and assessment methods have already determined. With learning objectives and assessments in hand, the instructor is well positioned to select the most strategies that align most closely with the stated course objectives and evaluation methods. For example, Bowen recommends posing the following questions to determine key elements of the course structure: (1) What enabling knowledge and skills will students need in order to perform effectively and achieve desired results? (2) What activities will equip students with the needed knowledge and skills? (3) What will need to be taught and coached, and how should it best be taught, in light of performance goals? and (4) What materials and resources are best suited to accomplish these goals?[16] These topics are explored in great depth in the following section.

Setting competencies and learning objectives should begin at the level of the overall course, but then these same strategies can be applied to each course session. A course syllabus then includes learning objectives not only for the course overall but for each class, along with readings and activities that support student mastery of the objectives. (A later section in this chapter on syllabi covers these notions in greater detail.) Instructors may find that crafting content for each class meeting will flow very naturally from the learning objectives for that session. It is possible that one of the most challenging aspects of applying this paradigm to course design is the temptation to "overstuff the sausage," trying to pack too much into the course or any one of its sessions. If this is an issue, the UbD approach helps faculty whittle down content by evaluating the extent to which any topic truly represents a "big idea" with "enduring value," lives at the "heart" of a discipline, requires facilitation for students to master, and presents potential for student engagement.[17,18] According to Smith et al., faculty who have applied these criteria to their courses have reported cutting anywhere from 25% to 33% of course content because that material does not pass muster.[19] Thus, backward design can help to hone the course, paring unnecessary or superfluous content and retaining and highlighting its most essential elements.

Crafting Meaningful Assessment Methods

Assessment methods should be designed to capture the extent to which students have mastered course competencies. Methods of evaluating learning can be direct or indirect. Direct methods of evaluation provide evidence of students' knowledge and skills, and include traditional measures such as scores on exams and quizzes, homework assignments, term papers, individual research projects, group projects, or observations of work in the field. Indirect measures typically focus on the reflections and perceptions of students on their learning; these might include student course ratings, student self-assessments of knowledge gained, perceived value of the course in meeting students' career goals, class participation rates, and number of hours spent on homework or class projects. While direct measures supply proof of new knowledge and skills gained, indirect measures point to the broader benefits to students and their educational and career goals.

By starting with competencies and measurable learning objectives, assessment methods can literally be mapped back to the individual learning objectives. To complete this mapping, an instructor might ask "What would a student need to know to perform this competency?" and "How will I know the students have met this learning goal?"[20] Some methods of assessment can be designed for in-class use, for use in a lab or recitation session, or for work completed independently outside of class. For example, in constructing assessment methods for the core course in biostatistics, students may be presented with a small data set and asked to compute and interpret the mean, median, standard deviation, quartiles, and range for a continuous measurement; this would provide proof of competency in generating descriptive statistics for summarizing public health data. Further evidence of this competency can be attained through targeted questions on an exam, such as a multiple-choice question regarding the best measure of central tendency for a skewed distribution. Similarly, in a research methods course designed to hone students' skills in seeking external funding, the draft of a grant application might be a useful final project to demonstrate grant-writing ability. Indirect measures, such as student self-perceptions of knowledge gained and overall course quality ratings, can also be useful to both the student and the instructor. Such reflections can aid the student in situating the course into the context of their overall learning in a given degree program, while the instructor can gain insights into what works well and what does not in terms of how well the course is meeting its overall goals and objectives (see later section in this chapter on course evaluations).

Determining Course Structure

Central to course design is course structure—how time will be used, in class and outside of it, to help students meet the course learning goals and demonstrate course competencies. Similar to the design of assessments, the elements of course planning can be mapped directly back to the learning outcomes set by the instructor. Specifically, in considering the course or session learning objectives, an instructor can craft strategies that seem most promising for uncovering new knowledge and practicing the application of that knowledge. Some approach this part of course design as setting the distribution of hearing, reading, and doing. The Cornell Center for Teaching Innovation has produced a decision guide for course planning that enumerates a range of strategies for achieving course goals.[21] The following are teaching strategies taken from the Cornell outline for achieving learning objectives, ranging from very traditional to highly innovative.

- Continuous series of lectures and reading assignments, periodically interrupted by one or two midterms.
- Sequence of reading, reflective writing, and whole class discussion.
- Start with lab work or fieldwork observations, followed by readings and whole class discussions.
- Present lectures, followed by fieldwork or lab observations.
- Students do assigned readings, followed by minitests done individually or in small groups, then move on to group-based application projects.
- Work through a series of developmental stages: build knowledge and/or skills (three to five weeks), work on small application projects (three to five weeks), and then work on larger, more complex projects (three to five weeks).
- Contract for a grade (e.g., read text and pass exams = C, + research paper = B, + extended project = A).

The decision guide also emphasizes the incorporation of activities, week by week, to support learning goals. The guide suggests specifying which activities should come first in the course, and which last, and then filling in steps along the pathway from start of the course to the finish. Another key consideration is student feedback; students must receive feedback on the assignments and activities they complete in order to integrate their new knowledge effectively.[22]

There is ample evidence from research studies that student engagement enhances learning, and that active learning strategies such as cooperative learning and problem-based learning increase individual achievement in terms of knowledge acquisition, retention, and accuracy, as well as ability to apply new knowledge.[23] Research by Astin has shown that two factors emerged as by far the most important in predicting positive change in students' academic development, personal development, and satisfaction: interactions among students and interactions among students and faculty.[24] While Astin's study focused on undergraduates, these conclusions likely extend to graduate student populations as well. Therefore, it makes sense in course design to build in, as much as possible, opportunities for student-faculty interactions. In small classes, this seems to be almost unavoidable, but interactions can also be fostered in large courses with careful planning. For example, the strategies of "think-pair-share," "tell-help-check," and problem-based learning allow for small-group experiences within classes with high enrollments.[25,26,27,28,29] A flipped classroom format, in which students complete readings or watch recorded lectures prior to class, can be used to ensure that more classroom time can be used for small-group experiences or other learner-centered interactive learning activities.[30,31]

Tying It All Together: The Course Syllabus

The course syllabus represents a sort of contract or informal memorandum of understanding between the instructor and the students, setting out a roadmap for how the course will proceed. The syllabus should include all the elements discussed previously: course goals, overall structure and tempo, competencies that students will acquire, learning objectives for the overall course and each class meeting, required readings and assignments, optional/supplemental readings, content and dates of exams and quizzes, and assessment methods and technique for computing final grades. A well-constructed syllabus will set expectations on the part of both the instructor and the student and can help to minimize misunderstandings that can derail a student's success in and satisfaction with a course.[32] A strong syllabus can also help the instructor to crystallize the course's goals and expectations, which has been shown to yield more robust student learning.[33] Some syllabi even describe an instructor's teaching philosophy and set the tone for learning, portraying the course as a shared endeavor to which everyone needs to contribute.[34]

Many universities have prepared manuals and guidelines for constructing a syllabus. The Columbia University Mailman School of Public Health teaching toolkit[35] provides a freely accessible public health syllabus template, as well as a 29-page syllabus toolkit to help assemble a new syllabus or revise an existing syllabus.[36] By breaking down the construction of a syllabus into a series of discrete steps, the syllabus toolkit makes the syllabus-crafting exercise at once both less daunting and more practicable.

Ensuring Quality: Course Evaluation and Response

The evaluation of a course can and should take many forms. The most familiar is the set of anonymous student ratings received at the end of the semester (or sometimes, midsemester). There has been fierce debate in the literature and the higher education press (and even the lay press) about the value of anonymous student ratings. Many faculty disdain these data, because of some literature that has shown their vulnerabilities. However, instructors know that student ratings data always reveal some new information that helps to improve a course in future offerings. How can these positions coexist?

There has been nearly 100 years of research on student ratings, so this is, in fact, a very well-studied subject. Although much of the research focuses on undergraduates, there is no strong reason to believe that it is not applicable to graduate students. And while some of the research is old, it addresses methods and concepts that are relevant to current learning situations. It also suggests that the negative image of student course ratings presented by the educational and lay press may be too one-sided (see blog posts by Barre).[37]

The research on student course readings suggests that validity is an important concern. To examine validity, many experts in this domain make several recommendations. First is to avoid using the term "course evaluations" in favor of "student ratings," since the latter term is more accurate. These surveys gather information on student perceptions of a course, which is not at all the same as a formal evaluation of an instructor's ability to teach. Having said that, this information can still be helpful to the instructor, if used appropriately.

A second clear recommendation from the literature is to use a properly validated scale for student ratings—a resource perhaps too few colleges and universities have invested in. A second recommendation is to brief colleagues on the appropriate design and use of course evaluations—recognizing their true nature as student perceptions and stating clearly how closely we can use them to evaluate student learning (which can arguably be thought of as the ultimate way to critique a course). Many faculty repeat an oft-stated claim in the press, as well as in some research studies, that course evaluations are hopelessly flawed because of their relationship to student grades, equating this correlation to professors "paying off" students for better reviews. While this assertion is often repeated, it is difficult to find colleagues who say that, when they were students, they themselves rewarded their own professors in this way. It may also be overly simplistic, as some studies have failed to find such a correlation.[38] And it ignores the possibility that a positive correlation could be explained by the fact that students who learned more may actually rate a course more highly—recognizing there is more than one explanation for any observed correlation. In fact, many studies have demonstrated a positive relationship between course difficulty and student ratings.

A third recommendation is that in summarizing student course ratings data, it may be important to control for or stratify by factors such as class size, course status (required or elective), and discipline (e.g., STEM versus humanities). Fourth, it may be wise to look at instructor characteristics (e.g., gender, race, or ethnicity) as factors, with some evidence showing correlations with these student ratings (in a variety of directions).

For those wishing to delve deeper into this topic, one key reference is a 1981 meta-analysis that took a very careful approach to summarizing many years of data and findings.[39] While this analysis indeed demonstrated differing findings from multiple studies, overall it demonstrated that in total, many more studies demonstrate the validity of student course ratings as opposed to their lack of validity. In addition, a recent paper provided detailed guidance to administrators and members of promotion and tenure committees on how (and how not) to interpret and apply student ratings in reviews of faculty members.[40] While far from a comprehensive list, both of these papers (along with the well-written blog posts by Barre, cited previously[41]) provide good starting points for understanding this area of inquiry.

If we accept that student course ratings have some merit, the next question is how to best use them to improve a particular course. To begin, instructors should be focusing on the primary messages delivered by most students, not the unusual statements made by a tiny number of students. There will always be odd comments in any set of student reviews, and they grab our attention because of their peculiarity. But it is a fool's errand to run after the rogue view as opposed to the clearer message from the majority. While many public health instructors are well aware of this fact due to their research training, many forget it in the face of having to read negative comments about their own teaching. We suggest first focusing on the quantitative ratings using a validated scale, and to scan the qualitative comments for suggestions from students who have thoughtfully contributed ideas for the future. In addition, it is probably advisable to pair each early career faculty member with a more seasoned colleague to leverage the senior faculty member's experience to learn how to glean the most useful information out of a set of student ratings. Also, student feedback need not be reserved for the end of the course. For one new educational program, we instituted an anonymous midterm evaluation, which we used not to evaluate course quality but rather to identify any issues that could be addressed before the semester ended. In one instance, the midterm evaluations revealed that quizzes conflicted with other student deadlines; rescheduling the quizzes made students feel less stressed and increased student satisfaction.

Special Considerations in Designing Public Health Courses

Leveraging the Relevance of Public Health Practice/Application

One of the best aspects of public health education is its immediate relevance to real-world problems. No one could deny the importance of the Institute of Medicine defining public health as "what we as a society do collectively to assure the conditions in which people can be healthy."[42] This seminal work advances the notion that public health requires a multisectoral workforce with widely varying skills. This translates to a unique advantage to public health professors—we are teaching a tremendously engaging and highly significant field that enables us to capture the imaginations of our students. Through the auspices of organizations such as the American Public Health Association, the Association of Schools and Programs of Public Health, and the Centers for Disease Control and Prevention, there are excellent websites that promote awareness of public health and its impact on society.[43,44,45] Websites like these and the abundant public health literature create opportunities to incorporate genuine examples of public health research and practice into our public health courses.

Preparing Students in Professional Schools for Success in the Workforce

Clearly one of the goals of public health education, and professional education more generally, is to prepare individuals to become effective members of the workforce. In contrast with graduate education more generally, professional studies tend to be more applied and less theoretical, with a strong emphasis on enabling the professional to contribute to the workforce after graduation. What are the knowledge and skills that will prepare public health students to do so?

Public health curricula have been undergoing dramatic change over the past five to ten years. Indeed, a host of experts has provided unique insights into how public health education needs to change to meet the challenges of the future.[46,47,48,49,50,51,52,53] Some institutions have gone so far as to implement significant curricular changes in response to these calls to action,[54,55,56] and some have even shared early evaluation data.[57] By and large, these curriculum renewal efforts have broadened the core curriculum for public health, including emerging topics such as globalization, life course studies, social determinations of health, systems thinking, and health economics in addition to the more "traditional" aspects of core public health education: ethics, human rights, biology of health, environmental health, health and behavior, comparative health systems, biostatistics, epidemiology, and program planning. Some institutions have also incorporated training in leadership for a range of experience levels, as well as case study methods for deeper learning on the practice of public health. These are critically important developments, many of which are now incorporated into the expectations of the Association of Schools and Programs of Public Health (www.aspph .org) and into the accreditation standards of the Council on Education for Public Health (www.ceph.org). For guidance on implementing radical curriculum change, two case studies may be especially useful.[58,59]

Another realm of this new public health education pertains to preparing students for careers as members (and leaders) of interdisciplinary teams. Exposure to and engagement with interdisciplinary teamwork is increasingly seen as a prerequisite for adequate public health training,[60,61,62] with some papers presenting strategies and approaches for nurturing interdisciplinary competencies among public health and other graduate students.[63,64,65] One of the best resources to share with students happens to be a freely available publication by experts at the National Institutes of Health titled "Collaboration and Team Science: A Field Guide."[66] This is a comprehensive but very practical "how-to" guide for young investigators embarking on careers involving interdisciplinary team science and could serve as an excellent text for any training efforts designed to build interdisciplinary capacity. This recognition of the importance of interdisciplinarity has also led other fields, such as biomedical and health informatics, to include public health methods and perspectives among their competencies.[67]

Diversity of Public Health Student Backgrounds

As noted previously, the knowledge and skills required for public health are extremely broad. One can pursue public health across a wide array of career types, ranging from lab scientist to policy expert to health advocate. Because of this, the students in our classes come from an astounding breadth of backgrounds and career experiences. While this diversity enhances the allure of public health, it also introduces a significant challenge in the classroom: an extensive variety of prior knowledge, experiences, and skills is represented in every public health class. Pitching course content to a class with major differences in background knowledge can be a difficult task. If one pitches the level of the class too low, the attention of the more experienced class members is lost; however, if one pitches the level of the class too high, there is a risk of losing the less experienced students along the way. How can public health educators navigate such treacherous waters?

Our first recommendation relates back to an earlier section of this chapter—always return to the learning goals and objectives that you have set for the course. These goals should be the polestar for any instructor. While some students will invariably have more experience than others on any given topic, the instructor can tackle this challenge by following the guidance set forth previously in the chapter—be sure to incorporate many actual public health examples in the course materials. The second recommendation is to employ multiple strategies for student engagement and active learning. Because most public health education involves adult students, familiarity with the research on how adults learn is invaluable. There are numerous, cutting-edge strategies that can engage learners at multiple levels with diverse experiences; these include active learning techniques,[68] problem-based learning,[69] the use of analogies and images in teaching,[70,71] and approaches for generating classroom discussion, even when the class is large.[72,73] The fourth and final recommendation is to remain vigilant; any instructor must keep a watchful eye on the class to try to gauge students' level of engagement and understanding. Facial expressions can be very telling in a class setting. In addition to simply watching their faces, monitoring can be aided by use of technological tools, such as online quizzes, as well as in-the-moment techniques, such as audience response systems. We have found the latter particularly useful for distinguishing between strong and weak levels of student comprehension, and for guiding lecture content to fill in gap areas in large, lecture-based public health classrooms.

Conclusion

Perhaps the most important principle of public health course design is that course design is never done. To remain current and relevant, all public health courses must be reviewed with a critical eye on a regular basis. Minor changes are required each and every time a course is offered; however, minor changes do not obviate the need for more significant change at wider intervals. As demonstrated by recent changes to public health education, we are constantly called on to reevaluate and renew the curricula we offer our students. The challenges in public health research and practice do not remain static, nor can any single public health class or degree program. Teaching in any domain is an iterative process, and change is the one constant. The most important attributes of a public health course designer are the ability to be self-critical, to discern the need for positive change from student ratings data, and to summon the energy and courage to modify already-existing course strategies and materials on a regular basis.

REFERENCES

1. Lapp, I., E. Bagiella, and L. Hooper. "Syllabus Development Toolkit." https://www.mailman.columbia.edu/sites/default/files/legacy/Mailman%20 School%20Syllabus%20Toolkit.pdf (accessed April 10, 2018).

2. https://registrar.stanford.edu/staff/courses-scheduling-and-bulletin/courses /what-course-description.

3. Nodine, T. R. "How Did We Get Here? A Brief History of Competency-Based Higher Education in the United States." *Competency-Based Education* 1 (2016): 5–11.

4. Eaton, J. S. "Accreditation and Competency-Based Education." *Competency-Based Education* 1 (2016): 12–16.

5. Valenta, A. L., E. A. Meagher, U. Tachinardi, and J. Starren. "Core Informatics Competencies for Clinical and Translational Scientists: What Do Our Customers and Collaborators Need to Know?" *Journal of the American Medical Informatics Association* 23, no. 4 (July 2016): 835–839.

6. Council on Education for Public Health. "Competencies and Learning Objectives." 2006. https://ceph.org/assets/Competencies.pdf (accessed April 10, 2018).

7. Bennett, C. J., and S. L. Walston. "Improving the Use of Competencies in Public Health Education." *American Journal of Public Health* 105, Suppl. 1 (2015): S65-S67.

8. Association of Schools of Public Health. "Master's Degree in Public Health Core Competency Development Project—Version 2.3." ASPH Education Committee. 2006. https://s3.amazonaws.com/aspph-wp-production/app/uploads/2014/04 /Version2.31_FINAL.pdf (accessed April 7, 2018).

9. Fink, L. D. "Integrated Course Design: IDEA Paper #42." IDEA Organization. https://www.ideaedu.org/Portals/0/Uploads/Documents/IDEA%20Papers /IDEA%20Papers/Idea_Paper_42.pdf (accessed April 10, 2018).

10. Hooper, L., M. D. Begg, and L. M. Sullivan. "Integrating Competencies and Learning Outcomes in Core Courses for Public Health." *Public Health Reports* 129 (2014): 376–381.

11. Hooper, Begg, and Sullivan, "Integrating Competencies and Learning Outcomes in Core Courses for Public Health."

12. Wiggins, G., and J. McTighe. *Understanding by Design (Expanded 2nd Edition)*. Alexandria, VA: ASCD, 2005.

13. Bloom, B. S. *Taxonomy of Educational Objectives: Handbook 1. Cognitive Domain*. New York: David McKay, 1956.

14. Lapp et al. "Syllabus Development Toolkit."

15. Hooper et al. "Integrating Competencies and Learning Outcomes in Core Courses for Public Health."

16. Bowen, R. S. "Understanding by Design." Vanderbilt Center for Teaching and Learning. 2017. https://cft.vanderbilt.edu/understanding-by-design (accessed April 10, 2018).

17. Wiggins and McTighe, *Understanding by Design*.

18. Smith, K. A., S. D. Sheppard, D. W. Johnson, and R. T. Johnson. "Pedagogies of Engagement: Classroom-Based Practices." *Journal of Engineering Education* 94, no. 1 (2005): 87–101.

19. Smith et al. "Pedagogies of Engagement."

20. Sullivan, L. M., L. Hooper, and M. D. Begg. "Effective Practices for Teaching the Biostatistics Core Course for the MPH Using a Competency-Based Approach." *Public Health Reports* 129, (2014): 381–392.

21. Cornell University. "Planning Your Course: A Decision Guide." Cornell Center for Teaching Innovation. https://teaching.cornell.edu/resource/planning-your -course-decision-guide (accessed November 10, 2018).

22. Hooper et al. "Integrating Competencies and Learning Outcomes in Core Courses for Public Health."

23. Smith et al. "Pedagogies of Engagement."

24. Astin, A. *What Matters in College? Four Critical Years Revisited.* San Francisco: Jossey-Bass, 1993.

25. Karge, B. D., K. M. Phillips, T. Jessee, and M. McCabe. "Effective Strategies for Engaging Adult Learners." *Journal of College Teaching and Learning* 8, no. 12 (2011): 53–56.

26. Lyman, F. "The Responsive Classroom Discussion." In *Mainstreaming Digest*, edited by A. S. Anderson, 109–113. College Park: University of Maryland College of Education, 1981.

27. Lyman, F. "Think-Pair-Share: An Expanding Teaching Technique." *MAA-CIE Cooperative News* 1 (1987): 1–2.

28. Archer, A., and M. Gleason. *Skills for School Success.* North Billerica, MA: Curriculum Associates, 1994.

29. Barrows, H. S., and R. M. Tamblyn. *Problem-Based Learning: An Approach to Medical Education.* New York: Springer, 1980.

30. Álvarez, B. "Flipping the Classroom: Homework in Class, Lessons at Home." *Education Digest* 77, no. 8 (2012): 18–21.

31. Crouch, C. H., and E. Mazur. "Peer Instruction: Ten Years of Experience and Results." *American Journal of Physics* 69, no. 9 (2001): 970–977.

32. Davis, B. D. *Tools for Teaching.* San Francisco: Jossey-Bass, 1993.

33. O'Brien, J. G., B. Millis, and M. Cohen. *The Course Syllabus: A Learning-Centered Approach.* San Francisco: Jossey-Bass, 2008.

34. Bart, M. "A Learner-Centered Syllabus Helps Set the Tone for Learning." *Faculty Focus.* July 29, 2015. https://www.facultyfocus.com/articles/effective -classroom-management/a-learner-centered-syllabus-helps-set-the-tone-for-learning.

35. Columbia University Mailman School of Public Health. "Teaching Toolkit." https://www.mailman.columbia.edu/information-for/teaching-learning/teaching -toolkit (accessed April 10, 2018).

36. Lapp et al. "Syllabus Development Toolkit."

37. Barre, E. "Do Student Evaluations of Teaching Really Get an 'F'?" Rice University Center for Teaching Excellence. 2015. http://cte.rice.edu/blogarchive /2015/07/09/studentevaluations (accessed April 10, 2018).

38. Griffin, T. J., J. Hilton, K. Plummer, and D. Barrett. "Correlation between Grade Point Averages and Student Evaluation of Teaching Scores: Taking a Closer Look." *Assessment and Evaluation in Higher Education* 39, no. 3 (2014): 339–348.

39. Cohen, P. A. "Student Ratings of Instruction and Student Achievement: A Meta-Analysis of Multisection Validity Studies." *Review of Educational Research* 51, no. 3 (1981): 281–309.

40. Linse, A. R. "Interpreting and Using Student Ratings Data: Guidance for Faculty Serving as Administrators and on Evaluation Committees." *Studies in Educational Evaluation* 54 (2017): 94–106.

41. Barre, "Do Student Evaluations of Teaching Really Get an 'F'?"

42. Institute of Medicine. *The Future of Public Health.* Washington, DC: National Academies Press, 1988.

43. American Public Health Association. "What Is Public Health?" https://www .apha.org/what-is-public-health (accessed April 10, 2018).

44. Association of Schools and Programs of Public Health. "This Is Public Health." https://thisispublichealth.org (accessed April 10, 2018).

45. Centers for Disease Control and Prevention. "Ten Great Public Health Achievements in the 20th Century." https://www.cdc.gov/mmwr/preview/mmwr html/00056796.htm (accessed November 10, 2018).

46. Sommer, A. "Toward a Better Educated Public Health Workforce." *American Journal of Public Health* 90, no. 8 (2000): 1194–1195.

47. Clark, N., and E. Weist. "Mastering the New Public Health." *American Journal of Public Health* 90, no. 8 (2000): 1202–1207.

48. Shortell, S. M., E. M. Weist, M. S. Sow, A. Foster, and R. Tahir. "Implementing the Institute of Medicine's Recommended Curriculum Content I Schools of Public Health: A Baseline Assessment." *American Journal of Public Health* 94, no. 10 (2004): 1671–1674.

49. Fineberg, H. V., G. M. Green, J. H. Ware, and B. L. Anderson. "Changing Public Health Training Needs: Professional Education and the Paradigm of Public Health." *Annual Reviews in Public Health* 15 (1994): 237–257.

50. Frenk, J., I. Chen, Z. A. Bhutta, et al. "Health Professionals for a New Century: Transforming Education to Strengthen Health Systems in an Interdependent World." *Lancet* 376, no. 9756 (2010): 1923–1958.

51. Institute of Medicine. "Who Will Keep the Public Healthy? Educating Public Health Professionals for the 21st Century." K. Gebbie, L. Rosenstock, and L. M. Hernandez, eds. Washington, DC: National Academies Press, 2003. http://www.nap.edu/openbook.php?record_id=10542 (accessed March 25, 2018).

52. Moser, J. M. "Core Academic Competencies for Master of Public Health Students: One Health Department Practitioner's Perspective." *American Journal of Public Health* 98, no. 9 (2008): 1559–1561.

53. Koh, H. K., J. M. Nowinsky, and J. J. Piotrowski. "A 2020 Vision for Education the Next Generation of Public Health Leaders." *American Journal of Preventive Medicine* 40, no. 2 (2011): 199–202.

54. Petersen, D. J., M. E. Hovinga, M. A. Pass, C. Kohler, R. K. Oesenstadt, and C. Katholi. "Assuming Public Health Professionals are Prepared for the Future: The UAB Public Health Integrated Core Curriculum." *Public Health Reports* 120, no. 5 (2005): 496–503.

55. Fried, L. P., M. D. Begg, R. Bayer, and S. Galea. "MPH Education for the 21st Century: Motivation, Rationale, and Key Principles of the New Columbia Public Health Curriculum." *American Journal of Public Health* 104, no. 1 (2014): 23–30.

56. Begg, M. D., S. Galea, R. Bayer, J. W. Walker, and L. P. Fried. "MPH Education for the 21st Century: Design of Columbia University's New Public Health Curriculum." *American Journal of Public Health* 104, no. 1 (2014): 30–36.

57. Begg, M. D., L. P. Fried, J. W. Glover, M. Delva, M. Wiggin, L. Hooper, R. Saxena, H. de Pinho, E. Slomin, J. R. Walker, and S. Galea. "Columbia Public Health Core Curriculum: Short-Term Impact." *American Journal of Public Health* 105, no. 12 (2015): e7-e13.

58. Galea, S., L. P. Fried, J. R. Walker, S. Rudenstine, J. W. Glover, and M. D. Begg. "Developing the New Columbia Core Curriculum: A Case Study in Radical Curriculum Change." *American Journal of Public Health* 105, Suppl. 1 (2015): S17-S21.

59. Yale University. "Yale School of Management Launches Innovative New MBA Curriculum." 2006. http://som.yale.edu/news/news/yale-school-management -launches-innovative-new-mba-curriculum (accessed April 10, 2018).

60. Committee on Facilitating Interdisciplinary Research, National Academy of Sciences, National Academy of Engineering, Institute of Medicine. *Facilitating Interdisciplinary Research*. Washington, DC: National Academies Press, 2004.

61. Gebbie, K. M., B. M. Meier, S. Bakken, et al. "Training for Interdisciplinary Health Research: Defining the Required Competencies." *Journal of Allied Health* 37, no. 2 (2008): 65–70.

62. Borrego, M., and L. K. Newswander. "Definitions of Interdisciplinary Research: Toward Graduate-Level Interdisciplinary Learning Outcomes. *Reviews in Higher Education* 34, no. 1 (2010): 61–84.

63. Begg, M. D., L. M. Bennett, L. Cicutto, H. Gadlin, M. Moss, J. Tentler, and E. Schoenbaum. "Graduate Education for the Future: New Models and Methods for the Clinical and Translational Workforce." *Clinical and Translational Science Journal* 8, no. 6 (2015): 787–792.

64. Begg, M. D., and R. D. Vaughan. "Are Biostatistics Students Prepared to Succeed in the Era of Interdisciplinary Science? (And How Will We Know?)" *American Statistician* 65, no. 2 (2011): 71–79.

65. Larson, E. L., T. F. Landers, and M. D. Begg. "Building Interdisciplinary Research Models: A Didactic Course to Prepare Interdisciplinary Scholars and Faculty." *Clinical and Translational Science Journal* 4, no. 1 (2011): 38–41.

66. Bennett, L. M., H. Gadlin, and S. Levine-Finley. *Collaboration and Team Science: A Field Guide*. Washington, DC: National Institutes of Health, 2010.

67. Valenta et al., "Core Informatics Competencies for Clinical and Translational Scientists."

68. Yeatts, K. B. "Active Learning by Design: An Undergraduate Introductory Public Health Course." *Frontiers in Public Health* 2 (December 2014): Article 284.

69. Barrows and Tamblyn, *Problem-Based Learning.*

70. Martin, M. A. "'It's Like . . . You Know': The Use of Analogies and Heuristics in Teaching Introductory Statistical Methods." *Journal of Statistics Education* 11, no. 2 (2003).

71. Ancker, J. S., and M. D. Begg. "Using Visual Analogies to Teach Introductory Statistical Concepts." *Numeracy* 10, no. 2 (2017): Article 7.

72. Smith et al. "Pedagogies of Engagement."

73. Karge et al. "Effective Strategies for Engaging Adult Learners."

Engaging the Public Health Student through Active and Collaborative Learning

KATHRYN M. CARDARELLI, ANGELA CARMAN, AND TREY CONATSER

THE LANDSCAPE OF higher education in the United States is changing in terms of rising tuition costs, shifting workforce demands, and a decline in the projected high school enrollment over the next decade in certain parts of the country—these changes are imparting strain on students, faculty, and administrators alike.[1] Additionally, the sociodemographic profile and communication preferences of today's university students have also dramatically shifted from those of just two decades ago. What has remained constant is the fact that student engagement continues to be an important predictor of retention and student success,[2] and active and collaborative learning environments can facilitate greater levels of engagement. This is particularly true in public health education, which strives to produce workforce-ready graduates who are able to engage with communities to improve population health.

Teaching in a discipline as broad as public health requires faculty who are proficient in a wide array of topics spanning scientific and behavioral content areas. Combining the breadth of public health as a discipline that covers both the "science and art" of health improvement[3] with the need for crosscutting skills, such as partnership building and infrastructure development, is a challenge for any public health instructor. The classroom may include students strong in analytical skills with a drive to pursue biostatistics or epidemiology as well as students intent on affecting unhealthy lifestyle choices and behaviors through community-based interventions, with a focus on human behavior skills. That same classroom may include students who are novices in the field as well as students with extensive professional experience. Our public health instructional methods must be sufficiently varied and flexible to affect students whose skills and interest levels vary. Instructional techniques that foster student engagement may be key to overcoming these challenges. In this chapter, we review the pedagogical theories and research that inform our understanding of student engagement in public health education. With that understanding, we outline best practices for a range of scenarios that engage students as motivated, active learners by modeling the values of social justice, citizenship, and equity on which public health rests.

Active and Collaborative Learning Techniques to Promote Student Engagement

Active learning has become the mantra of faculty development, curricular reform, and pedagogy in higher education. The benefits of active learning over traditional lecturing extend far beyond higher examination scores and lower failure rates. Freeman et al. make the provocative claim that if active learning experiments "had been conducted as randomized controlled trials of medical interventions, they may have been stopped for benefit—meaning that enrolling patients in the control condition might be discontinued because the treatment being tested was clearly more beneficial."[4] Moreover, they found that active learning "confers disproportionate benefits" for "disadvantaged" students and for women in the characteristically male-dominated STEM fields.[5] The case for active learning, from a research perspective, is well supported and has become increasingly clear and compelling.

Traditionally contrasted against rote learning and passive reception, active learning engages students in participatory roles and at higher levels of learning, such as analysis, evaluation, and creation. Yet, students may resist active learning and other innovative pedagogies, however empirically and intuitively superior they appear to instructors. In one analysis, the most significant barriers for student engagement in innovative learning environments were (1) a preference for conventional lectures, (2) unsatisfactory peer interactions or performances, and (3) a perception that innovative methods take too much time and lack relevance for overall educational and professional goals.[6] Active learning techniques do not guarantee student engagement in their own right. Researchers suggest the need for student-centered design in active learning pedagogy to maximize student engagement—the affective, qualitative, and individual experiences on which the efficacy of active learning depends. While engagement may signify the mere fact of student participation in active learning tasks, motivation is also required for students to reach learning objectives.[7]

As a collective of academic disciplines and professional practices dedicated to the equitable and sustainable deployment of health improvement and education, public health is uniquely positioned to move the discourse on student engagement to an ethical register, explicitly acknowledging active learning's implicit roots in critical pedagogy (described in the following paragraph). Drawing from theorists such as Paulo Freire, critical pedagogy seeks to develop a "critical consciousness."[8] This explicitly liberatory, ethical, and political pedagogy asks students to (1) explore how "contending forces and interests" shape the lived experiences of individuals and groups; (2) challenge doxa (common values, beliefs, behaviors, and practices) with context, analysis, and nuance; (3) question "power and inequality in the status quo" in order to expand the possibilities of human development; and (4) learn and effect positive change through "self-organiz[ation]" and "cooperative action."[9]

While critical pedagogy emerged as a challenge to the late capitalism of the mid-to-late twentieth century, it is no less urgent in the age of digital technologies and ubiquitous computing. Because digital technologies program the world and the possibilities for us to act in and on it, critical digital pedagogy "centers its practice on community and collaboration," especially "across cultural and political boundaries" in order to effect change "outside traditional institutions of education" with a polyvocal, democratic ethos.[10] Put more simply, the kind of critical student engagement that is most urgent for public health educators to foster and maximize is one of democratic, liberatory collaboration. Aligned with critical pedagogy, collaborative learning "encourages [polyvocal] dissent" as a meaningful and democratizing opportunity for growth in supportive environments.[11] Active learning and student engagement in public health education is not merely an instrumental question of knowledge and skill acquisition; rather, the implicit learning outcomes aim for students to make the world a better place. How students engage with their learning environments must align with these outcomes, and we offer the following approaches to active and collaborative learning techniques that seek to foster the kind of student engagement that the exigencies of public health demand.

Selected Scenarios to Maximize Student Engagement

Considering that meaningful student engagement occurs as a product of intrinsic and extrinsic motivation and active learning techniques that focus on critical literacies and collaboration, we offer the following selection of active and collaborative learning scenarios, organized from the most simple to the most complex. Researchers have suggested that educational scholarship ought to consider active learning not as an aggregate whole but rather as a constellation of strategies, scenarios, and formats—some of which will be more effective or appropriate for particular classroom situations.[12] Accordingly, we have attempted to frame strategies and activities for student engagement with respect to their usefulness in addressing particular kinds of issues in the public health classroom. All activities should focus on a concrete, "real-world public health issue or task" in order to maximize student engagement that otherwise has been shown to flag in the pursuit of "highly abstract material."[13]

Think-Pair-Share

Perhaps the most basic and classic form of collaborative learning—think-pair-share—represents a simple yet flexible strategy to engage students in the classroom by asking them to engage a question or problem first by themselves, then with a peer, and finally with the whole class. Class discussion can be engaging, but it may not always be democratic; moreover, an instructor may encounter moments when the class seems unable to generate and sustain momentum in a conversation. Beyond discussions, think-pair-share also works well for the interrupted lecture as an opportunity to engage students in response to difficult questions that require analysis and evaluation. This technique promotes student engagement best when questions allow a range of possible answers and require application and metacognition beyond factual recall.[14] Possible applications include determining the next best step in a case study or scenario; considering the best methodology or model to use for a given situation; evaluating two or more options and justifying a choice; interpreting difficult moments in a text; connecting course content with personal experiences; role-playing to demonstrate how a certain type of person would respond to a situation, phenomenon, or problem; and reflecting on the forces that shape a complex public health phenomenon as it manifests broadly or specifically.

However, to maximize student engagement in think-pair-share, it is important to give meaningful weight to the first and third steps of the process. To create a sense of equity among a variety of personalities, dispositions, cognitive processes, and neurotypes, students must be given time to think on their own without feeling pressured to speak before they are ready. A best practice for ensuring that all students are engaged in the initial step of the process is to do the thinking through writing. For challenging topics, about which students may be reluctant to engage in conversation with their peers in conversational exchange (i.e., the forces that shape racial health disparities or the pathological rhetoric that influences health policies related to nonheteronormative sexual behavior), the paired discussion may be structured so that one student is given time to speak while the other silently listens, and vice versa, after which they synthesize their reflections for sharing out. While this sharing can sometimes take the form of a large group discussion if a class is small enough, digital tools (e.g., classroom response systems and polling software) or collaborative spaces (e.g., Google Drive) can ensure that every group has the opportunity to share their insights with a real, embodied audience of their peers. Regardless of the method used for the share-out, the instructor should synthesize patterns, anomalies, and otherwise meaningful contributions to avoid the "pseudotransactionality" that can afflict student collaboration if it seems not to exert agency on the learning environment.[15]

Affinity Mapping

Underpinning critical pedagogy and collaboration is the ethical position that learning is polyvocal and democratic. Affinity mapping engages students in collaborative thinking for which identification, categorization, and the articulation of conceptual relationships are primary objectives. While traditional approaches, such as textbook reading, may simply present students with definitions, taxonomies, and concept maps, affinity mapping emphasizes that students are active coproducers of their own knowledge.

Affinity mapping is most appropriate at the initial stages of a learning unit or class meeting, when the aggregate whole of a field, discourse, theory, scenario, case, or problem needs to be segmented into more granular components for understanding and analysis. Individually or in teams, students write ideas on a shared space, such as a board at the front of the room or on portable paper such as sticky notes, in response to a question or prompt. Once all responses have been posted, the instructor facilitates a group conversion during which students take note of patterns, relationships, and categories that have emerged in their corpus of responses. This activity can also be done in small groups and reported out to the class as an embedded think-pair-share.

While affinity mapping itself models an ethos of critical pedagogy, it works especially well when confronting difficult or uncomfortable questions that occur frequently in the study and practice of public health. As an example, affinity mapping might allow students to wrestle with structural inequalities such as socioeconomic position in the context of public health. Given a case study with adequate data, students can categorize their responses from the essentialist and individually focused to the constructivist and socially focused. The structured reflection and taxonomical negotiations of affinity mapping provide space for dissent and growth in understanding a complex issue that may challenge, with kindness and academic rigor, the doxa that students bring to the classroom. In the context of public health education's commitment to social justice, citizenship, and equity, affinity mapping allows students to critique ideas as opposed to people by evaluating those ideas, as a network, in a public space to which all students have equal access and may exert agency.

Problem-Based Learning

Students may disengage from their learning because they feel that an exercise is artificial or that their engagement is irrelevant to the task at hand. A so-called active and collaborative learning exercise may fall flat because of an overwrought design by which predetermined procedures and solutions await student teams to unlock their secrets. To get the most out of exercises and to avoid counterproductive or confusing moments, instructors need to provide students with concrete situations and the resources needed to solve a problem.

For courses with learning objectives that emphasize research skills, information literacies, communication, and strategic thinking, problem-based learning does not negatively affect student recall of course content (in fact, it shows a minor increase compared to traditional formats), and it can greatly enhance the "integration of new knowledge with existing knowledge."[16] The instructor works as a consultant or facilitator who monitors student teams and provides feedback, prompts, and questions that keep them on track. Thus, problem-based learning is limited by student-teacher ratio, and instructors must carefully craft and peer review the problem scenarios for adequate complexity and alignment with course content and objectives. Problem-based learning aligns with best practices for student engagement, which can be enhanced even further with the integration of low-stakes writing tasks that promote inquiry and metacognition.[17]

Team-Based Learning

While team-based learning is popular in many disciplines, it is particularly suited to cultivate sustained student engagement in professional schools such as public health, whose governing competencies emphasize not just the recall of information but also its application to new situations (i.e., transfer of knowledge) in collaborative, multidisciplinary environments.[18] In order for team-based learning to work, four criteria must be met: (1) "properly formed and managed" groups, (2) a structured process to ensure both individual and team accountability, (3) frequent and timely feedback on student work and progress, and (4) assignments that "promote both learning and team development" equally.[19] Groups may be formed at the beginning of the term to include members of a variety of majors, achievement indicators, technical expertise, or other experiences or demographic characteristics. The academic term is then divided into multiweek units that begin with a brief "readiness assurance process," by which individual students and then teams are tested on assigned material. Following this process, teams collaborate (perhaps with specific, rotating roles assigned to team members) in order to address new situations using the information and methods assessed by the readiness assurance process.

When structuring the challenges for teams, instructors should balance content-based considerations equally with reflection on and self-assessment of teamwork and decision-making. As a strategy to maximize student engagement, team-based learning is most appropriate when the course learning outcomes involve communication and collaboration, as the explicit and sustained attention to team dynamics requires a significant amount of cognitive resources and time that otherwise might be used for content coverage. Digital platforms such as Google Drive and Slack allow flexibility for team collaboration as well as a way for instructors to track student progress toward specific goals.

Importance of Experiential Learning for Public Health Education

Active and experiential education allows learners to engage in questioning, solving problems, clarifying values, and developing skills to mutually benefit community partners. Experiences in the field are followed by reflection and discussion, resulting in learning that is personal and includes the importance of relationship building through an enhanced understanding of self, others, and the larger community.[20] Experiential learning can begin with a discussion of a public health issue such as environmental justice, during which students question the proximity of busy highways or industrial facilities to lower-income neighborhoods as compared to their own homes and neighborhoods. Instructors may add more hands-on experiential learning by touring particular neighborhoods, observing interviews with individuals receiving a public health intervention such as smoking cessation classes, or conducting environmental scans of services available to meet a community-identified need such as substance-use disorder treatment. Instructors may also coordinate with community partners who agree to host public health students in a work setting or allow students to observe or engage in a community-based intervention or research project.

Conclusion

Active and collaborative learning techniques to enhance student learning and engagement place instructors in the role of facilitator in the classroom. Because the fundamental determinants of population health are structural, social, and cultural in nature,[21] public health faculty often find themselves facilitating discussions not only about the empirical evidence as to how these factors shape health but also about the political, cultural, and social forces that shape these factors. Students bring a variety of identities, including their religion, gender identity, and political ideology, to the classroom, and the use of inclusive teaching practices can provide faculty with tools to navigate difficult, sometimes polarized, discussions. According to Ambrose et al.: "Even though some of us might wish to conceptualize our classrooms as culturally neutral or might choose to ignore the cultural dimensions, students cannot check their sociocultural identities at the door, nor can they instantly transcend their current level of development. . . . Therefore, it is important that the pedagogical strategies we employ in the classroom reflect an understanding of social identity development so that we can anticipate the tensions that might occur in the classroom and be proactive about them."[22]

There are potential benefits of inclusive teaching, including greater student engagement, a deeper understanding of the course materials, and mitigation of tension during conversations of controversial or heated topics. There are several techniques that may be particularly well suited to public health education, particularly in discussing the role of sociostructural factors producing inequitable health. For example, asking students to collectively decide on ground rules at the beginning of the semester allows them to fully understand the expectations of the instructor and their classmates.[23] It may also allow students to hold one another accountable to those rules and may prevent incivility. Following is a sample of communal agreements established recently by a graduate-level public health class on eliminating racial and ethnic health disparities—speak one at a time, pause and process before speaking, be open-minded, leverage the instructor to ask tough questions, freely share perspectives without burden, be empathetic in and out of class, and respect others. During a difficult conversation, the instructor may need to reiterate the ground rules to redirect the discourse.

Additional inclusive teaching practices include universal design, which allows for multiple means of representation (e.g., oral, visual, textual), attention to learning preferences, and evidence of meeting learning objectives to include as many learners as possible, including but not limited to students who self-identify as disabled.[24] Additionally, educators should encourage a growth mind-set in students. This approach fosters the notion that intelligence is not a fixed attribute but rather a capacity that can increase over time.[25] Instructors can encourage a growth mind-set by establishing that answering a question with an incorrect response is an important mechanism for deeper learning.

Regardless of the specific techniques used, public health education stands to promote student engagement not only as the instrumental means to an institutional end of retention, completion, and job placement—important criteria in their own right—but also as a model of social justice, citizenship, and equity, all of which underpin the scholarly and professional work of public health. By adapting these and other techniques, as well as explicitly conveying the rationale for their mechanics, educators may attune students to these values, which in turn become habits of mind as they become the next generation of leaders and practitioners in the field.

REFERENCES

1. Selingo, J. J. *The Future of the Degree: How Colleges Can Survive the New Credential Economy.* Washington, DC: Chronicle of Higher Education, 2017.

2. Tinto, V. "Research and Practice of Student Retention: What Next?" *Journal of College Student Retention* 8, no. 1 (2006): 1–19.

3. Winslow, C. E. A. "The Untilled Field of Public Health." *Modern Medicine* 2 (1920): 183–191.

4. Freeman, S., S. L. Eddy, M. McDonough, M. K. Smith, N. Okoroafor, H. Jordt, and M. P. Wenderoth. "Active Learning Increases Student Performance in Science, Engineering, and Mathematics." *Proceedings of the National Academy of Sciences of the United States of America* 111, no. 23 (2014): 8410–8415.

5. Freeman et al. "Active Learning Increases Student Performance in Science, Engineering, and Mathematics."

6. Ellis, D. E. "What Discourages Students from Engaging with Innovative Instructional Methods: Creating a Barrier Framework." *Innovative Higher Education* 40 (2015): 111–125.

7. Barkley, E. F. *Student Engagement Techniques: A Handbook for College Faculty.* San Francisco: Jossey-Bass, 2010.

8. Shor, I. *Empowering Education: Critical Teaching for Social Change.* Chicago: University of Chicago Press, 1992.

9. Shor, *Empowering Education.*

10. Stommel, J. "Critical Digital Pedagogy: A Definition." *Hybrid Pedagogy: A Digital Journal of Learning, Teaching, and Technology.* 2014. www.digital pedagogylab.com/hybridped/critical-digital-pedagogy-definition (accessed April 8, 2018).

11. Barkley, F. K., P. Cross, and C. H. Major. *Collaborative Learning Techniques: A Handbook for College Faculty.* San Francisco: Jossey-Bass, 2005.

12. Freeman et al. "Active Learning Increases Student Performance in Science, Engineering, and Mathematics."

13. Pinahs-Schultz, P., and B. Beck. "Development and Assessment of Signature Assignments to Increase Student Engagement in Undergraduate Public Health." *Pedagogy in Health Promotion* 2, no. 3 (2016): 206–213.

14. Prahl, K. "Best Practices for the Think-Pair-Share Active-Learning Technique." *American Biology Teacher* 79, no. 1 (2017): 3–8.

15. Petraglia, J. "Spinning Like a Kite: A Closer Look at the Pseudotransactional Function of Writing." *JAC: A Journal of Composition Theory* 15, no. 1 (1995): 19–33.

16. Allen, D. E., R. S. Donham, and S. A. Bernhardt. "Problem-Based Learning." *New Directions in Teaching and Learning* 128 (2011): 21–29.

17. Allen, Donham, and Bernhardt, "Problem-Based Learning."

18. Sibley, J., and D. X. Parmelee. "Knowledge Is No Longer Enough: Enhancing Professional Education with Team-Based Learning." *New Directions in Teaching and Learning* 116 (2008): 41–53.

19. Michaelsen, L. K., and M. Sweet. "The Essential Elements of Team-Based Learning." *New Directions in Teaching and Learning* 116 (2008): 7–27.

20. Association for Experiential Education. "What Is Experiential Education?" http://www.aee.org/what-is-ee (accessed October 30, 2017).

21. Cardarelli, K. M., J. S. de Moor, M. D. Low, and B. J. Low. "Fundamental Determinants of Population Health." In *Reinventing Public Health: Policies and Practices for a Healthy Nation,* edited by L. A. Aday, 35–64. San Francisco: Jossey-Bass, 2005.

22. Ambrose, S. A., M. W. Bridges, M. DiPietro, and M. Lovett. *How Learning Works: Seven Research-Based Principles for Smart Teaching.* San Francisco, CA: Jossey Bass, 2010.

23. Brookfield, S. D., and S. Preskill. *Discussion as a Way of Teaching and Techniques for Democratic Classrooms, 2nd Edition.* San Francisco, CA: Jossey-Bass; 2005.

24. Meyer, A., D. H. Rose, and D. Gordon. *Universal Design for Learning: Theory and Practice.* Wakefield, MA: CAST, 2014.

25. Dweck, C. *Mindset: The New Psychology of Success.* New York: Ballantine, 2006.

[13]

Teaching Cultural Competency for Twenty-First-Century Public Health Practice

LINDA ALEXANDER

CULTURAL COMPETENCE TRAINING for public health and medical students was the focus of a joint effort between the then Association of Schools of Public Health and the American Association of Medical Colleges, and provided the basis for a published report. This expert panel report utilized the following working definition of cultural competence: "Cultural competence is defined in the broader context of diversity and inclusion as 'the active, intentional, and ongoing engagement with diversity to increase one's awareness, content knowledge, cognitive sophistication, and empathic understanding of the complex ways individuals interact within systems and institutions.'"[1]

This definition acknowledges the importance of one's own needs related to cultural competence while simultaneously understanding the complexities between and among individuals, systems, and institutions. This report was also among the first to emphasize the significance of the individual's investment in becoming more culturally competent as opposed to directing and requiring change in populations of interest. A focus on student educational preparation in cultural competence was a marked shift away from creating what was analogous to so-called laundry lists attributed to change needs for those characterized by their race, ethnicity, sexual orientation, migration status, or gender.

Over the course of the past thirty years, several textbooks from a variety of fields have articulated the necessity to focus on the multicultural needs of patients, populations, systems, communities, and so forth, using a multicultural approach, lens, system, framework, and solution. A review of these proposed methods reveals an overemphasis on descriptors of populations, groups, systems, and institutions. The traditional checklist approach creates an overreliance on a bulleted list of population needs. Unintended consequences of this approach are stereotyping, unconscious bias, and limited preparation toward solutions. Checklists can provide insight into the multicultural patient, language barriers that influence patient access, and factors that optimize the clinical setting to reflect a diverse patient population, and can serve as supplemental resources useful for understanding the interdisciplinary nature of public health work. Contemporary public health training provides an appropriate layer of competency attainment for graduates of our programs and provides the opportunity to understand and practice cultural sensitivity, cultural humility, and the development and discovery of culturally appropriate interventions. A culturally competent public health workforce has the ability to influence, evaluate, and create change to reduce the burden of disease and to eliminate health disparities. The overarching focus of schools and programs of public health is the preparation of transformational leaders to tackle the health needs of contemporary society. The core disciplines of public health provide a framework for leading efforts to create desired change in population health through direct education, as well as the creation of policies, interventions, and programs that reduce the risk of exposure and disease. Graduates of public health, medicine, and other health-related disciplines must have a clear understanding of the historical context for economic, social, and political disadvantage, and how these factors contribute to disparate health outcomes.

Transformation occurs when the skill set required for a deep understanding of the social context for health disparities includes cultural competence. Therefore, innovation in teaching cultural competence begins with a comprehensive cultural immersion experience. Preliminary classroom preparation is essential for positive learning outcomes associated with the journey to cultural competency.

Putting on Your Own Mask First

The title of this section references the most common phrase uttered by flight attendants as part of the preparation for a safe flight. If you were deprived of oxygen, it would be difficult to render aid. Preparation is a key component of teaching cultural competence. This preparation allows you to anticipate students' cognitive struggles with information that may not necessarily be part of their own lived experience as well as information that may be counter to previous thoughts and beliefs about different subgroups. Public health students typically enter the academy with an overwhelming desire to effect change. While these students are likely to embrace the path forward to competence, they may have differential exposure to other cultures and population health needs via media soundbites, politically charged debates, and family influence. Therefore, those entering our classrooms may have a false sense of their comprehensive knowledge about what it means to be culturally competent and how to apply knowledge and skills toward solutions. Training in this area requires a methodical approach that is enhanced by putting in the time and effort needed in advance of the class start. As part of this process, it will be important to reflect on your own perceptions, biases, competencies, and readiness for change prior to instructing a captive audience. Additionally, an important step will be to embrace a teaching philosophy that acknowledges the students as cultural experts in their own right.

Part of embracing the appropriate philosophy is understanding the utility of the classroom as part of cultural competence education. Establishing an environment to enhance the learning experience is crucial to the successful teaching of cultural competency. The classroom, whether online or residential, provides an often-missed opportunity for teaching subject matter effectively. Participants enrolled in our courses bring a unique set of cultural experiences that can enhance learning for their peers and provide context for instruction. An optimal setting is one that allows for candid dialogue in a safe place to express unfiltered thoughts and interactive learning and to continually maximize the strengths of the learner.

The Classroom as a Cultural Experience

Defining culture is an important first step, setting the stage in the classroom for further learning. Regardless of your program, students most often equate culture with race. It will be important to provide a context for learning that continually references culture and cultural competency appropriately. Providing an opportunity to dialogue about what culture is and what it is not is a fundamental step in the learning process. An analogy can be as simple as having students understand that although there was a very distinct and much-touted 1970s culture in the United States, a public health practitioner would not develop a health intervention solely based on a person's style of clothing or taste in music.

Brislin has written extensively about culture and behavior. His writing provides a unique perspective about what constitutes culture. The following are highlighted examples that can move students beyond the notion of race[2]—culture consists of ideals, values, and assumptions about life that guide specific behaviors; culture allows people to fill in the blanks when presented with a basic sketch of familiar ideas; and there are emotional reactions when cultural values are violated or when a culture's expected behaviors are ignored.

I have used these types of examples to provide students with an opportunity to engage their peers in discussion about culture that moves away from racial and ethnic group behavior and toward a deeper understanding of shared meaning. Asking students to dialogue within this framework paired with examples from their own life experiences provides a more nuanced approach to the concept of health and culture. Today's classroom experience can help simulate the student's need to experience learning in the moment as part of the cultural competency process. The healthy tension created by fleshing out content as part of the classroom milieu is a fundamental step toward embracing a philosophy that will be a part of the student's arsenal of skills in this area. This innovation in teaching cultural competency content dictates the necessity of student involvement as part of learning. Online learning platforms that support peer inquiry and dialogue or the creation of virtual communities can enhance learning that transcends a cognitive exercise to an important feeling component. The following three quick and easy learning formats are illustrative of how to move students from passive to active participants in their own cultural journey. These activities can be enhanced or minimized to reflect baccalaureate versus graduate training.

Cultural Exchange Activities

Pair students in the class and have them identify family customs, rituals, and practices that someone from another culture may not understand. If necessary, prompt their thinking around holiday activities, birthday celebrations, death and bereavement, courtship and weddings, and caring for the elderly. This activity immediately places the student in the role of an expert about his or her cultural upbringing and provides the opportunity to begin to dialogue about differences without judgment or creating false categories for individuals. This process of exchanging differences also creates parity for students born outside of the United States who are often at a disadvantage when learning occurs almost exclusively in the context of the Western cultural experience.

Web-Based Dialogue

Utilizing the web-based platform your institution subscribes to is a convenient way to facilitate dialogue outside of the formal classroom environment. This practice also helps to establish the iterative process of attaining cultural competency skills. Create conversation starters around contemporary public health topics, have students respond to assigned topical readings focused on minority health issues, or facilitate a dialogue around a class discussion. Examples of contemporary provocative topics that call for sensitivity and empathy are the Black Lives Matter campaign, immigration reform, prescription drug abuse, transgender rights, reversal of women's rights, the Affordable Care Act, freedom of speech, gun laws, sexual assault on campus, and legalization of marijuana.

Minicultural Immersion Experience

Teaching students to be proactive in gathering information about a target population can be generalized from an experience of becoming familiar with campus resources with a social justice or inclusivity mission. Require students as part of a for-credit assignment to spend time becoming familiar with a campus or community group that represents a cultural group or cultural philosophy different from their own. This can be especially helpful for international students, who may assume that students born in the United States have a built-in cultural lens due to their birthplace. A cultural immersion experience is a great equalizer, especially if students are transitioned from merely attending a set of activities to interviewing, spending quality time, documenting, or journaling about the emotions and feelings associated with experiencing a different world.

Linking Cultural Competence to Public Health Education

As the accrediting body for schools and programs of public health, the Council on Education in Public Health, sets standards in the form of foundational competencies for required learning at the bachelor's, master's, and doctorate in public health degree levels.[3] It is important that cultural competence be viewed and taught as a part of the narrative around foundational competencies for students in public health and public health practice. These competencies also provide an opportunity to assess student's baseline knowledge of cultural competency in the context of other courses and learning experiences. The following selected foundational competencies for the Master of Public Health degree are among those that highlight the need for culturally competent public health practitioners: discuss the means by which structural bias, social inequities, and racism undermine health and create challenges to achieving health equity at organizational, community, and societal levels; assess population needs, assets, and capacities that affect communities' health; apply awareness of cultural values and practices to the design or implementation of public health policies or programs; propose strategies to identify stakeholders and build coalitions and partnerships for influencing public health outcomes; advocate for political, social, or economic policies and programs that will improve health in diverse populations; evaluate policies for their impact on public health and health equity; communicate audience-appropriate public health content, both in writing and through oral presentation; and describe the importance of cultural competence in communicating public health content.

Tying cultural competence proficiency to learning outcomes as part of the foundation of your students' preparation helps to frame the importance of cultural competence mastery. In addition to assessing students' course-specific knowledge through exam questions, group projects, written essays, and reports, students can assess their own development of cultural competency with questions about their learning in a cultural context. Sample items that might be included in a baseline or follow-up assessment of cultural knowledge are as follows:

- I can name cultural factors that contribute to overall health and wellness.
- I recognize that cultural competence alone does not address healthcare disparities.
- I am aware of my own strengths and learning needs as they relate to working with diverse populations.
- I can conduct culturally appropriate risk and asset assessments and communicate these with families and communities.
- I have gained considerable knowledge about racial and ethnic populations that will influence my public health practice after graduation.
- I appreciate how cultural competence contributes to the practice of public health and medicine.
- I am willing to go out on a limb to ensure that the institution or department that employs me offers culturally competent and relevant services.
- I am willing to continually assess my own biases and prejudices that may interfere with my work in effectively closing the gap in racial and ethnic disparities in health.

These kinds of questions are not designed to meet strict methodological constraints but rather to facilitate reflection and discussion for learning and as part of self-discovery for students.

Applying a Cultural Lens to Public Health Disciplines

Epidemiology and Biostatistics

A strong foundation in epidemiology and biostatistics remains the critical component of a public health program. However, it is equally important that students understand the need for better surveillance and tools to measure disparate health outcomes. Current methods and techniques to gather data may not capture comorbidities, genetic predispositions, or differential environmental exposures. The collapsing of cells to comply with power calculations and statistical methods creates an incomplete picture of some historically classified racial or ethnic groups, those who do not conform with socially prescribed gender identity, those who identify as bi or multiracial, and segments of populations bound by geographic or regional differences. Viewing data with a cultural lens can enhance the interpretation of data and acknowledge that traditional data collection may ignore important contextual factors. For example, an exhaustive list of published studies compares socially classified racial groups with Caucasian populations. Regardless of the inquiry in this type of comparative analysis, the difference between groups is highlighted as the most salient feature of the results. However, suppose you are actually interested in differences in risk behaviors for HIV/AIDS. It may be more important to look at differences between those who report sexual risk behaviors and those who do not. Setting up an analysis that focuses on the risk behavior of interest rather than comparing racial groups might yield important insight about protective factors. Applying a cultural lens also recognizes the value of understanding and incorporating other innovative methods of inquiry, such as social media-based techniques.

Environmental Health

The environmental justice movement of the 1960s provides a tremendous opportunity to view this particular public health discipline with a cultural perspective.[4] A historical perspective can frame health outcomes with an appropriate lens. Make certain that in addition to providing content on risk and exposure, students learn that segments of the population have endured years of institutionally sanctioned practices that have resulted in neighborhood segregation. Additionally, historical migration patterns have resulted in often-invisible geographic and regional boundaries. Applying a culturally sensitive approach dictates that it is important for students to be cognizant of the intergenerational effect of toxic exposures from air, water, and land, and how these might intersect with other health risk behaviors such as tobacco smoking or alcohol abuse.

Health Policy, Management, and Leadership

Not all populations benefit equally from policies designed to protect health. Coursework that requires students to understand the dynamics and interworking of creating effective policies enhances the likelihood that students will comprehend the often-unintended consequences of enforcing rules, laws, and regulations. Examples of policies that differentially affect vulnerable populations are found in tobacco legislation and smoking laws, sugar and sweetened beverage taxation, and employer health insurance incentive programs. In addition to providing students with the opportunity to understand the legislative process and to practice the techniques of policy writing, there are also opportunities for students to understand their role as an advocate for comprehensive laws that do not overly burden the poor. Cultural competency in this area prepares students to become the voice for those populations that are not represented in policy-making. A cultural lens in health policy requires students to consider how realities such as the rates of incarceration, percentage of people unemployed, number of welfare recipients, percentage with less than a high school education, and intergenerational poverty have an influence on which groups benefit and which groups do not from policies intended to promote great health for all.

Social and Behavioral Science

There are important contextual factors that influence the impact of prevention and other behavioral interventions. Traditional courses in health behavior often distinguish social determinants of health as a distinct method of applying and understanding theories in health behavior. Populations in the United States have suffered well-documented systematic and institutional racism over an identifiable period of health promotion and prevention activities. Yet, students are often taught that differences in health outcomes based on race, gender, and sexual orientation devoid of the important historical context and political realities facing targeted populations, migration patterns, neighborhood characteristics, zip codes, and environmental exposures provide a mandatory context when studying health outcomes. Health disparities are often viewed from a deficient perspective as opposed to a true characterization of laws, practices, and policies that were unjust, unfair, and avoidable.

Social and behavioral theories need to be taught to include contextual understanding of behavior as a function of an individual or group lived experience. Behavior related to health outcomes must be studied from a multilevel approach, taking advantage of the wealth of information provided by all five of public health's core disciplines.

Conclusion

Cultural competence is an ongoing process that requires career-long dedication. The suggestions in this chapter are designed to be used either in a stand-alone course or as part of an existing class. Regardless of the format or degree level, advanced course preparation, creation of safe space for candid dialogue, and a minicultural immersion experience are all necessary components. Faculty, staff, and students should be encouraged to seek formal training and embrace existing resources that provide more in-depth and ongoing practice of cultural competence.

REFERENCES

1. Expert Panel on Cultural Competence Education for Students in Medicine and Public Health. "Cultural Competence Education for Students in Medicine and Public Health: Report of an Expert Panel." Washington, DC: Association of American Medical Colleges and Association of Schools of Public Health, 2012.

2. Brislin, R. *Understanding Culture's Influence on Behavior*. New York: Harcourt College Publishers, 2000.

3. Council on Education for Public Health. "Accreditation Criteria: Schools and Programs of Public Health." Silver Spring, MD: CEPH, 2016. https://ceph.org/assets/2016.Criteria.pdf (accessed March 25, 2018).

4. Carlson, R. *Silent Spring*. New York: Houghton Mifflin Company, 1962.

[14]

Teaching in a Diverse Classroom

A Student-Centered Approach

LORRAINE M. CONROY, SUSAN ALTFELD, JENNIFER HEBERT-BEIRNE,
JYOTSNA JAGAI, AND UCHECHI MITCHELL

OVER THE PAST few decades, we have seen a paradigm shift in teaching, from providing instruction to producing learning. A focus on producing learning requires the institution, the instructor, and the student to engage in the collaborative production of learning.[1] A significant amount of research related to student-centered active learning is available for elementary, secondary, and undergraduate education. Research specific to graduate education is limited but confirms that methods and approaches shown to be effective at the undergraduate level are also effective in graduate and professional education programs.[2]

The US population is becoming increasingly multicultural, a trend also reflected in enrollments in higher education. The US minority population more than doubled from 1970 to 2016 and is projected to represent more than 50% of the population by 2042.[3] Barriers have existed for racial and ethnic minorities as well as other underrepresented groups in higher education,[4] but there have been improvements over the past few decades, with a two-and-a-half-fold increase of underrepresented minority (URM) students enrolled in higher education and a tripling of URM students enrolled in graduate and professional programs.[5] However, URM students continue to be underrepresented in science and engineering, where they comprise approximately 20%, 14.5%, and 8% of bachelor's, master's, and doctoral degree recipients, respectively, although they comprise 37% of the college-aged population.[6,7] In schools of public health, the patterns of enrollment are similar; URM students comprise 19.8% of graduates from accredited schools and programs belonging to the Association of Schools and Programs of Public Health.[8] The diversity gap is more pronounced among college and university faculty, with URM individuals comprising only 10% of all faculty[9] and 13% of public health faculty.[10] The relatively low proportion of minority faculty in schools of public health adds more complexity and challenge as the field aims to meet the needs of a diverse study body.

While the term "diverse" is often used to refer to racial and ethnic minorities, in this chapter we use the phrase "diverse classroom" to refer to a classroom of learners who are different in terms of social identity, which includes characteristics such as sexual orientation and gender identity, age, ability, political orientation, and economic and educational disadvantage.

Learning requires individual transformation and involves fitting, extending, and, in many cases, supplanting older understanding and knowledge with new knowledge, understanding, and experiences.[11] Student-centered learning places an emphasis on connecting new knowledge and skills to previous experiences,[12,13] requires respect for diversity and different ways of learning,[14] provides adequate contact between students and instructors and among students, fosters engagement of students,[15,16] and provides necessary supports.[17] It also involves setting high but well-defined expectations and providing meaningful feedback.[18]

A culturally responsive and inclusive classroom links classroom content to student experiences and requires cultural humility with respect to students' lived experiences. For students to succeed, the instructor must bring these experiences into the classroom and recognize the social capital and expertise students bring with them.[19,20] The goal is to build a community of learners, where students are active partners rather than marginalized, passive vehicles who absorb information and knowledge and regurgitate information on request,[21] and where the instructor is also a learner. This requires instructors to recognize how their positionality and behaviors influence their students' learning in both positive and negative ways,[22] to reject deficit-based thinking and banking education models in which students are receptacles of information, and to appreciate the assets that students bring to the classroom.[23,24]

Instructors' social identities and experiences as well as the space they make for other identities is key to culturally relevant instruction. This space includes how students are greeted—using welcoming preferred pronouns and names—and ensures inclusivity of topics, voices, experiences, and expertise. Culturally relevant pedagogy requires a focus on achievement, cultural humility rather than assimilation, and sociopolitical consciousness, and can result in a deeper understanding of and appreciation for the role of culture,[25] including the culture of higher education, in the learning process. This pedagogy requires a social justice approach that not only celebrates diversity but examines why and how education is unjust for some students, analyzes policies and practices that privilege some students and disadvantage others,[26] and engages in critical dialogue about historical and contemporary issues such as entrenched disparities and institutional racism.[27]

Developmental and educational theories describe social interaction as necessary to elicit cognitive disequilibrium, which in turn leads to learning.[28] Diversity in the student body provides the discontinuity necessary for more active thinking and for students to move beyond their embedded worldviews.[29] Campus and classroom practices that help integrate learning, build new knowledge on previous experiences, and increase skills in intergroup relations can transform the thinking of all students. This results in students with more skill in critical inquiry, better ability to constructively consider multiple perspectives,[30] and increased pluralistic orientation, including an interest in poverty issues and concern for the public good.[31] Diverse perspectives are critical for problem-solving (particularly for problems requiring innovation), public policy,[32] and public health advocacy.

URM students often express doubts about their ability to succeed, and higher education systems can knowingly and unknowing invalidate students by discounting their life experiences, detaching faculty from students, and promoting competitive classroom environments. Students who do not feel validated in the classroom will rely on out-of-classroom validation, which may be more limited for URM students.[33] However, active intervention by an instructor that affirms the academic capability of the student can help URM students succeed. Merely offering opportunities for involvement is not sufficient, particularly for students with limited experience with these kinds of opportunities. Examples of in-class validation include demonstrating a genuine interest in teaching students, structuring learning experiences that demonstrate confidence that students are capable of learning, working individually with students, and providing meaningful feedback,[34] as well as selecting course material that is inclusive of diverse experiences and recognizing diverse kinds of expertise and ways of knowing.[35]

While all students appear to benefit from active learning approaches, economically and educationally disadvantaged students appear to benefit the most.[36,37,38,39] These approaches have been successful in large classrooms—and can improve performance of all students while also reducing the achievement gap—and require limited additional resources compared to programs traditionally used to assist students from disadvantaged educational backgrounds (e.g., tutoring and other individualized support programs).[40]

Quality of education is enhanced when faculty and administrators engage in continuous improvement strategies.[41] Ultimately, the key to a successful learning environment is trust—trusting the students to do their part but also trusting that instructors will be fair and understanding of circumstances. Instructors must understand that learners from economically and educationally disadvantaged backgrounds have a greater number and severity of circumstances that may interfere with academic success, as measured by traditional metrics.

There is compelling evidence that culturally responsive pedagogy, engagement, and active learning approaches improve outcomes for all students while also closing the achievement gap.[42] However, universities and faculty have been slow in adopting these approaches. Instructors may not know about the evidence-based benefits of active learning, some may distrust the evidence because they see scientists and scholars who have succeeded with the current approach, others may feel intimidated by the challenge of learning new teaching methods, and still others may fear that being identified as a committed teacher will reduce their credibility as a researcher.[43] It may also be that instructors are afraid to appear vulnerable in the classroom and want to maintain the control and safety that the front of the classroom provides.

Student-centered active learning approaches require a considerable amount of effort and resources. Adoption of these practices may be a function of the financial and administrative climate in higher education rather than faculty preferences.[44] Institutions have long established expectations for faculty productivity and evaluation, specifically for promotion and tenure, financial arrangements and funding streams, classroom design and scheduling, decision-making policies, and a host of other systems that support and require instruction. The institution may not provide space nor support for redesigned learning environments or for experimenting with alternative learning technologies or course structures.[45] This will need to change, in some cases in very dramatic ways, to fully implement a student-centered learning approach that better serves the needs of an increasingly diverse student body.

Case Study: Teaching Public Health and Health Equity to a Diverse Student Body

Our home institution is a public research university designated as a Minority Serving Institution and has received awards for its commitment to and support of a diverse student body.[46] The demographics of Master of Public Health (MPH) students are approximately 29% URM, 76% female, an average age of 27 years, and 31% first-generation college graduates.[47] Data on sexual orientation/gender identity, economic disadvantage, and students with disabilities are currently not available.

In 2008, our School of Public Health began an academic strategic planning initiative to address what faculty saw as deficiencies in students' ability to retain core knowledge and skills, and to apply knowledge and skills to more complicated problems associated with advanced coursework and capstone projects. Similar efforts were being initiated at other schools of public health (e.g., see Begg et al.[48] and Sullivan et al.[49]). Our initiative involved revising the MPH core curriculum to move away from discipline-specific core courses to a three-course, team-taught, integrated core curriculum. The curriculum uses a cohort approach, where groups of approximately 60 students participate in the same section of all three core courses over the course of the first year in the program. There are currently two full-time on-site cohorts and one online cohort, which includes distance and part-time students.

An extensive mixed methods evaluation of the courses and student outcomes was conducted in the first two years and found improvements in several important metrics—for example, preparation for subsequent courses, applying theory and models to public health problems, performing data analysis, and reported higher satisfaction with peer group support, class activities, and team-based instruction (unpublished data).

Here we describe the initial development, implementation, and ongoing evaluation of one MPH core on-site course, Determinants of Population Health (see table 14.1), and interrogate this course against the best practices for meeting the educational needs of diverse learners. Specifically, we attempt to answer four questions: Is the course designed and delivered in a way that fosters engagement and collaborative and active learning? Do we set high and well-defined expectations and provide regular and meaningful feedback? Do we seek feedback from students and others and respond to that feedback? Is the curriculum culturally responsive?

For this course, we adapted a culturally responsive pedagogical approach using engagement, active learning, and a flexible course plan. The course uses small group discussion-based learning to facilitate understanding and integration of key concepts and to enhance skill development, followed by short presentations from the small groups. An instructor-facilitated class discussion follows, where instructors or guests often provide examples of their research and advocacy to the class. A small-group, problem-based exercise is included during each class period. Each class session ends with students reflecting on the class content and experience in an online journal that instructors read and use to adapt instruction.

The large class size makes it challenging to ensure that all students are participating and that the small group discussions are productive. A few students have indicated in their journals that they find the small group discussion less effective than the instructor-facilitated discussion, while other students report that the small group discussion allows everyone to participate rather than a few, more assertive students who speak during the large group discussion. More explicit products from the small group discussions and report-back may improve student satisfaction.

Three of the authors have been involved in developing and teaching the course since its inception, and the other two joined the team with the addition of the second on-site cohort. The course has two-to-three teaching assistants (TAs) who are shared across sections. The instructor team meets frequently to ensure fidelity of student learning experience. Instructors' expertise is leveraged across both cohorts, exposing the students to a broader spectrum of faculty expertise. After the initial

TABLE 14.1. Determinants of Population Health Course Development Timeline

Academic Year	Building Infrastructure	Faculty Development	Course Implementation and Evaluation
2012–2013	Faculty identification ▪ Cross-discipline ▪ 2 EOHS, 2 CHS ▪ Codeveloped ▪ Compensated	Case-based discussion learning ▪ Faculty trained ▪ Train the trainer approach	
2013–2014		Dialogue initiative ▪ Promoting dialogue, not debate ▪ Focus on inclusion/respect	Launched pilot ▪ 1 section ▪ 2 instructors ▪ Organized: where one is born, lives, works, plays, prays
2014–2015	Added second section ▪ Additional instructors and expertise		Pilot evaluation ▪ Mixed methods ▪ Strong qualitative
2015–2016		Course Design Institute ▪ 3-day course ▪ Backward course design ▪ Active learning ▪ Seminars ▪ Student-centered teaching	
2016–2017	Added online section		Evaluation ▪ Input from faculty, students, Radical Public Health ▪ Reconfigured course
2017–2018			Launched revised course ▪ Focus on structural drivers of health inequity as well as social determinants ▪ Emphasis on experiential learning ▪ Increased emphasis on other ways of knowing

offering, we reviewed our experiences with the course, both as a team and with input from students. To improve our teaching, we sought consultation from the Dialogue Initiative (https://dialogue.uic.edu), a campus resource that recognizes inclusion and differences as fundamental to learning in a pluralistic society. The Dialogue Initiative staff provided instructor training to more sensitively address issues of student identity and inclusiveness in the classroom. We established the dialogue guidelines described later in the chapter.

Specifically, we establish clear expectations for preparation before class, participation in class, and graded assignments. We require a number of low-stakes, low-point assignments spread out throughout the semester, which include a mix of individual and group assignments. A grading rubric providing detailed expectations is provided to students prior to completing each assignment, and the completed rubric with instructor or TA feedback is provided on completion of each assignment. The class also establishes a set of agreed-upon ground rules related to group work, including behaviors they agree to engage in (i.e., being accountable and responsible, meeting deadlines, respecting other members' time, respecting the contributions of all members) as well as behaviors they agree to avoid (i.e., not contributing their fair share or dominating the work such that others feel they cannot contribute).

In response to initial course offerings in which the students were not completely prepared for discussion-based learning, we adapted the assignments to require a written summary of the assigned readings by the evening before class. The purpose of the summary was to prepare the student for discussion learning, thus we accepted a wide range of summaries to match the different styles of learners.

One major goal of the course is to study the roots of health inequity in the United States and globally. We initially developed the course using a place-based (where one is born, lives, works, plays, prays, and ages) approach to our understanding of the determinants of health.[50] In the spring of 2017, we reviewed our experiences with the course as well as students' experiences and met with representatives of Radical Public Health, an association of students, alumni, faculty, and staff at our institution committed to addressing the systemic underlying causes of public health challenges within School of Public Health learning, research, and practice (http://publichealth.uic.edu/current-students/rph). The course instructors and Radical Public Health representatives felt that this course needed to move away from the focus on place and bring its attention further upstream, with more emphasis on economic and political determinants of health. A major restructuring of the course was conducted for the Fall 2017 semester. The course now follows the World Health Organization's Conceptual Framework for Action on the Social Determinants of Health, which places greater influence on socioeconomic and political drivers of health inequities,[51] rather than more proximal (downstream) determinants of health, such as health behaviors.

We use a variety of class materials, such as peer-reviewed literature, TED talks, newspaper and magazine articles, and music, and also incorporate material from the Roots of Health Inequity[52] interface to describe historical perspectives and current examples of discrimination and oppression as well as their relationships to ongoing health inequities.

Part of critical analysis is questioning our own (students' and instructors') biases, examining and synthesizing evidence to reach a conclusion, and developing strategies and approaches to solving problems. As instructors, we acknowledge that we are not neutral observers but advocates for improving public health, and that our biases influence the selected topics and course materials. We explicitly encourage students to challenge these biases in our class discussions and to suggest relevant, additional, or alternative material.

We also recognize that public health deals with controversial issues and that consideration of these issues may cause disagreements or may evoke strong personal feelings, depending on individual experiences, histories, identities, and worldviews. Recently, there has been much public discourse about trigger warnings and safe spaces versus free speech.[53] We have taken the stance that these are not mutually exclusive. It is important to create a safe space for deliberate, thoughtful dialogue on so-called difficult topics. It is important to face the politics of public health. We feel we need to teach students to be comfortable with the uncomfortable, and we spend time at the beginning of the course reviewing guidelines for respectful and productive dialogue. These guidelines include maintaining confidentiality in order to create a safe atmosphere for open, honest exchange; committing to learn from each other; listening to each other and not talking at each other; acknowledging differences among us in backgrounds, skills, interests, and values, and realizing that these differences will increase our awareness and understanding; not demeaning or devaluing people for their experiences, lack of experience, or different interpretation of those experiences; trusting that people are always doing the best they can; challenging the idea, not the person; speaking our discomfort, as our emotional reactions to this process often offer the most valuable learning opportunities; and being mindful of taking up much more space than others and being empowered to speak up when others are dominating the conversation.

Almost every time the course is taught, an unanticipated issue emerges based on student concerns. In our pilot offering, a transgender student was initiating the process of transitioning during the first semester of graduate school. He asked for faculty support to educate his classmates about gender and sexual minorities, and shared his own plans for transitioning with the cohort. The next year, students involved in Black Lives Matter struggled with their commitments to school as they dealt with broader political and societal events demanding their time. Faculty struggled with how to balance respect for students' activism with their obligation to cover the material in the syllabus. Most recently, we have been called on to be more inclusive of disability issues. We worked together to provide some flexibility in class attendance with a responsibility for those involved to share their personal perspectives and experiences. Additionally, we have ensured academic accommodation for students struggling with homelessness and other difficult personal circumstances. Grappling with these issues has helped us greatly improve our course offerings. Course plans are designed to be flexible, to bring real-time issues into the class as they emerge. Current political events, often paired with divisive rhetoric, have provided the class with weekly case studies in the political determinants of health inequities. This past year alone, we were afforded the opportunity to engage in active learning on the disparities in disaster relief for Houston versus Puerto Rico, the roots of the opioid epidemic, health impacts of trickle-down economics, freedom of speech and civil liberties from those kneeling for social justice in the National Football League, white supremacists, and changes in the US Census and the importance of being counted.

Conclusion

The increasing diversity of the student population in public health programs provides both challenges and opportunities. Recognizing the diverse backgrounds, experiences, and worldviews of students and integrating their contributions can enrich our teaching and contribute to the development of a respectful and responsive classroom climate. We adopted a student-centered, active learning model in our newly developed MPH core curriculum. In our experience, this model has demonstrated benefits for both students and faculty. The teaching team continues to learn from our students as each new cohort comes with its own characteristics and the environment in which we live, work, and practice continues to evolve. We believe that this engaged learning better prepares our students as public health professionals and leaders in an increasingly complex and diverse world.

REFERENCES

1. Barr, R. B., and J. Tagg. "From Teaching to Learning—A New Paradigm for Undergraduate Education." *Change* 27, no. 6 (1995): 13–26.

2. Bonwell, C. C., and J. A. Eison. "Active Learning: Creating Excitement in the Classroom—ASHE-ERIC Higher Education Report No. 1." Washington, DC: George Washington University, School of Education and Human Development, 1991.

3. United States Census Bureau. "A Look at the 1940 Census." https://www.census.gov/newsroom/cspan/1940census/CSPAN_1940slides.pdf (accessed April 9, 2018).

4. United States Department of Education. "Advancing Diversity and Inclusion in Higher Education, Key Data Highlights Focusing on Race and Ethnicity and Ethnicity and Promising Practices." 2016. https://www2.ed.gov/rschstat/research/pubs/advancing-diversity-inclusion.pdf (accessed April 9, 2018).

5. United States Department of Education. "Fall Enrollment in Colleges and Universities Surveys." https://nces.ed.gov/programs/digest/d15/tables/dt15_306.10.asp?current=yes (accessed April 9, 2018).

6. United States Census Bureau. "A Look at the 1940 Census."

7. National Science Foundation. "Women, Minorities, and Persons with Disabilities in Science and Engineering." 2014. https://www.nsf.gov/statistics/2017/nsf17310/digest/fod-minorities/degree-share.cfm (accessed April 9, 2018).

8. Association of Schools and Programs in Public Health. "ASPPH Graduate Employment 2014 Common Questions Pilot Project." 2015. https://s3.amazonaws.com/aspph-wp-production/app/uploads/2015/07/ASPPH_Graduate_Employment_Pilot_Project_Report_May2015.pdf (accessed April 9, 2018).

9. Meyers, B. "Where are the Minority Professors?" *Chronicle of Higher Education.* 2016. https://www.chronicle.com/interactives/where-are-the-minority-professors (accessed April 9, 2018).

10. Association for Schools and Programs in Public Health. "Data Center." https://data.aspph.org (accessed December 19, 2017).

11. Fry, H., S. Ketteridge, and S. Marshall. "Understanding Student Learning." In *A Handbook for Teaching and Learning in Higher Education—Enhancing*

Academic Practice, 3rd Edition, edited by H. Fry, S. Ketteridge, and S. Marshall, 8–26. New York: Routledge, 2009.

12. Kolb, A. Y., and D. A. Kolb. "Learning Styles and Learning Spaces: Enhancing Experiential Learning in Higher Education." *Academy of Management Learning and Education* 4, no. 2 (2005): 193–212.

13. Lea, S. J., D. Stephenson, and J. Troy. "Higher Education Students' Attitudes to Student-Centered Learning: Beyond 'Educational Bulimia'?" *Studies in Higher Education* 28, no. 3 (2003): 321–334.

14. Banks, J., M. Cochran-Smith, L. Moll, A. Richert, K. Zeichner, P. LePage, L. Darling-Hammond, H. Duffy, and M. McDonald. "Teaching Diverse Learners." In *Preparing Teachers for a Changing World: What Teachers Should Learn and Be Able to Do*, edited by L. Darling-Hammond and J. Bransford, 232–274. San Francisco: Jossey-Bass, 2005.

15. Chickering, A. W., and Z. F. Gamson. "Seven Principles for Good Practice in Undergraduate Education." *AAHE Bulletin* (1987): 3–7.

16. Study Group on the Conditions of Excellence in American Higher Education. "Involvement in Learning: Realizing the Potential of American Higher Education." Washington DC: National Institute of Education, US Department of Education, 1984.

17. Gosling, D. "Supporting Student Learning." In *A Handbook for Teaching and Learning in Higher Education—Enhancing Academic Practice, 3rd Edition*, edited by H. Fry, S. Ketteridge, and S. Marshall, 113–131. New York: Routledge, 2009.

18. Banks, "Teaching Diverse Learners."

19. Kolb and Kolb, "Learning Styles and Learning Spaces."

20. Study Group, "Involvement in Learning: Realizing the Potential of American Higher Education."

21. Gosling, "Supporting Student Learning."

22. Howard, T. C. "Relevant Pedagogy: Ingredients for Critical Teacher Reflection." *Theory into Practice* 42, no. 3 (2003): 195–202.

23. Freire, P. *Pedagogy of the Oppressed, 30th Anniversary*. New York: Bloomsbury Academic, 2000.

24. Ladson-Billings, G. "Culturally Relevant Pedagogy 2.0: A.k.a. the Remix." *Harvard Educational Review* 84, no.1 (2014): 74–84.

25. Ladson-Billings, "Culturally Relevant Pedagogy 2.0."

26. Nieto, S. "Placing Equity Front and Center: Some Thoughts on Transforming Teacher Education for a New Century." *Journal of Teacher Education* 51, no. 3 (2000): 180–187.

27. Lopez-Littleton, V. "Critical Dialogue and Discussions of Race in the Public Administration Classroom." *Administrative Theory and Praxis* 38 (2016): 285–295.

28. Hurtado, S. "Linking Diversity with the Educational and Civic Missions of Higher Education." *Review of Higher Education* 30, no. 2 (2007): 185–196.

29. Gurin, P., E. L. Dey, S. Hyrtado, and G. Gurin. "Diversity and Higher Education: Theory and Impact on Educational Outcomes." *Harvard Educational Review* 72, no. 3 (2002): 330–366.

30. Nagda, B. A., P. Gurin, and G. E. Lopez. "Transformative Pedagogy for Democracy and Social Justice." *Race Ethnicity and Education* 6, no. 2 (2003): 165–191.

31. Hurtado, "Linking Diversity with the Educational and Civic Missions of Higher Education."

32. Page, S. E. *The Difference—How the Power of Diversity Creates Better Groups, Firms, Schools, and Societies.* Princeton, NJ: Princeton University Press, 2007.

33. Rendon, L. I. "Validating Culturally Diverse Students: Toward a New Model of Learning and Student Development." *Innovative Higher Education* 19, no. 1 (1994): 33–51.

34. Rendon, "Validating Culturally Diverse Students."

35. Hooks, B. *Teaching to Transgress: Education as the Practice of Freedom.* New York: Routledge, 1994.

36. Cabrera, A. F., J. L. Crissman, E. M. Bernal, A. Nora, P. T. Terenzini, and E. T. Pascarella. "Collaborative Learning: Its Impact on College Students' Development and Diversity." *Journal of College Student Development* 43, no. 1 (2002): 20–34.

37. Freeman, S., D. Haak, and M. P. Wenderoth. "Increased Course Structure Improves Performance in Introductory Biology." *CBE Life Sciences Education* 10 (2011): 175–186.

38. Haak, D. C., J. Hillerislambers, E. Pitre, and S. Freeman. "Increased Structure and Active Learning Reduce the Achievement Gap in Introductory Biology." *Science* 332, no. 6034 (2011): 1213–1216.

39. Eddy, S. L., and K. A. Hogan. "Getting under the Hood: How and for Whom Does Increasing Course Structure Work?" *CBE Life Sciences Education* 13 (2014): 453–468.

40. Haak et al. "Increased Structure and Active Learning Reduce the Achievement Gap in Introductory Biology."

41. Study Group, "Involvement in Learning: Realizing the Potential of American Higher Education."

42. Haak et al., "Increased Structure and Active Learning Reduce the Achievement Gap in Introductory Biology."

43. Handelsman, J., et al. "Scientific Teaching." *Science* 304, no. 5670 (2004): 521–522.

44. Lea, Stephenson, and Troy, "Higher Education Students' Attitudes to Student-Centered Learning."

45. Fry, Ketteridge, and Marshall, "Understanding Student Learning."

46. University of Illinois at Chicago. "Minority Serving Institution Status." https://research.uic.edu/minority-serving-institution-status (accessed April 9, 2018).

47. University of Illinois at Chicago. "UIC Office of Institutional Research." http://www.oir.uic.edu/?q=StudentDataBookPage2 (accessed April 9, 2018).

48. Begg, M. D., S. Galea, R. Bayer, J. R. Walker, and L. P. Fried. "MPH Education for the 21st Century: Design of Columbia University's New Public

Health Curriculum." *American Journal of Public Health* 104, no. 1 (2014): 30–36.

49. Sullivan, L. M., A. Velez, V. B. Edouard, and S. Galea. "Realigning the Master of Public Health (MPH) to Meet the Evolving Needs of the Workforce." *Pedagogy in Health Promotion* (2017): 1–11.

50. World Health Organization. "Social Determinants of Health." http://www.who.int/social_determinants/sdh_definition/en/ (accessed April 9, 2018).

51. Solar, O., and A. Irwin. *A Conceptual Framework for Action on the Social Determinants of Health—Social Determinants of Health Discussion Paper 2 (Policy and Practice).* Geneva, Switzerland: WHO Press, 2010.

52. National Association of County and City Health Organizations. "Roots of Health Inequity." http://rootsofhealthinequity.org/about-project.php (accessed April 9, 2018).

53. Pérez-Peña, R., M. Smith, and S. Saul. "University of Chicago Strikes Back against Campus Political Correctness." *New York Times.* August 26, 2016. https://www.nytimes.com/2016/08/27/us/university-of-chicago-strikes-back-gainst-campus-political-correctness.html.

[15]

Innovative Active Learning in Public Health

DAVID G. KLEINBAUM

THIS CHAPTER EXPLORES mechanics of public health education that employ active learning, a teaching approach that strives to more directly get students to participate in the learning process, rather than passively listening.[1] The learning process is typically enhanced if students read, write, discuss, or are engaged in solving problems as well as enjoy, or at least appreciate, their learning experience. What is taught is as important as how it is taught. Doing and thinking are components of active learning. Introducing active approaches to learning can enhance the overall learning experience and can help make learning fun, even for difficult subject material. Techniques to promote active learning can be organized into four general categories. Each is discussed in some detail in the following sections.

Create a Relaxed, Friendly Classroom Environment That Positively Influences Student Motivation for Taking and Remaining in the Course

This issue is fundamental to public health courses in any area (not just biostatistics, as discussed later on) because successful teaching can rarely be accomplished without students and their instructors working together in a harmonious class environment. Issues with overall student motivation have occurred in biostatistics courses among nonbiostatistics public health students who are frightened by not being mathematically prepared to understand the course material. Additionally, they may be worried about the discipline's notorious reputation for poor instructors. This problem is not as widespread today in introductory biostatistics courses thanks to better-prepared, application-oriented instructors; improved instructional materials; and recent computer technology. However, the problem continues in higher-level quantitative courses as well as in other areas of public health. To help ensure a harmonious classroom environment, instructors should consider the following.

Make a Positive First Impression by Trying to Learn Students' Names, No Matter How Large the Class

If available, study a face book of student photos a week or two before the semester begins. (If a face book is not provided by your school, lobby your technical support office to create this as a permanent computer option available for all scheduled courses.) Then, greet students by name at the first class. You will not get them all right (especially in a large class), but many students are delighted to learn that you were interested enough in them to learn their names and recognize them. It builds rapport! Additionally, because students realize the instructor has taken the time to learn who they are, it can motivate them to be more interactive, work harder, do the homework on time, attend the teaching assistants' (TAs) labs, and so forth.

Be Friendly, Humorous, and Receptive to Questions Both In and Out of the Classroom

Students learn better if the learning environment is relaxed and enjoyable. This does not mean telling a joke that you think is funny but that has nothing to do with the class material. Instead, bring humor into the context of what you are teaching. For example, you could say something that is blatantly incorrect about the material being covered, make exaggerated facial or vocal expressions, and make fun of yourself, including telling stories about yourself or past teaching experiences. It is important to proactively provide friendly interaction with the students during and after class, and to ensure course material is relevant to student lives, especially as everyone, including students, experiences health and medical problems to which they can relate.

Learn to Improvise during Your Lecture

Flexibility and improvisation are important ingredients in how one teaches. I have often had to improvise how or what I am teaching to make it more relevant and interesting for the class. This is not easy to do well, but it is worth trying. The more you try, hopefully the better you can make improvisation enliven the classroom atmosphere.

Be Conscious of Using Clear and Simple Communication

A grandiose and flamboyant speechmaking approach never worked for me, although instructors with such talent should incorporate this into their teaching. When you are speaking to an audience, no matter how large, speak directly as if you are talking to an individual or small group of friends, rather than a large theater audience. You want your students to have an enjoyable and understandable learning experience. Some teachers take their subject matter so seriously that the classroom environment becomes a serious reflection of the teacher's lack of effort for promoting active student learning.

Create Alternative Approaches to Teaching a Class Rather Than Using a Standard Lecture Format

Small Group Discussions in the Classroom

This is not very easy to accomplish in large classes of less than two hours with more than 40 students that rely on mathematical understanding of the course material. However, it works well when focusing on a reading assignment that involves a practical application of a public health study. It can also be used for conceptual/theoretical issues in any public health area. Brief discussions of five minutes interspersed throughout the class session can be well worth the investment of time.

This approach allows active learning in journal club and smaller classes on any public health topic. A typical format is to assign the class to review a topic or application such as a published paper in advance.

State questions to be discussed about the reading either before or at the beginning of class. Divide the class into subgroups of six to ten students, each of which will be assigned to discuss within the subgroup one of the questions for about 10 minutes. Then have one or two students from each subgroup lead a brief class discussion of the subgroup's question. Finally, the instructor, TAs, or a student will summarize overall conclusions derived from earlier subgroup discussions.

Student Take-Home Final Exam Projects with Abbreviated Summary Presentations by Project Groups to the Entire Class

This approach can take slightly different forms depending on the course topic, quantitative level, and class size. In my Epidemiologic Modeling course (class size 130 to 150 students), student final grades are primarily determined from two types of exams taken during the course.

The first exam type involves one or two in-class midterms and an in-class final exam with short-answer questions (multiple-choice, fill-in-the-blank, true-false, and open-ended questions requiring brief answers). Students take these exams individually and receive individual grades on each exam.

The second exam type is a take-home part of the final exam in which students work within self-selected groups of up to three persons to analyze a real or realistic data set involving an epidemiologic research question (though epidemiology PhD students are required to work individually on the take-home final).

This take-home project involves a (typically abbreviated) description of an epidemiologic research study. Students are then required to answer approximately 15 questions about various methodologic features of the study. Answers typically require data analysis methods using computer procedures and analysis strategies covered in the course. The same data set in the same computer file is provided to every student group. Students are prohibited from consulting any students outside their group but can question the TAs and instructors.

Assigned during the last three weeks, the take-home project emphasizes material taught during the second half of the course. Each group turns in a single group report at the end of the semester, detailing the analysis used and conclusions reached from their project work. The group report also should include an appendix describing the use of computer code to answer questions.

This group assignment is a valuable example of active learning because students work together outside of class and experience working with a team of colleagues to combine ideas, knowledge, and experience similar to what they will experience in the real world of public health research. Although giving an alternative form of final exam with only short-answer questions is much easier to grade, the active learning in a group project provides a valuable real-world experience for students.

Grading group project reports is a time-consuming task for instructors. To reduce the grading burden, the instructor can select a specific subset (without advanced notice) of the 15 questions to grade. The same subset is graded for each project group; therefore, each student in a given group gets the same overall (numerical) grade on the take-home exam. A student's overall final course grade also reflects a weighted average of all the grades from exams taken individually together with the grade on the take-home final completed by the group.

I have used a second type of project format in my highly quantitative Analysis of Correlated Data Course (35 to 55 students). In this course, there are no midterm exams but rather a single take-home project. Students work in groups of up to four persons and must provide both written and oral final reports. Each group determines its own topic and submits a short project plan by midsemester for review. Each student's final grade is decided by the combined performance on the group's final report and presentation, as well as on class participation. This course requires a more sophisticated active learning experience than Epidemiologic Modeling because students choose their own topics, work with more difficult course content, and give an oral presentation similar to what they might do later in their career.

Peer Instruction or Peer-to-Peer Approach

A third project format, often referred to as a "peer-to-peer" approach, involves students individually giving abbreviated presentations during the course to the entire class.[2] This works best for small class sizes (fewer than 20 students). The instructor assigns either individuals or small groups of students to discuss a topic or research paper introduced in class and present any debatable interpretations or complexities of interest in 10 to 20 minutes.

As an example, in Teaching Epidemiology (about 12 students), each student is asked to give a 15-to-20-minute presentation to the class. This is followed by a few minutes of feedback and questions from the entire class. Student presentations can use media/computer support such as PowerPoint presentations prepared in advance.

In another exercise, each student is asked without advance notice to give a five-minute extemporaneous description of an epidemiologic term, concept, or analysis method. This illustrates active learning using improvisation.

Flipped Approach to Classroom Teaching

A flipped classroom is an instructional approach that reverses the traditional learning process by delivering instruction content outside the classroom—often online. Activities that have traditionally been considered homework are moved into the classroom. When using the flipped approach, students typically watch online lectures prior to class, collaborate in online discussions during the class, or discuss concepts and exercises during the class with instructor guidance. This approach was initially suggested by King[3] and further detailed by Lage, Platt and Treglia,[4] and Sams.[5]

The flipped classroom intentionally shifts instruction so that online videos or text readings are used to deliver content outside the classroom. In-class activities are redefined to include traditional homework problems to actively engage students in the content. In-class activities can also include emerging mathematical technologies, in-depth laboratory experiments, debate or individual presentations, current event discussions, peer reviewing, and project-based learning. Because these types of active learning allow for highly differentiated instruction, more time can be spent in class on higher-order thinking skills such as study design, problem-solving, and group work. The teacher's interaction with students in a flipped classroom can be more personalized and less didactic.

Challenges in the flipped classroom approach include: (1) developing content for students with varying levels of learning, (2) creating high-quality videos or instructor-prepared PowerPoint narrations requiring significant time and effort, and (3) creating opportunities for students to ask questions during class time, as a traditional lecturer is not available for questions when students rely on videos or text readings at home.

Provide Mechanisms for Reinforcing Learning Outside the Regular Classroom

Higher-Level Students as Teaching Assistants

In classes of all sizes, interaction between students and TAs is invaluable for enhancing learning as well as providing career development experience for the TAs. In addition to regularly scheduled class lectures, the class is divided into subgroups (lab sections) that meet weekly but are optional for each student. In each lab, the TA can answer questions and discuss class material, homework assignments, upcoming exams, new examples, or relevant applications. For each scheduled exam, instructors can provide as least one practice exam (with answers), which TAs can discuss in a separate (optional) class session before the scheduled exam. Additionally, each TA should schedule weekly office hours to meet individually with students wanting more assistance (again, optional for students).

Learning Management Systems

Online network systems known as learning management systems (LMSs) became available in the early 1990s.[6] They provide convenient organization and administration of all instructional course features. Two popular LMSs are Blackboard and Canvas. LMSs are widely used throughout the United States and internationally because they help the instructor deliver material to the students, administer tests and other assignments, track student progress, and manage record-keeping. Key features include announcement folders, easy access to an up-to-date syllabus, contact information for instructors and TAs, assignments, data sets and other computer files, lecture material such as PowerPoint, recommended additional instructional material, lecture recording videos, lab/TA materials, communication tools for email and student enrollment, grade lists, discussion and chat folders for students and instructors, references, and library reserve resources.

Lecture Recording Videos

Lecture recordings are an important benefit of LMSs and allow students to access lectures, replaying them as often as they wish to review sections that they find difficult to understand. While not every student uses these recordings, some students prefer looking at recordings instead of attending class. Ideally, offering both classes and recordings can enhance learning.

Distance Learning

This approach, which typically requires online learning, has become quite common within the past decade in a variety of fields. A key limitation is the absence of the traditional classroom lecture environment, which provides students with timely personal face-to-face interaction with the instructor. Some universities schedule on-campus time at the beginning and end of the course schedule, thereby allowing students to have some face-to-face contact with the instructor. The online-only limitation can be partially offset when instructors incorporate personally prepared PowerPoint material or relevant third-party multimedia, provide ongoing discussion formats for online communication involving students and instructor(s), require graded homework assignments, and give exams that are graded. Its success further depends on the teaching quality and creativity of the online instructional material. Even with its limitations, distance learning is clearly a valuable resource that lets students worldwide conveniently obtain instruction from home.

Incorporate Multimedia Instructional Materials to Promote Active Learning

Multimedia teaching approaches have become more sophisticated in recent decades. This section discusses techniques to incorporate multimedia materials to stimulate active learning.

From Classroom Blackboard to Overhead Transparencies

In the early 1970s, most instructors (particularly in mathematically oriented courses) used chalk on blackboard. Presentations could be more effective if the instructor provided handouts so that the students would have something to take with them, or possibly add notes to, rather than spending time copying from the blackboard. This simple but effective approach of providing handouts contributed to active learning before more sophisticated technologies were developed.

When overhead transparencies came into use in the early 1980s, many teachers, including myself, used them instead of chalk on blackboard. At first, transparencies were not prepared in advance but rather were written on during class—not much different from using chalk on blackboard. However, eventually instructors realized that learning could be enhanced by preparing transparencies in advance and by providing copies to students prior to the lecture. This can be further modified by using two overhead transparencies and two projectors. For example, simultaneously showing a formula on one screen and an example on the other, thereby clarifying the explanation with a realistic application.

Multimedia Approach for Teaching Probability Using Transparencies

One difficult topic to teach in an introductory biostatistics course typically has been probability, including permutations and combinations as well as rules of probability. Many students struggle to understand this topic and how useful it is in the real (including public health) world. To address this issue, in the 1970s, I developed a multimedia pedagogical approach based on a realistic example involving numerical data for teaching probability. Working with an instructional designer, I designed a 1-hour module for teaching probability that contained 20 colorful transparencies. The introductory transparency illustrates a sample of 20 persons observed on 2 variables (smoking status and lung illness status). This leads directly to introducing the term "probability" (estimate) in the context of a two-way data layout. Additional transparencies were used to visually help illustrate basic rules of probability, including the difference between observed and expected probabilities.[7] This provided the foundation for introducing the chi-square statistic for testing the independence between two variables.

In 2012, the probability transparency module was converted into audio and nonaudio PowerPoint presentations with an updated viewing study guide, now freely accessible on YouTube.[8] Instructors can lecture from the nonaudio presentation while students can use the audio presentations for self-study.

Slide-Tape Presentation on Fundamentals of Statistical Inference

Another pre-PowerPoint multimedia innovation I developed in the 1970s was a collection of seven slide-tape presentations to describe the properties of the binomial and normal distributions as well as statistical inference fundamentals, such as hypothesis testing and interval estimation. Each had colorful slides, an audiotape, and a viewing study guide. The guide included a summary of the material, a practice exercise, and a posttest. Students were assigned to work individually through these materials, which were available in the library. This took approximately an hour of a student's time in contrast to what was covered briefly in 10 to 15 minutes in the classroom. In 2012, the slide-tape presentations were converted into narrated PowerPoint presentations with updated viewing study guides. These introductory biostatistics presentations and accompanying guides are now freely accessible on the author's "Visual Archive," found at https://www.youtube.com/channel/UCOf1Em8o8thYcQZAsF7F84Q.

PowerPoint Texts Prior to PowerPoint Presentations

In 1994 and 1998, I published two textbooks, coauthored with Mitchel Klein.[9,10] They were essentially written in PowerPoint format before PowerPoint exploded on the scene. The left side of each page contained what would be the slides. The right side contained the text written as if it were an in-class lecture. This approach has been effective for creating an active and clearly readable feature not typically used in textbooks.

ActivEpi: The First Multimedia Epidemiology Textbook

ActivEpi was originally developed as a CD-ROM in 2003 and updated in 2008.[11] In 2010, the ActivEpi CD-ROM was converted to an online (electronic) multimedia textbook, ActivEpi Web, which was completed in 2015.[12] ActivEpi Web represents a unique twenty-first-century update of my 1982 textbook on modern epidemiologic research.[13] The link for signing up for ActivEpi Web is http://activepi.herokuapp.com—it is free and available to all. As of October 2018, there are more than 12,200 registrants from more than 100 countries.

A supplement to the ActivEpi Web is the *ActivEpi Companion Textbook*.[14] This book provides convenient access to the textual information in all 15 lessons. The supplement, however, is not a substitute for the narrated and animated presentations on the website, which provide the primary learning material.

ActivEpi Web is first and foremost a unique multimedia textbook covering the conceptual and methodological fundamentals of epidemiology research. It is not simply a computer software package. ActivEpi Web incorporates short, narrated instructional presentations that include video and animation, interactive study questions, quizzes (answers provided), homework exercises, and point-and-click footnotes covering extra new material and textual clarifications of narrated expositions. The homework answers are purposefully unavailable on the ActivEpi website to allow instructors the option of using them for graded homework exercises and exams. However, instructors and self-study ActivEpi users can get the answers by emailing the author at dkleinb@emory.edu.

Because ActivEpi Web is freely accessible, multimedia, pedagogically authored, and interactive, it can be valuable for teaching epidemiology in all kinds of learning environments. This includes instruction for classrooms, distance learning, and self-instruction. ActivEpi Web is intended to appeal to all audience sizes, age groups, and education levels (including high schools) in locations throughout the world.

The author's website (http://www.activepi.com) provides descriptions and contact information of many features of ActivEpi Web as well as other useful resources, some of which are free. They include free downloadable PowerPoint presentations covering all 15 lessons, which faculty can use and modify. The author's website also provides free access to ActivEpi Español, the Spanish translation of ActivEpi (for Windows only)[15] and the *ActivEpi Español Companion Text*, the Spanish text translation that accompanies the software.[16] The Pan American World Health Organization also cosponsors ActivEpi Español for use by its member countries through its website (www.paho.org).

Conclusion

Active learning can enhance student enjoyment and, consequently, understanding and knowledge. Many strategies such as creating an enjoyable classroom environment, using alternative lecture and exam formats, and introducing multimedia instruction are available. Instructors should consider these approaches when preparing and carrying out their teaching plan in almost any course environment. Active learning approaches are particularly useful in courses that are quantitatively oriented, such as courses in biostatistics and epidemiology, because the mathematical preparedness of the students can inhibit student learning and motivation. It is my hope that the total passive listening format using chalk on blackboard is permanently obsolete.

REFERENCES

1. Bonwell, C. C., and J. A. Eison. "Active Learning: Creating Excitement in the Classroom—ASHE-ERIC Higher Education Report No. 1." Washington, DC: George Washington University, School of Education and Human Development, 1991.

2. Mazur, E. *Peer Instruction: A User's Manual Series in Educational Innovation.* Upper Saddle River, NJ: Prentice Hall, 1997.

3. King, A. "From Sage on the Stage to Guide on the Side." *College Teaching* 41, no. 1 (1993): 30–35.

4. Lage, M., G. Platt, and M. Treglia. "Inverting the Classroom: A Gateway to Creating an Inclusive Learning Environment." *Journal of Economic Education* 31, no. 1 (2000): 30–43.

5. Sams, A. "The Flipped Class: Shedding Light on the Confusion, Critique, and Hype." *Daily Riff.* 2011. http://www.thedailyriff.com/articles/the-flipped-class -shedding-light-on-the-confusion-critique-and-hype-801.php (accessed April 9, 2018).

6. Gilhooly, K. "Making E-Learning Effective." *Computerworld* 35, no. 29 (2001): 52–53.

7. Kleinbaum, D. G., and A. P. Kleinbaum. 1976. "A Team Approach for Systematic Design and Evaluation of Visually Oriented Modules." In *Report of the American Statistical Association Study of Modular Instruction in Statistics*, edited by J. R. O'Fallon and J. Service, 115–121. Washington, DC: American Statistical Association, 1976.

8. Kleinbaum, D. G. "Probability Concept and Rules." YouTube. 2018. https://www.youtube.com/channel/UCOf1Em808thYcQZAsF7F84Q.

9. Kleinbaum, D. G., and M. Klein. *Logistic Regression—A Self-Learning Text: Third Edition.* New York: Springer Publishers, 2010.

10. Kleinbaum, D. G., and M. Klein. *Survival Analysis—A Self-Learning Text: Third Edition.* New York: Springer Publishers, 2012.

11. Kleinbaum, D. G. *ActivEpi CD ROM.* 2nd edition. Springer Publishers, 2008.

12. Kleinbaum, D. G. *ActivEpi Web.* Self-published, 2015. http://activepi .herokuapp.com.

13. Kleinbaum, D. G., L. L. Kupper, and H. Morgenstern. *Epidemiologic Research: Principles and Quantitative Methods.* New York: John Wiley and Sons, 1982.

14. Kleinbaum, D. G., K. M. Sullivan, and N. D. Barker. *ActivEpi Companion Text, Second Edition.* Springer Publishers, 2013.

15. Kleinbaum, D. G., and D. L. Calles. *ActivEpi Espanol, 2nd Edition.* Self-published, 2018, http://www.activepi.com.

16. Kleinbaum, D. G., K. M. Sullivan, and D. L. Calles. *ActivEpi Español Companion Text.* Self-published, 2018, http://www.activepi.com and www.paho .org.

Practice-Based Teaching in Public Health

JACEY A. GREECE AND JAMES WOLFF

Accreditation standards related to achievement of foundational and concentration competencies have accelerated the need for schools and programs of public health (SPPH) to ground professional public health education in the real world[1,2,3] and to provide educational experiences allowing Master of Public Health (MPH) students to develop skills and competencies through applied public health practice.[4] Preferable to classroom-only instruction or a structured, skills-only practicum setting,[5] practice-based teaching (PBT) is a pedagogical approach that fosters student learning through both course instruction and opportunities to work on real problems for a public health agency. Successful use of PBT relies on an understanding of the elements of PBT and a framework for designing, implementing, and evaluating the pedagogy.

Defining PBT for Public Health

PBT is "a transdisciplinary, collaborative process that . . . enable[s] students to critically reflect and synthesize learning to enhance professional competence."[6] PBT is recommended for students in MPH,[7] Master of Science, and Doctor of Public Health programs, and integrates elements of traditional instructor-centered learning, student-centered learning, and project-based learning. In PBT courses, students work with public health agencies and, by extension, the communities they serve. Working with these agencies offers students the opportunity to reinforce classroom learning, to apply acquired knowledge, to practice skills, to create tangible end products and deliverables,[8] and to negotiate real-life work issues that build professional confidence.[9]

Instead of traditional educational terminology, PBT borrows language from both public health practice and consulting. Collaborating public health agencies are often referred to as clients, and student work groups are referred to as consultant teams. PBT deliverables, also called scopes of work, contain elements of traditional course assignments, such as papers and reports, literature reviews, spreadsheet models, and course projects, but are developed for practical use by the client—thus, the deliverables are tailored and specific to the collaborating agency's needs. PBT deliverables receive a course grade, as in traditional courses, but the grade is assigned with consideration for the utility to the agency and the quality of teamwork to produce it.

Benefits and Challenges of Practice-Based Teaching

There are numerous benefits of PBT for all stakeholders involved (figure 16.1). For a public health school, PBT can increase reputational capital, build interdisciplinary collaboration among faculty, provide a means for public health activism, and, in some cases, generate financial resources. PBT allows faculty to expand and deepen their relationships with public health agencies, offer professional opportunities,[10] and integrate practice and research activities.[11]

PBT courses expose students to real-life problems facing the field, provide opportunities to build technical knowledge and professional skills, expand their professional networks, refine their career goals,[12] and can result in practicum placements or part-time work opportunities for students. Working on a consulting team provides experience in leadership, managing client relationships, and applying public health skills in a specific community, organization, or population. While working with a public health agency, students can generate work products that can be used for future employers or for a practicum or part-time job.[13]

Public health agencies benefit from the collaboration by introducing an academic, evidenced-based perspective into their organization. They

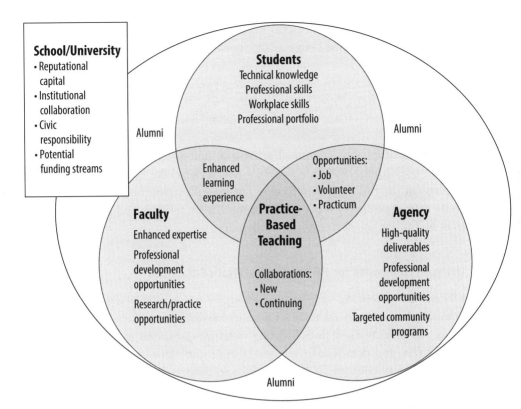

Figure 16.1. Stakeholders and Benefits of Practice-Based Teaching. Greece, Jacey A., William DeJong, Jonina Gorenstein Schonfeld, Ming Sun, and Donna McGrath. "Practice-Based Teaching and Public Health Training: Bringing Real-World Projects to the Classroom to Teach Intervention Planning and Communication Strategies." *Pedagogy in Health Promotion* (2018): https://doi.org/10.1177/2373379918760929.

also receive high-quality and tailored deliverables at no cost and within a relatively short time frame, and initiate and maintain relationships with trained academics and researchers, which may provide opportunities for access to current research or future collaborations.[14,15] Working with a student consulting team also gives agency partners an opportunity to assess a group of talented potential new hires.

PBT courses involve substantial work outside of class for both students and faculty. For students working in teams, scheduling constraints make meeting outside of class difficult and completing deliverables on time challenging. For faculty, real-time issues require immediate attention and time to readjust course components. In addition, faculty should be prepared to provide further training and guidance to inexperienced students so that they can be successful in a professional setting[16] and to manage the agency's expectations of the students. An agency's competing priorities can impact the course's timeline and level of agency staff engagement.

SPPH are typically organized around public health disciplines that limit interdisciplinary collaboration,[17] which can make PBT difficult to implement. In addition, faculty may not have flexible, robust relationships with organizations providing public health services and products, making finding agency partners challenging.

Using a Framework for PBT in Public Health Education

PBT involves three aspects—planning, implementation, and evaluation. Planning begins with creation of a course syllabus that details course goals and objectives, defines learning outcomes, specifies materials for instruction, and details assessments. During implementation of a PBT course, faculty coordinate with agencies to ensure that the course design (as specified in the syllabus)[18] accurately and continually reflects the collaboration planned[19] and that the final deliverables are appropriate. Finally, evaluation should encompass not only assessment of student learning and teaching effectiveness but also the quality of the faculty, student, and agency collaboration.

Frameworks for effective PBT can be helpful for schools and faculty ready to implement PBT pedagogy who are uncertain about how to begin. The PBT STEPS framework, developed by the authors, provides a foundation for the development and design of a PBT course and its implementation through securing partnerships (S), technology and training (T), engagement and implementation (E), presenting deliverables (P), and sizing up results (S)[20] (figure 16.2). The PBT STEPS framework ensures that a PBT course builds technical knowledge, integrates existing knowledge and experience, develops and strengthens public health skills and competencies through working with real-world situations, and realizes the benefits of PBT to all stakeholders.

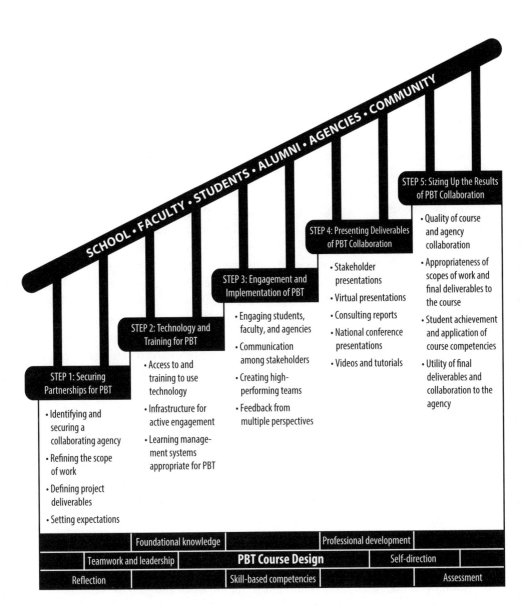

SCHOOL · FACULTY · STUDENTS · ALUMNI · AGENCIES · COMMUNITY

STEP 1: Securing Partnerships for PBT

- Identifying and securing a collaborating agency
- Refining the scope of work
- Defining project deliverables
- Setting expectations

STEP 2: Technology and Training for PBT

- Access to and training to use technology
- Infrastructure for active engagement
- Learning management systems appropriate for PBT

STEP 3: Engagement and Implementation of PBT

- Engaging students, faculty, and agencies
- Communication among stakeholders
- Creating high-performing teams
- Feedback from multiple perspectives

STEP 4: Presenting Deliverables of PBT Collaboration

- Stakeholder presentations
- Virtual presentations
- Consulting reports
- National conference presentations
- Videos and tutorials

STEP 5: Sizing Up the Results of PBT Collaboration

- Quality of course and agency collaboration
- Appropriateness of scopes of work and final deliverables to the course
- Student achievement and application of course competencies
- Utility of final deliverables and collaboration to the agency

Foundational knowledge		Professional development	
Teamwork and leadership	**PBT Course Design**		Self-direction
Reflection	Skill-based competencies		Assessment

Figure 16.2. PBT STEPS Framework. © 2017 Jacey A. Greece and James Wolff. All rights reserved.

PBT Course Design

At its core, PBT provides an exceptional opportunity for experiential, active, and student-centered learning. The work that students perform for their client agency constitutes the central learning experience and is complemented by various student learning opportunities, including: (1) information dissemination through lectures, readings, and guest speakers; (2) active learning through class exercises, case studies, and simulations; (3) just-in-time learning associated with meeting the needs of the agency, student group, and class; and (4) professional interactions with key stakeholders, including the agency and its constituents.

A common element of all PBT courses is that students work with public health organizations on a deliverable that meets a priority need for the public health agency. PBT courses are designed to address real-life problems in challenging real-world situations. Consequently, PBT courses should provide the foundational knowledge and analytical frameworks to directly support the work that the students do for their clients while refining skills for application in professional settings after the course is over.

All PBT courses should integrate opportunities for students to reflect on their experience in the course, their relationship with their client, their team's performance, and the individual leadership skills they developed. Finally, PBT courses should provide timely, regular, and frequent feedback from multiple perspectives that can be used to evaluate the effectiveness of PBT to improve deliverables for the agency and to provide a mechanism for agency feedback on the utility of deliverables.

Securing Partnerships for PBT (Step 1)

The first step in effective PBT involves (1) identifying and securing a collaborating agency, (2) refining a scope of work that aligns with the course objectives and the agency's needs, (3) defining project deliverables that benefit all stakeholders, and (4) setting expectations of time engagement, communication, and collaboration.

Advance planning with potential agency partners to discuss the benefits of collaboration should begin six months before the start of the course to allow time to identify suitable partners and to secure their collaboration for the semester. At a minimum, partner agencies should understand the design of the course, course objectives and schedule, types of deliverables required by the course to meet the objectives, and specific roles and responsibilities of the agency during the course. Unfortunately, there is no guarantee that all conversations will result in agency collaboration.

Faculty can find potential agencies using their own networks, their colleagues' networks, the school's career services department, and alumni. Agencies that have previously participated in a PBT course, collaborated on research projects, or offered internships or practicums through the school are often interested in PBT collaborations. Successful implementation of PBT requires that the faculty and the agency work collaboratively to develop specific, feasible, and clear scopes of work with challenging and educationally appropriate deliverables that are a priority for the agency. Providing scopes of work from past collaborations as a template is useful. The final scope of work should give students adequate information on which to base their efforts.

Execution of a well-crafted scope of work should result in achievement of course objectives and learning outcomes as well as project deliverables that are beneficial to the agency. Rubrics should be developed by the faculty in consultation with the client for each deliverable to assess student performance. Rubrics are effective for setting expectations of student performance regarding the quality and content expected for the deliverable. Deliverables can be assessed by both faculty and agencies for quality, content, and utility, though the grade is ultimately assigned by the faculty. With appropriate permission, students can use all or part of the deliverables as evidence of mastery of competencies for job interviews, as writing samples for further educational endeavors, or for other professional development opportunities.

Faculty must set expectations for a mutually beneficial collaboration. Partnership guidelines, a letter of engagement, or a simple contract can provide guidance to the agency concerning their roles and responsibilities in the course and avenues for conflict resolution, if necessary.

Technology and Training for PBT (Step 2)

PBT courses require technology and support to ensure seamless collaboration with the agency, regardless of their geographic location and proximity to the school. Technology and support needs include: (1) access to and training for technologies that streamline communication, (2) infrastructure within the classroom that promotes active engagement of students and agencies, and (3) learning management systems (LMSs) that are comprehensive and flexible to support the different stakeholder needs and communication approaches.

Communication technology for PBT is essential for streamlining student, faculty, and agency collaboration, and for gaining insight into team process. Students can use Skype, Adobe Connect, and Google Hangouts for communicating with clients and among themselves as well as project management software such as Trello and Slack to manage their work. These technologies may require some level of training and support for faculty, students, and agencies.

Physical classroom space and resources are important in creating a structural environment that promotes active engagement. To facilitate in-class collaboration for consulting teams of three to six students, the classroom should have moveable tables and chairs. Students use their personal computers in the classroom to engage in the course content, use communication technologies and project management software, and access online resources—thus, reliable internet access is imperative.

PBT courses use all of the traditional features of an LMS, such as document posting, assignment submission, quizzes and surveys, and discussion groups. However, a PBT LMS should additionally support student and agency interaction with functionality for client communication and feedback. Clients should have access to LMS functionality that includes brainstorming ideas, collecting and sharing feedback on the performance of the team, monitoring student experience through surveys and evaluations, and facilitating a structured assessment of student deliverables. Portfolio software for journaling and reflection can be integrated into the LMS or used separately to facilitate, track, and share student reflections.

Engagement and Implementation of PBT (Step 3)

Successful implementation of PBT requires (1) exceptional engagement from students, faculty, and agencies; (2) robust communication among stakeholders; (3) high-performing teams; and (4) ongoing and consistent feedback from multiple perspectives on aspects of the course.

Active and positive engagement is a necessary component of success-ful PBT implementation. A PBT course demands consistent and enthu-siastic engagement from students, faculty, and agency partners. Positive engagement begins with the faculty and agency before the semester, with a shared vision of PBT culture, course goals, and objectives and collab-orative development of scopes of work and deliverables. Engagement of students with the agency continues during the semester, and acces-sibility of agency partners to respond to student needs maximizes the potential for useful and tailored deliverables. Engagement is motivated throughout the semester by the benefits perceived by the students of working with an agency and the anticipation of useful deliverables at the end of the course by the agency.

Direct, open, effective, and regular faculty-agency communication to discuss the direction of the project and the quality of student work en-sures seamless collaboration during the semester. Faculty can facilitate student-agency communication by helping to resolve communication difficulties that students may experience with their agencies; providing students the foundational knowledge and skills to problem-solve and to think critically about development of deliverables; and giving con-structive feedback on team performance, leadership, and team deliver-ables. In addition, faculty can facilitate focus groups, surveys, and interviews in the community, when appropriate, to help students engage with their client's target population.

Most public health work is done in interdisciplinary teams comprised of people with different knowledge, skills, and interests. Working ef-fectively in a team is one of the fundamental components of a PBT course. Most PBT scopes of work are complex and require deliverables that exceed the capacity of a single individual to complete successfully. Consequently, there is considerable pressure to function as a high-performing team that can successfully navigate in an intense, deadline-driven, and stressful environment. PBT faculty can assign students to teams randomly or use a set of criteria to ensure balance.

Faculty should facilitate and foster team cohesion and collaboration, and provide constructive feedback to individual students to help them develop their own capacity to function as an effective team member. In-dividual and team feedback provided in the safe setting of a course under the supervision of faculty can have long-term impacts on students' professional success. Given that learning in a PBT course involves higher orders of cognitive domains,[21] assessments in courses based on PBT use consulting team products and deliverables as the principal assessments for evaluating learning outcomes.

Formative assessments in PBT provide information that students can use in real time to assess and improve their performance as managers and leaders, improve their deliverables, and enrich and deepen their ability to reflect on and learn from their experience. The faculty, the client, the students, and other stakeholders can contribute to assessments. Formative assessments can include 360 peer evaluations of team and leadership performance, faculty and client reviews of team deliverables, student and faculty in-class critiques of presentations, portfolios or other journaling techniques, team performance evaluations, individual leadership development evaluations, and faculty and student feedback on reflections. Whether graded or not, feedback from these assessments is critical to improve student performance and to refine deliverables.

Summative assessments should be based on issues, problems, or decisions that are similar to those required in the client scopes of work. To simulate a real-world situation, questions should be open and unstructured and should test professional and technical skills that the students are developing in the course. Both qualitative and quantitative metrics are useful to assess professional and technical skills.

Presenting Deliverables of PBT Collaboration (Step 4)

PBT courses are designed to provide multiple opportunities for students to disseminate their work and deliverables through a variety of modalities, including: (1) in-person oral presentations or meetings; (2) web-based presentations or meetings via use of communication technologies; (3) written reports, slide decks, and manuals; (4) national dissemination opportunities such as webinars and conferences: and (5) prerecorded videos. Preparing for these varied dissemination activities requires learning and refining professional presentation and writing skills; multiple presentation opportunities are ideal.

Oral and virtual presentations, written reports, slide decks, and opportunities to respond publicly to questions in real time can be integrated into the course. Virtual presentations allow agencies to participate in presentations remotely. In addition, they provide an opportunity to showcase deliverables such as videos, mHealth apps, slide decks, and website wireframes. National dissemination opportunities such as webinars for the client's stakeholders or presentations at major research conferences provide students a chance to enhance presentation skills in a professional setting and can deliver awareness and recognition of the agency and its work.

The principal deliverable of a PBT course is usually a written report, which provides a tangible product that the agency can show to their stakeholders and eventually implement to benefit their constituents. As creating a unified deliverable from work of multiple authors is a perennial challenge for students, coaching from faculty to organize the writing, editing, formatting, and proofreading of written deliverables specifically tailored to the agency is essential.

Sizing Up the Results of PBT Collaboration (Step 5)

Evaluation of courses involving PBT should focus on (1) quality of course and agency collaboration, (2) appropriateness of scopes of work and final deliverables to the course, (3) student achievement and application of course competencies, and (4) utility of final deliverables and collaboration to the agency.

While the quality of agency collaboration should be assessed throughout the semester for purposes of course correction, troubleshooting, and refining deliverables, evaluation after the course provides an opportunity to reflect on the entire experience of collaboration. Debriefing discussions, interviews, focus groups, and identified or anonymous surveys can assess frequency and modes of communication across stakeholders, access and ease of use of technology, and resources and support available during the semester.

Much of the success of a PBT course rests on the initial scope of work and whether it allowed for the development and application of skills and achievement of course objectives and competencies. Cross-checking the deliverables with the course objectives to ensure that each objective was met through the development of targeted deliverables provides an opportunity to assess the competencies and the learning outcomes of the students. Faculty can discuss the initial scope of work and quality of the final deliverable with the client. In consultation with clients, faculty can develop rubrics that are assignment-specific, provide a structured opportunity for feedback, and contribute to the faculty-assigned course grade. Faculty and the school can also elicit feedback from students, agencies, and faculty through focus groups, stakeholder interviews, and postcourse surveys.

A student's level of professional and technical knowledge and skills can be evaluated at baseline, after the course, and after graduation with standard surveys. Qualitative assessments are useful to explore specific activities that led to achievement and application of competencies and to identify areas where competencies were expected but not achieved.

For partner agencies, high-quality, practical deliverables can have substantial value and impact, but the benefits are not always recognized immediately. Long-term follow-up with the agency is important to assess whether the resources needed for the agency to implement the deliverables are available, whether the deliverables are being used, and to develop a deeper understanding of the impact of the collaboration on the agency and community.

Sustaining PBT Collaborations

To make PBT a continuous and sustainable teaching methodology requires (1) institutional support for PBT, (2) developing and maintaining a cadre of faculty equipped with the skills to develop and implement PBT, and (3) establishing a continuous flow of agencies for collaboration. In particular, several factors should be considered for successful sustainability. These include institutional support for the use of communication technologies; investment in an LMS that facilitates agency-student communication and exchange; increased time and resources for PBT faculty; access to resources to support special events where students' work is presented; a public website showcasing student work, testimonials from clients, and benefits of agency-school collaboration; and use of school publications and social media to connect alumni and their organizations with PBT faculty.

Conclusion

SPPH must prepare graduates by identifying the knowledge and skills needed for future employment and by ensuring that graduates are adequately trained to utilize the knowledge and skills to be successful in the public health workforce. PBT offers SPPH an opportunity to foster student learning through both course instruction and the opportunity to work on current public health problems for a public health agency. PBT provides MPH students with an engaging way to meet competency requirements and offers students the opportunity to practice those competencies and to build professional confidence in public health practice settings. A successful PBT course in public health relies on an understanding of the elements of PBT and a framework for designing, implementing, and evaluating the pedagogy. SPPH faculty can use a five-step framework, PBT STEPS, to develop a practice-based curriculum.

REFERENCES

1. Institute of Medicine. *The Future of Public Health*. Washington, DC: National Academy Press, 1988.

2. Association of Schools and Programs of Public Health. "Public Health Trends and Redesigned Education—Blue Ribbon Public Health Employers' Advisory Board: Summary of Interviews." September 6, 2013. http://s3.amazonaws.com /aspph-wp-production/app/uploads/2017/10/BlueRibbonPublicHealthEmployers AdvisoryBoard_Report_FINAL_09.06.13-SJC.pdf.

3. Council on Education for Public Health. "Accreditation Criteria: Schools and Programs of Public Health." Silver Spring, MD: CEPH, 2016. https://ceph.org /assets/2016.Criteria.pdf (accessed March 25, 2018).

4. Hilliard, T. M., and M. L. Boulton. "Public Health Workforce Research in Review: A 25-Year Retrospective." *American Journal of Preventive Medicine* 42, no. 5 (2012): S17-S28.

5. Rutkow, L., M. B. Levin, and T. A. Burke. "Meeting Local Needs While Developing Public Health Practice Skills: A Model Community-Academic Partnership." *Journal of Public Health Management and Practice* 15, no. 5 (2009): 425–431.

6. Association of Schools and Programs of Public Health, Council of Public Health Practice Coordinators. c October 2004. https://s3.amazonaws.com/aspph -wp-production/app/uploads/2014/06/Demonstrating-Excellence_Practice-Based -Teaching.pdf.

7. Calhoun, J. G., C. A. Wrobel, and J. R. Finnegan. "Current State in US Public Health Competency-Based Graduate Education." *Public Health Reviews* 33, no. 1 (2011): 148–167.

8. Breny, J. M. "Developing Agreements and Delineating Tasks: Creating Successful Community-Engaged Service Learning Projects." *Journal for Civic Commitment* 19 (2012): 1–14.

9. Pollard, C. E. "Lessons Learned from Client Projects in an Undergraduate Project Management Course." *Journal of Information Systems Education* 23, no. 3 (2012): 271–282.

10. Kegler, M. C., A. Lifflander, J. Buehler, D. Collins, J. Wells, H. Davidson, and P. Hishamuddin. "Multiple Perspectives on Collaboration between Schools of

Public Health and Public Health Agencies." *Public Health Reports* 121, no. 5 (2006): 634–639.

11. Association of Schools and Programs of Public Health, Council of Public Health Practice Coordinators, "Demonstrating Excellence in Practice-Based Teaching for Public Health."

12. Hartwig, K. A., K. Pham, and E. Anderson. "Multiple Perspectives on Collaboration between Schools of Public Health and Public Health Agencies." *Public Health Reports* 119, no. 1 (2004): 102–109.

13. Association of Schools and Programs of Public Health, "Public Health Trends and Redesigned Education."

14. Breny, "Developing Agreements and Delineating Tasks."

15. Kegler et al., "Multiple Perspectives on Collaboration between Schools of Public Health and Public Health Agencies."

16. Hartwig, Pham, and Anderson, "Multiple Perspectives on Collaboration between Schools of Public Health and Public Health Agencies."

17. Kegler et al., "Multiple Perspectives on Collaboration between Schools of Public Health and Public Health Agencies."

18. Nilson, L. B. *Teaching at Its Best: A Research-Based Resource for College Instructors.* San Francisco: Jossey-Bass, 2010.

19. Anderson, L. S., M. O. Royster, N. Bailey, and K. Reed. "Integrating Service-Learning into an MPH Curriculum for Future Public Health Practitioners: Strengthening Community-Campus Partnerships." *Journal of Public Health Management and Practice* 17, no. 4 (2011): 324–327.

20. Greece, J. A., J. Wolff, and D. McGrath. "A Framework for Practice-Based Teaching in Public Health." Journal of Public Health Management Practice (August 31, 2018): https://doi.org/10.1097/PHH.0000000000000863.

21. Bloom, B. S. *Taxonomy of Educational Objectives, Handbook I: The Cognitive Domain.* New York: David McKay, 1956.

[17]

Teaching Public Health by the Case Method

NANCY KANE

Tell me and I will forget, show me and I may remember, involve me and I will understand.—*Ancient Chinese Proverb*

IN 2014, the Association of Schools and Programs of Public Health published "Framing the Future: A Master of Public Health Degree for the 21st Century," establishing thirteen foundational areas of public health, including knowledge, skills, and attitudes for the Master of Public Health (MPH) core.[1] The association recommended that the core could be taught as an integrated learning experience rather than as distinct courses in the traditional five core disciplines. In a related document, the Council on Education for Public Health identified a case-based curriculum as one way to efficiently integrate the core.[2] These changes have sparked heightened interest in adapting case-based learning—already a tradition in business, medicine, and law curricula—into public health.[3]

Meanwhile, research on learning over the past 20 to 30 years has firmly established that active learning methods are better for achieving certain learning goals than the traditional lecture, despite the lecture's predominance in education since Plato's Academy of ancient Greece. While good lectures can be effective for communicating the most up-to-date knowledge in a cogent, well-synthesized manner by an expert instructor modeling scholarly behavior, lectures are criticized for promoting intellectual passivity and poor retention among students while failing to cultivate problem-solving skills, interest in lifelong learning, or the ability to transfer information to new situations.[4] The lecture alone is unlikely to effectively teach the new MPH core, which puts developing problem-solving and other skills such as analysis, decision-making, planning, and execution on par with transferring traditional public health knowledge. Schools of public health are looking to adopt a range of active learning approaches to effectively and efficiently deliver the twenty-first-century MPH foundational knowledge, skills, and attitudes.

Research Supporting Active Engagement and Case-Based Discussion in Adult Learning

A triangular "cone of learning" concept evolved from a 1969 study that ranked how well students retained material based on instructional method.[5] Students were asked to recall information that had been taught six weeks earlier; findings indicated that the least effective method was lecture, with only 4–8% retention. Reading worked only slightly better, at 6–10% retention. Lecture with visuals achieved 12–18% retention, while demonstration resulted in 20–45% retention. Only active engagement methods achieved student retention above 50%: students in cooperative learning groups retained 60–80% of the material, and students teaching one another retained 80–98%. Dale's research has been replicated by others with consistent results.[6,7] A meta-analysis of learning methods for students in science, engineering, and math found that a wide range of active learning methods produced superior learning compared to traditional lectures.[8] The meta-analysis found that active learning increased student performance on exams by half a grade, and that students in traditional lecture courses were one and a half times more likely to fail than students in courses employing active learning methods.

Discussion is a component of cooperative learning, where students work together to achieve a common goal.[9] A case presents a complex problem for which no obvious or single answer exists. Students explore and debate concepts, ideas, and opinions among peers. Peer discussion has been found to enhance understanding and retention in part by facilitating the integration of new information with prior knowledge.[10] Verbal discussion fosters persuasive speaking and critical listening skills.[11]

Cases are invaluable tools for structuring real-life problems that engage and excite students, and are used in a wide variety of fields, including quantitative sciences. One study evaluated the effectiveness of teaching biostatistics and epidemiology to medical students using cases and found that the approach maintained good student mastery of the material, as demonstrated both in course exams and national board scores in the subject areas; it also significantly improved student ratings of the course.[12] A survey of 101 faculty teaching science at universities found that case teaching, as compared to traditional lecture, resulted in stronger critical thinking skills, a better ability to make connections across multiple content areas, deeper understanding of content, and more engagement in the class.[13] A meta-analysis examining problem-based learning (a version of case-based learning used in medical schools) as compared to lecture found that it showed significantly better results for critical thinking and skills-related assessments, but no differences in accumulated knowledge.[14] Cases are often used with lectures, labs, readings, and problem sets to ensure that students know how to apply the knowledge, concepts, and techniques to a wide range of problems. For instance, in the biostatistics and epidemiology evaluation described earlier, students were given the option to attend three traditional lectures followed by a multiple-choice exam before moving into the case discussion module of the course.[15]

Getting to a Good Case Discussion

It is not hard to answer "What makes a bad discussion?"—the question generally elicits a flurry of hands among faculty and students, who consistently make some or all of the following observations.

- A few students dominate discussion time
- Students compete for "air time" rather than with thoughtful contributions
- Quiet students never speak up
- Some students are distracted by their own or their neighbors' use of electronic devices
- Students arrive late or leave early

- Students go on tangents, off topic
- Students do not prepare for the discussion
- Students become overly defensive of their positions
- No one responds to instructor questions
- The instructor has not established clear learning objectives
- The discussion rambles without direction
- The instructor dominates
- The instructor does not wait for responses to questions before answering herself
- Nonnative or less articulate speakers cannot be understood
- Mistakes and errors are not corrected
- The discussion becomes disrespectful

Good case discussion—the opposite of the aforementioned bad discussion behaviors—requires extra instructor effort, beyond content mastery, in selecting the case and devising a teaching plan, as well as developing the skills of facilitating classroom discussion. To mitigate or avoid bad discussion, the instructor must conscientiously set expectations (addressing the first eight points in the previous list), plan class time (the next three), and master good discussion facilitation technique (the last eight). Each of these case-teaching skills is described in more detail in the following sections.

Setting Expectations

When case discussion is not the school norm, the rules of classroom behavior must be made clear from day one. These can be articulated in the syllabus, as well as discussed in the introductory session of the course and reinforced in subsequent classes.

The syllabus can help set expectations for classroom discussion by specifying desired class preparation, attendance, and participation behavior. The following is an example of such language in a syllabus.

> Classroom participation: Students are expected to be active participants in classroom discussions. This includes attending all classes, being prepared by having read and analyzed the assignments ahead of class time, and being ready to offer analyses and insights to the class. Listening to and offering constructive comments regarding the thoughts and analyses

of others in the classroom is an important component of class participation. Tiers of participation in ascending order of quality:

1 Respond to something the professor says or asks
2 Respond to comments of other students by building on or disagreeing with their points
3 Initiate a relevant line of discussion that provokes other students to respond and join in the conversation

Distracting behaviors include the use of electronic devices during class time, tardiness, and early departures. Students often express a desire to take notes on their devices, but research has established that typing notes on a laptop is less effective than taking notes by hand in terms of learning or retention.[16] To replace note-taking, the instructor can use the blackboard for recording key parts of the class discussion, and then take pictures of the board to upload to the course website for student review. Another increasingly common excuse to keep laptops open is that cases and course reading material are stored on them; instructors should consider requiring students to print out their cases before coming to class, or producing a hard-copy packet of the cases for all students taking the course.

Tardiness and early departures may also require explicit policies. If there are good reasons for tardiness or early departure (e.g., child care responsibilities or not enough time between classes), then the instructor might want to use the beginning and end of class for brief lectures, announcements, or summary thoughts. If there are no good reasons for tardiness or early departures, one option is to penalize unexcused tardiness, early departure, or unexcused absences by lowering the classroom participation component of the course grade for chronic violators. Policies regarding student presence in class should reinforce the concept that class discussion time is meaningful and important to their learning in the course.

Finally, participation expectations can be actively discussed during class. On day one, the instructor can facilitate a discussion of what constitutes good versus bad discussion, and build that into an ongoing evaluation tool to assess the class as a whole (discussed in the following section). Case discussion is a team sport, and, as such, team players need to appreciate their respective roles.

Planning and Facilitating Classroom Discussion

The time needed to plan for each class is often underestimated by novice discussion leaders. Each class session requires its own learning objectives that are clearly tied to overall course objectives. These can be presented in the syllabus as well as at the beginning of each class. Before class begins, the instructor writes down a teaching plan that includes opening and follow-up questions in each topic that the instructor wants the class to explore. Thinking about questions and possible responses as well as how to organize them with a board plan are the key elements of classroom planning.

The case discussion leader must master the essential skills of question, listen, and respond.[17] Good questions—generally no more than five or six for a 90-minute discussion—should push students to analyze the situation using the conceptual frameworks underlying the course, come to judgment or decision on what the protagonist should do, debate alternatives, and recommend a course of action. The questions should focus on what students think of the situation in the case (analysis, synthesis, evaluation) rather than on what the situation is in the case (black-and-white facts). It is best to avoid questions that require very precise answers, unless you plan to use them to ask students to explain how they got there or to ask others if they came to a different conclusion and why.

Listening, an often-overlooked skill of discussion facilitation, is one of the hardest to master, especially when moving from the role of lecturer to discussion leader. Many instructors will answer their own question as part of the asking or will not give students sufficient time to reflect on the question before becoming anxious or impatient.[18] The instructor may need to count slowly to 10, maintain an open and interested expression, and take comfort that silence can mean students are thinking about how to respond. Listening can be even more difficult if the points made do not seem responsive to the question. Patience, looking around the room for more volunteers, and trying to understand what a student means (sometimes paraphrasing can help) are critical to good discussion facilitation.

Finally, the instructor needs to anticipate possible student responses and how they might be organized to facilitate learning. A board plan for recording relevant comments under meaningful headings or as annotations to figures and graphs that reinforce course concepts can be very helpful for indicating how student responses relate to key course concepts. Besides writing down key words on the board, the instructor can ask for further clarification, look to others for comment, paraphrase what is heard, and politely interrupt and redirect when the response is tangential. Managing spontaneity requires self-reflection and practice. Observation of classroom performance by an experienced case teacher who can give constructive feedback can be invaluable in the learning process for new case teachers.

Maintaining a Safe and Positive Learning Community

A fundamental principle underlying successful case discussion is the maintenance of a safe, positive learning community.[19] Setting and maintaining this tone is the instructor's responsibility and involves judgments around how much physical and psychological distance the instructor maintains from students, how well the instructor gets to know the students, and how thoughtfully the instructor manages the discussion and listens to students. Instructor body language, movement around the classroom, and facial expression can affect the quality of the learning community culture. A peer observer or a videotape of the instructor leading a class discussion reviewed by a coach can be very helpful.

One of the most challenging aspects of maintaining a positive learning community is managing the diversity of students in the class, particularly with respect to active participation in case-based discussion. Some students have language or cultural barriers to speaking up, or a natural tendency toward being the observer rather than the active speaker. Rather than allow the quiet student to withdraw into passive class observation, the instructor must present alternative avenues for engagement. The instructor can maintain a record of who is not speaking so that if one of those students does have a hand up to speak, the instructor will make an effort to call on that student. Small group discussions during class bring out quieter students, as do group presentations of case "solutions." During large group discussion, the instructor can use "warm calls," in which the students are given advance warning that they may be called on to address a specific issue.

Evaluating Individual Classroom Performance

Most case discussion instructors allocate some share of the course grade to class participation. This reinforces the importance of active engagement and provides opportunities for feedback. How much of the grade to base on class participation depends on the overall course structure, but given the relatively more subjective nature of this type of grading, it is unusual to weight it for more than 50% of the grade. Students appreciate multiple avenues to demonstrate their learning, including presentations and written assignments as well as exams that can generally be graded more objectively, using detailed grading rubrics.

There are several approaches to evaluating class participation, from self-assessment at multiple points in the course, to instructor/teaching assistant (TA) tracking and grading individual comments during every class, to peer evaluation of each other or the group as a whole. More than one approach can be employed simultaneously. Multiple attributes can be evaluated, including presence (physical presence, on-time arrival and departure, use of electronic devices), preparation (cites case facts in comments), listening behavior (not distracted, hands down when others are talking, comments reflect contributions of others), as well as verbal contributions (quantity, quality).

Self-assessment involves setting individual goals for class participation; quieter students may set a goal of speaking in the large group at least once a week; more confident speakers may set a goal of limiting their comments to no more than twice per class. To advance listening skills, students may set goals of commenting on the contribution of others at least half of the time. Initial self-assessments can be turned in for instructor review and enhancement; middle and end-of-course assessments can also be reviewed, and the instructor may weigh in with her own observations of a student's strengths and areas needing improvement. The "grade" may be based on the degree of effort or improvement noted (with instructor agreement), or simply a "pass" if all components appear to have been completed in good faith.

The instructor may opt to formally evaluate individual performance during class. This can be done several ways and depends on the size of the class, how well the instructor knows each student, and whether or not the course has a TA who can attend every class. A TA can maintain a class roster on which quantity and well as quality of student contributions are noted; various presence and preparation attributes can also be noted. At the end of class, the instructor can review this document with the TA and adjust where necessary. Ideally, such evaluations should be provided to students at the midpoint of the course to allow for improvement.

An alternative is for the instructor—and TA, if available—to try to remember who said what after class. This is the least intimidating but most subjective approach to grading student participation. It is subject to instructor or TA bias, which can be counterproductive toward maintaining a safe and positive learning environment for all participants. For instance, at Harvard Business School, where case teaching is gospel, in 2011 the school installed scribes and a software tool for monitoring student participation in classrooms to reduce recall bias of professors, as part of a larger (and apparently successful) effort to address grade disparities for female students.[20]

Peer evaluation of group participation can be used as part or all of the class participation component of a course grade. Based on consensus of what makes a good discussion, a rubric can be constructed that is given to one or two students in the class to observe and evaluate each day's discussion. Responsibility for evaluation can rotate among the students to increase awareness as well as compliance. Observers summarize their evaluation in the last two to three minutes of class time. The result may be quantified into a group grade for participation. This exercise reinforces the student's responsibility for effective class discussions.[21]

Conclusion

Teaching one's own disciplinary content and skills using case discussion is challenging, but a much bigger challenge is teaching a case-based integrated core. It requires more extensive advance planning, engagement in interdepartmental politics, and development of team-teaching skills among the faculty. It is not hard to develop cases that address multidimensional public health problems, as public health problems by their very nature require a multidisciplinary approach. A good resource for public health cases can be found at https://caseresources.hsph.harvard.edu, which provides links to cases and case collections at Harvard and other schools of public health. But developing an integrated curriculum involves several critical steps that are not needed when teaching a traditional, disciplinary-based course.

The first step is obtaining the active, visible support of the school's senior leadership. Many schools of public health are organized by disciplinary-based departments that do not often cross organizational boundaries to work together on professional educational innovation. Unsticking those boundaries requires leadership from the top.

The second step is to identify a course leadership team committed to professional education and willing to marshal the course through several years of development and implementation. Ideally, some members of the team have successfully taught using case discussion within their own discipline, so that they can guide curriculum development, class planning and coordination, in-class teaching skills, and student evaluation methods to reinforce the goals of an integrated, case-based public health core.

The third step is for the leadership team to negotiate which of the foundational areas will be included in the case-based course. A common area of faculty concern is that of "public health data analysis and interpretation," which generally covers both theoretical and applied biostatistics and epidemiology concepts and methods. More generally, any part of the foundational core that requires knowledge transfer of content may be best taught using methods other than case discussion, such as in-person or online lectures, readings, tutorials, and lab exercises. They can be taught in a separate course, or incorporated within an integrated course. The case discussion is most appropriate for developing skills and attitudes as well as applying tools and concepts introduced in lectures or readings. Some core areas may be best taught in field practice.

For the fourth step, the leadership team must determine specific competencies in each foundational area as well as the relative weight or class time to assign each competency. This will reflect both the perceived need for the competency and the school's own faculty expertise. These competencies may also need to meet the prerequisite requirements for students to advance to higher-level courses in their selected concentrations.

The final step is developing a disciplined project management approach to ensuring faculty training in case discussion leadership, curriculum development, and communication with students to bring the course to reality. The logistics of team-teaching across disciplines are far more complicated than solo teaching in one area; regular group meetings to discuss the syllabus, teaching plans, assignments, and grading rubrics are required, and must start months before the course is first offered.

The challenge of delivering an integrated, case-based core is leadership, faculty commitment, and resources. The benefits of a well-delivered course are worth the effort—students who are better prepared for interdisciplinary analysis, decision-making, and execution in public health practice.

REFERENCES

1. Association of Schools and Programs of Public Health. "Master of Public Health Degree for the 21st Century: Key Considerations, Design Features, and Critical Content of the Core." November 3, 2014. https://www.aspph.org/teach -research/models/mph-degree-report/.

2. Council on Education for Public Health. "PowerPoint Presentation." https://ceph.org/assets/comparison_charts_diagrams.pdf (accessed October 17, 2017).

3. Garvin, D. A. "Making the Case: Professional Education for the World of Practice." *Harvard Magazine*. September–October 2003. http://harvardmagazine .com/2003/09/making-the-case-html.

4. Bland, M., G. Saunders, and J. K. Frisch. "In Defense of the Lecture." *Journal of College Science Teaching* 37, no. 2 (2007): 10–13.

5. Dale, E. *Audio-Visual Methods in Teaching*. New York: Dryden Press, 1969.

6. Cross, K. P., and T. A. Angelo. *Classroom Assessment Techniques: A Handbook for Faculty*. Ann Arbor: National Center for Research to Improve Postsecondary Teaching and Learning, University of Michigan, 1988.

7. Lord, T. "Society for College Science Teachers: Revisiting the Cone of Learning—Is It a Reliable Way to Link Instruction Method with Knowledge Recall?" *Journal of College Science Teaching* 37, no. 2 (2007): 14–17.

8. Freeman, S., S. L. Eddy, M. McDonough, M. K. Smith, N. Okoroafor, H. Jordt, and M. P. Wenderoth. "Active Learning Increases Student Performance in Science, Engineering, and Mathematics." *Proceedings of the National Academy of Sciences* 111, no. 23 (2014): 8410–8415.

9. Shen, D. "Discussion." https://ablconnect.harvard.edu/discussion-research (accessed October 17, 2017).

10. Schmidt, H. G., M. L. De Volder, W. S. De Grave, J. H. C. Moust, and V. L. Patel. "Explanatory Models in the Processing of Science Text: The Role of Prior Knowledge Activation through Small-Group Discussion." *Journal of Educational Psychology* 81, no. 4 (1989): 610.

11. Smith, M. K., W. B. Wood, W. K. Adams, C. Wieman, J. K. Knight, N. Guild, and T. T. Su. "Why Peer Discussion Improves Student Performance on In-Class Concept Questions." *Science* 323, no. 5910 (2009): 122–124.

12. Marantz, P. R., W. Burton, and P. Steiner-Grossman. "Using the Case-Discussion Method to Teach Epidemiology and Biostatistics." *Academic Medicine* 78, no. 4 (2003): 365–371.

13. Yadav, A., M. Lundeberg, M. DeSchryver, and K. Dirkin. "Teaching Science with Case Studies: A National Survey of Faculty Perceptions of the Benefits and Challenges of Using Cases." *Journal of College Science Teaching* 37, no. 1 (2007): 34.

14. Lundeberg, M. A., and A. Yadav. "Assessment of Case Study Teaching: Where Do We Go from Here? Part II." *Journal of College Science Teaching* 35, no. 6 (2006): 8–13.

15. Marantz, Burton, and Steiner-Grossman, "Using the Case-Discussion Method to Teach Epidemiology and Biostatistics."

16. Dynarski, S. M. "For Better Learning in College Lecture, Lay Down the Laptop and Pick Up a Pen." Brookings Institute. August 10, 2017. https://www.brookings.edu/research/for-better-learning-in-college-lectures-lay-down-the-laptop-and-pick-up-a-pen.

17. Barnes, L. B., C. R. Christensen, and A. Hansen. "Premises and Practices of Discussion Teaching." In *Teaching and the Case Method*, edited by L. B. Barnes, C. R. Christensen, and A. Hansen, 23–33. Boston: Harvard Business School Press, 1994.

18. Napell, S. M. "Six Common Non-Facilitating Teaching Behaviors." In *Teaching and the Case Method*, edited by L. B. Barnes, C. R. Christensen, and A. Hansen, 199–202. Boston: Harvard Business School Press, 1994.

19. Barnes, Christensen, and Hansen, *Teaching and the Case Method*.

20. Fondas, N. "First Step to Fixing Gender Bias in Business School: Admit the Problem." *Atlantic*. September 17, 2013. https://www.theatlantic.com/education/archive/2013/09/first-step-to-fixing-gender-bias-in-business-school-admit-the-problem/279740.

21. Hollander, J. A. "Learning to Discuss: Strategies for Improving the Quality of Class Discussion." *Teaching Sociology* 30, no. 3 (2002): 317–327.

Group-Based Service Learning Teaching Approaches

LAURA LINNAN, MEG LANDFRIED, ELIZABETH FRENCH, AND BETH MORACCO

IN THIS CHAPTER, we provide an overview of a service learning group education teaching method, including principles, strengths, and challenges of this approach. We then illustrate the approach with an example and summarize, including future directions for this teaching approach.

Group Education Teaching Method

Group education teaching methods are widely used in universities as a strategy for deepening student content knowledge and skills, leveraging benefits of peer-to-peer instruction while meeting the needs of different learning styles and providing students with real-world experience by working in teams to complete major projects. In this approach, all students in a group are able to apply their own new and existing knowledge and experience to a problem in a group setting with the result that, collectively, they arrive at a new or richer understanding and skill set.[1]

When designed thoughtfully, group-based projects can also help students develop skills that are critical to the public health workforce. Recent blue-ribbon reports have stressed the need for Master of Public Health (MPH) graduates skilled in working in teams and in partnership with communities to solve public health problems.[2,3] Group-based teaching and service learning approaches can help students build such skills by providing hands-on learning experiences that contribute to the work and impact of local community-based organizations; interdisciplinary, group-based projects that model what they will experience in their careers; opportunities to explore areas of professional interest, to network, and to develop or revise career goals; extensive mentorship from public health professionals; and opportunities to develop a myriad of products and skills that are directly relevant for job interviews and career opportunities.

For their part, community members can also benefit significantly from group teaching approaches. Such educational approaches can provide community partners with community-driven products or services that are responsive to the partner organization's needs and that help advance their organizational mission; significant in-kind services, staffing, and expertise that might not be available in the local organization; an extensive commitment of student time and effort that allows for a deep scope of work on a wide array of topics; exposure to students with the most current public health training and skills; energy and enthusiasm for addressing issues that students are uniquely able to bring to an organization; technical expertise from faculty advisors; and university resources and supports (e.g., the Institutional Review Board, access to library resources).

Likewise, group-based service learning educational approaches benefit faculty by providing opportunities to stay up-to-date with needs in the field, translate research into practice, build practice-based evidence, fill gaps in their expertise, keep grounded in practice, gain exposure to local organizations, enhance campus-community partnerships, and strengthen their advising portfolios.

The considerable direct and indirect benefits to students, community organizations, and faculty offered by a dedicated group-based service learning experience outweighs the extensive planning and support they require. We have found this to be particularly true when group-based learning opportunities are structured as a capstone experience for groups of students. The capstone group-based service learning approach gives students an opportunity to synthesize knowledge and skills learned through their academic courses while providing the academic program an effective means of allowing students to plan, implement, and evaluate real-world deliverables within a system that provides ongoing student mentoring and evaluation.

Principles for Group-Based Teaching Approaches: The Capstone within Health Behavior

Developing and sustaining a major group-based service learning educational opportunity or course requires significant investment to ensure a high-quality experience for students as well as sustainable relationships with community partners. As an example, the Department of Health Behavior (HB) at the authors' home institution, a large public university with more than 1,500 students enrolled, has a yearlong, group-based, mentored service learning course that gives student teams an opportunity to apply knowledge and skills gained through the HB MPH curriculum to real-world public health problems identified by local organizations and to develop solutions in partnership with them. Over the course of an academic year (August–April), a group of four to six MPH students works with a partner organization and its stakeholders to produce a set of deliverables (e.g., products such as reports, plans, evaluations, curricula, databases, and other materials) that serve one overarching goal and enhance the partner organization's mission.

Here we crystalize lessons learned from eight years of teaching the HB Capstone course to provide key principles, approaches, and examples for maximizing beneficial results on students, faculty, and the communities using a group-based service learning approach. It is best to "nest" group-based education approaches within a service learning course to deepen and extend positive effects to students while ensuring that the course equally benefits community partners. Group-based education provides students with opportunities to synthesize information, develop new skills, and solve complex problems. Doing so within a service learning course extends this impact exponentially by providing students with a real-world context where they can experience the immediate effect of their work, even as they gain skills in working with groups and communities. Moreover, because students are still learning while working with community partners, we have found that it is essential to provide classroom-based time for discussion and processing as well as specific exercises and activities that provide students with needed support to ensure a beneficial experience for all participants in this collaborative partnership. In the case of HB Capstone, course designers strive to balance benefits to both students and community partners while simultaneously balancing a focus on the service and learning

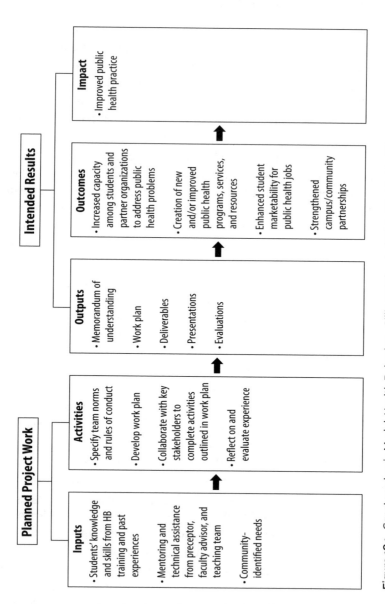

Figure 18.1. Capstone Logic Model, Health Behavior—Gillings School of Global Public Health

aspects of the experience. Students complete HB Capstone in the second year of the program, after demonstrating an initial mastery of competencies through coursework and comprehensive exams. Along with monitoring and ongoing support, this timing helps ensure a "do no harm" value when working with community partners. The result is a course with multiple, mutually reinforcing aims—increasing student and organizational capacity to address public health problems; creating new or improved public health programs, services, and resources; enhancing student marketability; and strengthening campus-community partnerships (figure 18.1).

Cultivate Authentic Partnerships and Plan Projects with Partners Carefully for Consistent Quality and Depth of Opportunities

In the HB Capstone course, partner organizations work with faculty to define the scope of project work. This approach prioritizes their specific needs and gives students an opportunity to do applied public health work on a range of topics and settings with diverse populations under the guidance of a practitioner.

This approach benefits community partners and provides a platform for sustainability, yet it also requires significant planning. In HB Capstone, planning begins in the fall of the previous academic year, when we send out email announcements requesting capstone project proposals to current, former, and potential local community partners. Organizations interested in submitting a proposal must meet or speak with the course instructor to discuss project ideas. This process promotes consistent quality and depth of opportunities across proposals and helps course instructors obtain insights about an organization's capacity to support a student team and the prospective preceptor's communication, work, and leadership styles. Based on our experience, specific criteria to consider when reviewing project proposals include the following.

Project Feasibility
Are key stakeholders located within driving time of the students? Is the proposed timeline for project work appropriate and does it fit within the academic calendar? Will students have adequate time to familiarize themselves with the subject matter through formative research?

Deliverables

Do proposed deliverables have clear purposes and steps, are they inter-related, and do they connect to the overall project goal? Projects are most manageable when all deliverables relate to one overarching goal. Otherwise, project work feels disjointed and students find the work less meaningful. Are the breadth and depth of deliverables appropriate for four to six students? Do deliverables allow for knowledge and skills acquisition that will enhance students' marketability as public health practitioners? Meeting both of these needs assures students that this investment in their education is worthwhile.

Mentorship

Is the preceptor known to have the time, expertise, and interest needed to mentor MPH students? An effective preceptor is key to a successful group-based service learning course. In our experience, successful preceptors need to have a keen interest in mentoring students, prior experience working with public health graduate students, and, ideally, have participated in a field-based experience in their own training. We require a support letter as part of the HB Capstone project proposal application to help ensure adequate motivation and resources to support a student team for a yearlong project.

Organizational Capacity

Is the partner organization known to have (or demonstrate capacity to) support a team of four to six students? Organizations that employ fewer people than there are students on a team may not have the needed capacity to support the venture or might be suited for working individually with a student in a practicum or some other volunteer arrangement.

Engagement

Is project work informed by and responsive to project stakeholders? Will students have an opportunity to interact with the priority population(s) associated with the project work? We have learned to make sure that students have a chance to work with the community partner and the community members they represent. This type of stakeholder engagement provides a capstone team with access that is of greatest interest to our students, provides them with rich learning opportunities, and helps them develop the widest possible opportunities to implement technical skills in complex settings.

Screening capstone opportunities for all the aforementioned criteria, in conjunction with phone calls and meetings with prospective partner organizations, helps ensure excellent learning opportunities and projects that yield greatest benefits to students, community partners, and faculty.

Give Students a Choice in Selecting Projects

This gives students agency and improves student morale and investment in their own learning and service contributions. In the HB Capstone, we provide students with this input at capstone "Pitch Day," an annual event held in March, when we invite preceptors associated with the top 15 to 17 highest-scoring proposals to present their project ideas to students. After hearing brief overviews of project ideas and associated deliverables, students rank their top five capstone project choices. Based on student rankings, the HB Capstone teaching team assembles student teams and works with the MPH program director and department chair to match faculty to the capstone teams/projects. The HB Capstone course instructor announces selected projects and team composition in early April. Student teams meet with the mentoring team once before summer break to draft work plans and memoranda of understanding (MOUs). The HB Capstone teaching team reviews draft work plans and MOUs over summer and troubleshoots with preceptors so that teams can begin work as soon as classes commence in the fall.

Provide Students with a Mentoring Team

In keeping with a group-based, real-world approach to education, providing students with a mentoring team means that they get feedback, insights, and evaluative input from multiple perspectives. This rigorous, multiangled approach to assessing work products and processes pushes students to meet high standards from a range of perspectives. In HB Capstone, a highly coordinated group of experts serves as the mentoring team for student groups. Specifically, each team works with an HB faculty advisor, who provides technical expertise and support. A preceptor (e.g., on-site supervisor/mentor) at the partner organization plans, designs, and supervises the HB Capstone project work. The HB Capstone teaching team (e.g., course instructor and teaching assistants) oversees all project work, establishes intentional processes and structures, promotes authentic partnerships, and facilitates critical reflection, all of which support a mutually beneficial capstone experience. On-call experts complete the mentoring team—including faculty or individuals with specific content expertise from the department, school, or larger community, who are also identified and available to student teams.

Establish Intentional Structures and Processes to Promote Authentic Partnerships and Encourage Reflection

Such approaches help ensure balanced benefits to students and community partners. In HB Capstone, two documents provide the foundation for such structures and processes (1) the MOU and (2) the work plan.

The Memorandum of Understanding

The success of capstone projects hinges on how well students and the mentoring team work together. MOUs promote effective partnerships by establishing a team culture (group norms) and clarifying behavioral expectations (rules of conduct) for meetings, communication between and among stakeholders, decision-making, managing tasks, and managing relationships. Capstone teams revisit MOUs at the midpoints and end points of each semester and modify them as necessary to maintain positive group dynamics.

The Work Plan

Just as the MOU helps to clarify expectations, so does the work plan. Each group's work plan provides a detailed account of how and when they plan to accomplish the HB Capstone project goal, including specific deliverables within specified timelines. Each student group sends structured, weekly email updates to the mentoring team to keep them informed of and engaged in work plan progress. These emails are also a useful cue to action when students need assistance.

The 360-Degree Evaluation

Finally, the teaching team administers 360-degree evaluations (e.g., all members of the student, community partner, and mentoring teams evaluate all members of their own student, community partner, and mentoring teams) at the mid- and end points of each semester to assess how projects are going and to facilitate opportunities for feedback and constructive dialogue. This effort actively supports a continuous quality improvement approach to the work the HB Capstone team undertakes with the community partners.

Provide Ample, Structured Team Time throughout the Semester

"Team time" in the group-based teaching approach gives students an opportunity to make progress on project work, deepen learning, receive guidance from mentors, and be out in the community. In HB Capstone, we also provide time for monthly student-led reflection sessions, in which a representative from each group helps facilitate class discussions and activities designed to promote critical reflection and sharing of best practices learned across projects. Such sessions can also help students recalibrate group dynamics to help ensure that they continue collaborating effectively.

Create a Culminating Event That Celebrates the Accomplishments/Impact of the Partnership

A celebration event provides all stakeholders with the opportunity to fully recognize the depth and breadth of learning and service that was accomplished over a semester or academic year. In HB Capstone, the course culminates with a "Celebration Day"—an event where teams present insights and impacts of their capstone project experiences to preceptors and other community partners, faculty, staff, alumni, and other students. This honors the work and the relationship while offering an opportunity for critical reflection on the yearlong project.

Principles in Action: Developing Authentic Relationships, Solving Real-World Problems

In our eight years of implementing the HB Capstone, 82 teams have worked with 49 partner organizations to produce 319 deliverables, contributing an estimated $2,009,016 worth of in-kind service to our partner organizations. Sixteen organizations have had more than one team, with the number of multiple teams per organization ranging from two to six. HB Capstone teams have addressed a wide array of public health topics and have produced deliverables that include assessment, planning, development, implementation, and evaluation tasks, using a variety of strategies, including asset mapping, photo voice, GIS mapping, surveys, and focus groups. Settings have included worksites, hospitals, schools, nonprofit organizations, and more, in rural and urban locales, and have served populations across the life span.

One example of how group-based, yearlong capstone projects can maximally benefit students, community partners, and faculty can be seen in the highly productive and impactful partnership between our HB department and the Orange County Department on Aging (OCDOA) (see table 18.1). The OCDOA's mission is to "provide leadership in planning and operating a system of integrated aging services through state-of-the-art senior centers, serving as focal points for coordinated community and individualized programs designed to educate seniors and their families and maximize the health, well-being, community engagement, and independence of older adults at all functional levels."[4] In 2011–2012, the OCDOA solicited an HB Capstone team to help develop the 2012–2017 Orange County, North Carolina, Master Aging Plan (MAP). The team organized and facilitated a community forum, coordinated a public comment period, and worked with the MAP management and MAP steering committee to develop objectives and strategies in five areas: (1) health and wellness, (2) housing, (3) navigation and transportation, (4) community engagement, and (5) aging in place. The team's work on the MAP was recognized by the Marvin Collins Planning Award for Graduate Student Project Planning, presented by the North Carolina chapter of the American Planning Association.

The following year (2012–2013), a team built on the work of the previous year's team by focusing on one key MAP component, developing expanded communication networks and information dissemination methods for health promotion among older adults in Orange County. In 2013–2014, a third HB Capstone team provided additional continuity by working with OCDOA to help address two MAP goals—(1) information dissemination and (2) service gap resolution—by implementing and evaluating a program that trains senior leaders to become resource leaders for their communities. Finally, in 2015–2016, a fourth HB Capstone team worked with OCDOA to create research-based organizational and marketing strategies to foster healthy aging and quality of life among 50-to-70-year-olds in Orange County.

Capstone teams' work with OCDOA over the years has strengthened the partnership between the university and a community-based organization, significantly contributed to OCDOA's capacity to address public health concerns, and served as a model for similar collaborations. Indeed, in 2017–2018, a neighboring county's Council on Aging worked with an HB Capstone team to develop their "optimal aging" plan using OCDOA Capstone teams' work as a guide.

Conclusion

Semester-long or yearlong group-based service learning educational programs and courses, when well designed and thoughtfully implemented, have enormous potential to significantly deepen student learning and skills development as they strengthen partnerships and provide enduring benefits to communities. The HB Capstone service learning, group-based education approach is now the centerpiece of the authors' HB MPH training. Implemented over eight consecutive years, with 354 students and 49 partner organizations, HB Capstone teams have helped build the capacity of organizations to do their work more efficiently and effectively while students gain real-world, mentored experience that serves them extremely well on the job market.

Our school has a commitment to continuous quality improvement of the capstone experience for all key stakeholders. We continue to refine our evaluation of the capstone from the perspective of students (current and prospective), alumni, faculty, preceptors, and other community partners. We also want to pursue opportunities and funding to allow our students to travel to global settings for their capstone projects and to work with interprofessional teams. As constructed, elements of the

TABLE 18.1. Sample Capstone Projects, Health Behavior, Gillings School of Global Public Health

Partner Organization	Year	Project Goal	Deliverables
Orange County Department on Aging	2011–2012	To produce a master aging plan for Orange County, NC	1. Community forum report 2. Community engagement toolkit 3. Master aging plan
	2012–2013	To develop improved and expanded communication networks and information dissemination methods for health promotion among older adults in Orange County, NC	1. Evidence tables 2. Assessment tools 3. Summary of findings report 4. Recommendations report 5. Dissemination plan
	2013–2014	To address two major goals of the master aging plan—(1) information dissemination and (2) service gap resolution—by implementing Project EngAGE, a program that trains senior leaders to become resource leaders who address concerns in their communities	1. Recruitment materials 2. Revised curriculum 3. Event plan 4. Evaluation plan 5. Evaluation report
	2015–2016	To create research-based organizational and marketing strategies to foster healthy aging and quality of life among 50-to-70-year-olds in Orange County, NC	1. Literature review 2. Formative research report 3. Recommendations 4. Marketing plan
North Carolina Harm Reduction Coalition (NCHRC)	2012–2013	To recommend policy solutions to reduce accidental drug overdoses in NC to legislators and policy think tanks	1. Literature review 2. Policy recommendations 3. Policy briefs 4. Summit materials

Organization	Year	Objective	Products/deliverables
	2013–2014	To evaluate SB 20, legislation that provides legal protection for those who call for medical help in the case of a drug overdose, and HB 850, legislation enacted to reduce the spread of blood-borne diseases by providing legal protection for those who declare a clean syringe to a law enforcement officer prior to being searched, to understand their impact in the populations they are intended to benefit; and to advocate for revision of the University of North Carolina's system-wide drug policy to reflect the intent of the newly enacted laws	1. IRB applications 2. Literature review 3. Key informant interview guides 4. Policy brief 5. Manuscript 6. Overdose Prevention Awareness Day event
	2014–2015	To assist NCHRC with (1) legislative advocacy, (2) strengthening and diversifying its media portfolio, and (3) engaging with stakeholders to create events that advocate for legislative changes	1. Policy advocacy packet 2. Media portfolio 3. Event planning
Art Therapy Institute of North Carolina (ATI)	2012–2013	To measure program effectiveness and improve the sustainability of the Burma Art Therapy Program (BATP), an art therapy program designed to help address complex trauma, increase self-esteem, and build social support among child and adolescent refugees from Burma in Chapel Hill and Carrboro, NC	1. Outcome evaluation plan 2. Funding toolkit 3. Assessment tools 4. Grant proposal 5. Evaluation report
	2013–2014	To fill gaps in the literature regarding art therapy, to improve ATI's capacity to attract funding, and to ensure sustainability of the BATP	1. Data management user guide 2. Evaluation report 3. Manuscript 4. Grant proposal
	2016–2017	To garner support and increased funding for expanding ATI's pediatric oncology art therapy program at Duke Hospital	1. Literature review 2. Funding toolkit 3. Evaluation plan and instruments 4. Evaluation report 5. Project presentation for stakeholders 6. Grant proposal

HB Capstone fulfill Council on Education for Public Health (CEPH) requirements related to the Integrative Learning Experience and the Applied Practice Experience.[5] The Integrative Learning Experience requires students to demonstrate synthesis of foundational and concentration competencies through a high-quality written product, while the Applied Practice Experience requires that students master at least five specified competencies (three of them foundational CEPH competencies) within an applied setting. As we work to comply with 2016 CEPH requirements, we believe that this capstone group-based learning experience is not only a hallmark of our MPH training program but may serve as a model for group-based service learning for other schools that aim to enhance their academic mission and strengthen relationships with community organizations and practitioners.

REFERENCES

1. Bransford, J. D., A. L. Brown, and R. R. Cocking, eds. *How People Learn: Brain, Mind, Experience, and School.* Washington, DC: National Academy Press, 1999.

2. Association of Schools and Programs of Public Health. "Public Health Trends and Redesigned Education—Blue Ribbon Public Health Employers' Advisory Board: Summary of Interviews." September 6, 2013. http://s3.amazonaws.com/aspph-wp -production/app/uploads/2017/10/BlueRibbonPublicHealthEmployersAdvisory Board_Report_FINAL_09.06.13-SJC.pdf.

3. United States Agency for International Development. "Survey of Major Employers of Global Health Personnel—Executive Summary." 2015. https://docplayer.net /14109619-Survey-of-major-employers-of-global-health-personnel-executive-summary .html (accessed November 29, 2018).

4. Orange County Department of Health. "Aging." http://www.orangecountync .gov/departments/aging (accessed April 9, 2018).

5. Council on Education for Public Health. "Accreditation Criteria: Schools and Programs of Public Health." Silver Spring, MD: CEPH, 2016. https://ceph.org /assets/2016.Criteria.pdf (accessed March 25, 2018).

[19]

Effective Collaborative Learning Experiences

It Is All in the Design

LUANN WHITE AND ANGELA BRECKENRIDGE

COLLABORATIVE LEARNING IS an educational method that employs teams of students to advance learning, develop new ideas, solve problems, cocreate new products, or carry out an assignment or task. When designed and used effectively, collaborative learning experiences enhance individual students' mastery of course material, achievement of learning objectives, and the development of practical and collaborative skills.[1,2,3] Fried et al. argue for a dramatic change in public health curricula in order to prepare graduates to learn, work, and problem-solve as interdependent contributors to collaborative teams capable of understanding and addressing large-scale forces influencing population health. They write,

> Recognizing the centrality of collaborative work as a key ingredient in the solution to complex problems, it is vital that a public health education of the future incorporate a strong element of learning that prepares students for team-based research and practice. Although, increasingly, large teams are most effective at competing for research grants and tackling high-level research questions, educational initiatives have been slow to teach students both the value and the skills to be effective team members. Knowing how to effectively work in a team is a pivotal part of becoming a successful public health professional, and it falls to public

health schools to train students in the skills needed for effective teamwork.[4]

The practical aspects of integrating collaborative learning experiences in the classroom or for interprofessional projects pose significant challenges for implementation.[5] The effectiveness of instructor-designed collaborative learning experiences is often constrained by prior experiences that influence attitudes and willingness to engage in group activities. These challenges set a negative precedent for engagement in collaborative learning and undermine the potential for developing team-building and interpersonal skills through collaborative methods.[6] The extent to which the instructor has adequate knowledge of the evidence-based theory and experience with the pedagogy of collaborative learning can limit the implementation of effective collaborative learning. Difficulties arise when the instructor does not understand how to structure and carry out the fundamental components of collaborative learning for the classroom or assignment. However, with appropriate structural design and instructor training, collaborative learning is an effective means of achieving learning goals.

Selecting a Collaborative Learning Experience

Collaborative methods are flexible enough to be used for all learning goals with all types and levels of learners. However, not every collaborative method or activity is appropriate for every learning situation. Appropriate selection of a collaborative activity depends on the complexity of the desired learning goal and the degree of interactivity required to achieve it. There are essentially four categories of collaborative learning experiences that can be tailored to attain a variety of desired learning goals: (1) in-class activities, (2) formal group assignments, (3) team-based learning, and (4) interprofessional projects.[7] We describe each in detail in the following sections.

In-Class Activities

In-class activities engage students with one another, the course material, and the instructor. In-class activities advance a single lesson through short, interactive exchanges in small groups of two or three students and typically result in a brief written response. This approach works well for small group discussion, listing key points of an assigned reading, or summarizing key points in a lecture.[8] These are low-risk activities that may or may not be scheduled or even graded. This activity itself may take only a few minutes, but it is effective in preparing the class as a whole for moving on with the lesson, for clarifying important points, and for engaging students with one another. Because this type of active learning does not depend on group cohesion, self-assessment, or peer assessment to be effective, the groups can be randomly assigned or formed by the students themselves.

Formal Group Assignments

Formal group assignments involve tasks that are assigned to larger groups of students for the purposes of accomplishing a learning objective in the course, advancing understanding of key issues, and developing interdisciplinary skills by cocreating knowledge through interdependent collaboration. Formal group assignments are more structured, may require a specified process, often span multiple class sessions, involve out-of-class coordination of the group, and include individual roles with unique accountabilities. These types of collaborative assignments work well with groups of at least four but no more than six students and ideally include students with different strengths. Groups embarking on a formal assignment together should be formed by the instructor in order to ensure heterogeneity, divergent thinking, and interdependent capabilities.

Team-Based Learning

Team-based learning is a formal methodology and structural framework imbedded in the course curricula and designed to achieve specific learning objectives, augment disciplinary learning, and develop collaborative skills. The method has been used successfully across disciplines, from business to health and social sciences.[9] In a team-based activity or project, learning teams are formed by the instructor at the beginning of the term and are the central learning unit for processing course material, analyzing real-world case studies, and strengthening skills in critical thinking, innovation, and problem-solving for the duration of the course. This method is effective for applying discipline-specific content through simulated scenarios or problem-based projects, as well as for developing interpersonal skills, leadership, critical thinking, and collaborative solutions.[10] Team-based learning is a viable approach to preparing public health graduates for collaborative conversations central to advancing population health.

Interprofessional Projects

Interprofessional projects allow students to demonstrate acquired knowledge, skills, and abilities within a professional context through collaborative work with practicing public health professionals and professionals from related fields such as medicine, nursing, pharmacy, social work, or private business. Public health educators incorporate interprofessional experiences into the curriculum to prepare students for the rapidly evolving complexities they will encounter in their future careers.[11] Students join a group of professionals in a collaborative work team to develop a real-world solution, product, or intervention. Collaborative learning on interprofessional teams has been shown to increase student proficiency across all public health core competencies.[12] These learning experiences allow students to expand their core knowledge through the exchange of perspectives, approaches, and vocabulary used among related professionals in the field.

Evidence-Based Design for Collaborative Learning

In order to realize the benefits of collaboration on individual student learning, the experience has to stimulate cooperative interactions among the group members. Research on social interdependence provides valuable insight into what makes collaboration work and informs evidence-based design principles for structuring collaborative learning experiences.[13] It is essential that instructors make informed design choices that foster the positive interdependence required for effective collaboration. Even previous experiences that faculty or students may have had with dysfunctional work groups can be mitigated through intentional design practices that optimize social interdependence. Design factors to consider (discussed in in the following sections) include: how groups are formed (group formation); how groups work together to achieve a common goal (group dynamics); and how to assess contributions of individuals to the group process and final product (evaluation and grading).

Group Formation

Who forms groups for collaborative activities? Who should be in which group? How big or small should each group be? Collaborative learning groups can be formed in a variety of ways—by students, by the instructor, by random assignment, or by shared common interests. While students may prefer to form their own groups, the typical homogeneity that results from student-formed groups can negatively impact the desired learning goal, create a lack of divergent thinking, and increase the likelihood of subgroups within the group.[14] In-class small group activities provide the most appropriate setting for students to form their own groups or for randomized group formation based on counting off or drawing names. In general, a smaller group produces better results for in-class activities, where partners or triads are able to make decisions quickly for simple tasks that relate to the immediate topic.

For formal group assignments, team-based learning, and interprofessional collaborations, larger groups formed by instructors consistently perform better as collaborative teams than those formed by students or by randomization. In the case of formal group assignments or more complex and lengthy projects, groups need sufficient resources to adequately perform the task—no fewer than four members—but not so many that it would make coordinating the group difficult or encourage freeloading (no more than six members). However collaborative groups are formed, the process of selecting individuals for a work group must be transparent and appear fair to students.[15]

Group Dynamics

How do you prevent freeloaders? Social loafing? Negative stereotyping? Interpersonal conflict? Preparing students to learn and work effectively in a collaborative learning situation takes commitment and dedicated class time, and it is the most influential contributing factor to achieving successful collaborative outcomes and developing essential collaborative skills required for public health professionals. Preemptive actions such as determining ground rules, formalizing a group contract, and role-playing effective behaviors in collaborative scenarios can prepare groups to function effectively and prevent counterproductive activities such as freeloading or social loafing, the most commonly identified student concerns related to group activities.[16]

Ground rules provide a common understanding of expected conduct and cooperation by each member of the group in order to accomplish the desired outcome. One approach to setting ground rules is for the class to discuss how effective collaboration works, drawing from published research as well as students' previous experiences with group projects. These discussions will produce a list of behaviors that promote or detract from collaborative learning, and that prevent or address potential conflicts that could impede the group's agenda. Positive behaviors typically include contributing good ideas, listening to others, taking initiative, being on time, and doing one's share of the work. The class discussion itself may serve as a positive example of effective collaboration in reaching consensus on a code of conduct that includes individual contribution and the interdependence necessary for achieving the desired result.

Formalizing the ground rules through a group contract may further deter conflict. While Thompson is among those who believe that group conflict is an opportunity to strengthen interpersonal communication,[17] most find the opposite to be true when conflict occurs in collaborative learning experiences, especially for group members who are just beginning to develop collaborative skills. Conflict can and often does demoralize and demotivate individuals. Starting with consensus on goals, ground rules, and group norms significantly decreases these odds that conflicts will arise.

In addition to ground rules and group contracts, instructor-led role-playing allows students to anticipate types of conflict by practicing strategies for handling conflict and recognizing behaviors that underlie it.[18] In scenarios where functional and dysfunctional teams are faced with a conflict to resolve, students play out familiar roles such as the coordinator, who distributes tasks and materials and facilitates team discussion; the devil's advocate, who poses arguments from another perspective; and the overachiever, who does everybody else's job without discussion.[19] Group members take on roles such as these to practice strategies for listening, engaging, and acknowledging issues in scenarios that require them to reach a final resolution together. This type of exercise can be instrumental in dispelling preexisting beliefs and attitudes that often sabotage collaborative learning efforts.

Students who have had negative experiences with group learning often require more structure than students who have had positive experiences. Structure may include guidance on assignment of roles within the group, early individual feedback with interim checkpoints, and feedback on early drafts of work products. Feedback provides a means to keep the activities moving forward productively.

Once formed and prepared for the task at hand, student groups must determine how to achieve their given task. If the activity is not designed to integrate individual work into the group process and the final product, individual contributions may be reduced to isolated tasks rather than a collaborative learning process. This often occurs when traditional assignments typically designed for an individual are used in a collaborative context and assigned to a group without proper modifications for collaboration. The research paper is an infamous example of a group activity or task susceptible to being divvied up, allocated to individual group members as parts of projects, and produced in isolation (i.e., the "divide and conquer" approach). But this is not collaboration or even cocreation. In fact, this absence of interdependence undermines the group's ability to accomplish intended collaborative outcomes. Collaborative learning activities must be equipped with mechanisms for interdependent contribution. Otherwise, the benefits of collaborative learning are rendered futile.[20]

Evaluation and Grading

Why is my grade dependent on team members who do not do their share of the work? How can I evaluate both individual contributions to the group product as well as the ability of the group to function as a team? Grading collaborative learning experiences fairly and thoroughly is complex. What is particularly challenging is separating an individual student's grade from that assigned to the final product presented by the group and representing the overall group performance. This inevitably raises the issue of fairness and equity—the single most common concern about collaborative activities shared by both students and faculty.

Complicating the issue of fairness is the fact that neither group processes nor individual contribution are necessarily evident in the final product. Designing assessments for group interdependence and individual performance are key to assigning grades equitably.[21] Carefully designed assessments address concerns of top-notch students who feel that their own success is dependent on team members who do not do their share of work or who do not have an equal level of commitment. Students need to see the breakdown of their final grade that clearly indicates proportions for individual contribution, group performance, and the final work product.

One method for determining individual contribution is with peer assessments in which each member of the group provides feedback on the other members as well as themselves. Instructor observations may also contribute to the grade for both individual contribution and the overall group performance grade.[22] Observing group process when the group is working together in class or even in an out-of-class group meeting provides instructors with a view into group dynamics and collaborative processes. These observations should always be conducted with a quality rubric that standardizes evaluation across groups and over class periods. The standard measures demonstrate fairness and account for different types of interactions and personalities within the group. Separating the scores for contribution and process from that of the final work product helps to address concerns.

Conclusion

Public health graduates need to be prepared to contribute to teams and work collaboratively to address the changing landscape of population health. Collaborative skills are not innate in most people and must be developed to produce high-performing and innovative public health professionals. Collaborative learning pedagogy is a means to produce highly competent professionals who are better prepared to solve the public health challenges in evolving roles and job responsibilities. If we are to incorporate collaborative learning effectively into public health curricula, faculty need to be prepared to successfully implement these methods. We would suggest, in conclusion, the following recommendations to promote effective collaborative learning experiences.

- Emphasize development of collaborative skills as a course objective. Many students focus only on the content of the final product without understanding the process for building collaborative skills.
- Tailor the type of collaborative activity and method to the learning objective. Types of activities range from short-term in-class activities to more structured formal group assignments and onto longer-term team-based learning. Select the appropriate method to foster interdependent learning to achieve specific course objectives.
- Include dedicated time for students to develop ground rules and to identify positive and negative behaviors prior to launching collaborative learning activities.
- Prepare students to undertake collaborative learning. Allow in-class time to establish ground rules and role-play to understand productive and nonproductive behaviors that contribute to successful learning experiences.
- Grade both individual and group performance. Carefully and thoroughly lay out the component parts of the final grade for individual students and use standardized grading rubrics for consistency and transparency.
- Understand the body of evidence-based research to effectively design courses and activities that will achieve interdependent learning and foster collaboration.

REFERENCES

1. Cohen, E. G. "Restructuring the Classroom: Conditions for Productive Small Groups." *Review of Educational Research* 64, no. 1 (1994): 1–35.

2. Johnson, D. W., and R. T. Johnson. *Cooperation and Competition: Theory and Research*. Edina, MN: Interaction Book Company, 1989.

3. Slavin, R. E. *Cooperative Learning: Theory, Research, and Practice, 2nd Edition*. Boston: Allyn and Bacon, 1995.

4. Fried, L. P., M. D. Begg, R. Bayer, and S. Galea. "MPH Education for the 21st Century: Motivation, Rationale, and Key Principles for the New Columbia Public Health Curriculum." *American Journal of Public Health* 104, no. 1 (2014): 23–30.

5. Smith, K. A. "Cooperative Learning: Making 'Groupwork' Work." *New Directions for Teaching and Learning* 67 (1996): 71–82.

6. De Hei, M. S. A., J. Stijbos, E. Sjoer, and W. Admiraal. "Collaborative Learning in Higher Education: Lecturers' Practices and Beliefs." *Research Papers in Education* 30, no. 2 (2015): 232–247.

7. Smith, "Cooperative Learning."

8. Johnson, D. W., R. T. Johnson, and E. Holubec. *Cooperation in the Classroom.* Edina, MN: Interaction Book Company, 2008.

9. Michaelson, L., T. O. Peterson, and M. Sweet. "Building Learning Teams: The Key to Harnessing the Power of Small Groups in Management Education." In *The SAGE Handbook of Management Learning, Education, and Development*, edited by S. J. Armstrong and C. V. Fukami, 325–343. London: SAGE Publications, 2009.

10. Michaelson, L. K., A. K. Bauman, and L. D. Fink. *Team-Based Learning: A Transformative Use of Small Groups in College Teaching.* Sterling, VA: Stylus, 2004.

11. Hammick, M., L. Olckers, and C. Campion-Smith. "Learning in Interprofessional Teams: AMEE Guide No 38." *Medical Teacher* 31, no. 1 (2009): 1–12.

12. Wallar, L., and A. Papadopoulos. "Collaboration, Competencies, and the Classroom: A Public Health Approach." *Canadian Journal for the Scholarship or Teaching and Learning* 6, no. 1 (2015): http://ir.lib.uwo.ca/cjsotl_rcacea/vol6/iss1/6.

13. Johnson, D. W., and R. T. Johnson. "Social Interdependence Theory and Cooperative Learning: The Teacher's Role." In *The Teacher's Role in Implementing Cooperative Learning in the Classroom*, edited by D. W. Johnson and R. T. Johnson, 10–38. Boston: Springer, 2008.

14. Mills, B. J. "Enhancing Learning—and More!—through Cooperative Learning—Idea Paper #38." IDEA Center. 2002. https://www.ideaedu.org/Portals/0/Uploads/Documents/IDEA%20Papers/IDEA%20Papers/IDEA_Paper_38.pdf (accessed April 9, 2018).

15. Hall, D., and S. Buzwell. "The Problem of Free-Riding in Group Projects: Looking Beyond Social Loafing as Reason for Non-Contribution." *Active Learning in Higher Education* 14, no. 1 (2012): 37–49.

16. Forehand, J. W., K. H. Leigh, R. G. Farrell, and A. Y. Spurlock. "Social Dynamics in Group Work." *Teaching and Learning in Nursing* 11, no. 2 (2016): 62–66.

17. Leigh, T. *Making the Team: A Guide for Managers.* Upper Saddle River, NJ: Pearson Education, 2014.

18. Hansen, R. S. "Benefits and Problems with Student Teams: Suggestions for Improving Team Projects." *Journal of Education for Business* 82, no. 1 (2006): 11–19.

19. Barkley, E. F., K. P. Cross, and C. H. Major. *Collaborative Learning Techniques: A Handbook for College Faculty.* San Francisco: Jossey-Bass, 2014.

20. Feichtner, S. B. "Why Some Groups Fail: A Survey of Students' Experiences with Learning Groups." *Journal of Management Education* 9, no. 4 (1984): 58–73.

21. Johnson, D. W., R. T. Johnson, and K. A. Smith. *Active Learning: Cooperation in the College Classroom.* Edina, MN: Interaction Book Company, 1998.

22. Michaelsen, L., T. O. Peterson, and M. Sweet. "Building Learning Teams: The Key to Harnessing the Power of Small Groups in Management Education." In *The SAGE Handbook of Management Learning, Education and Development*, edited by S. J. Armstrong and C. V. Fukami, 325–343. London: SAGE Publications, 2009.

Navigating Difficult Conversations in Public Health Classrooms

YVETTE C. COZIER AND SOPHIE GODLEY

These are rancorous times, characterized by a divided country, and, increasingly, a divided world. The present climate has generated plenty of heat, but often little light. Schools operating within universities can lend clarity to the public debate by allowing for discussion and a free exchange of competing, data-informed ideas.—*Dr. Sandro Galea, dean of the Boston University School of Public Health, July 2017*

What Are Difficult Conversations, and Why Are There Difficult Conversations in Public Health Classrooms?

Public health is an inherently diverse and multidisciplinary field. Diversity is critical to our success. A diverse community is by definition heterogeneous and includes students with very different perspectives and life experiences. These different perspectives and experiences can often result in differences of opinions and perspectives that can make for difficult conversations in the public health classroom.

The term "difficult conversations" is perhaps self-explanatory and is very likely something all public health faculty, researchers, and practitioners experience at some point in their career. Difficult conversations involve an element of confrontation—either in defense of oneself or another person, as a means of corrective action for improper or inappropriate behaviors, or, most commonly, to clear up what one may view as a misunderstanding or miscommunication.

The subject of difficult conversations can range tremendously. For example, in classrooms, difficult conversations may involve confronting a student about using a cell phone during class or addressing a group of students working together on a project who are experiencing conflict. Regardless of the topic, difficult conversations make most people uncomfortable. When the scenarios include an element of difference or "otherness," this discomfort may be heightened. For example, if students working on a group project are having issues that appear to be dividing domestic and international students, faculty might fear that involvement will be interpreted as being biased toward one side or the other. So how, then, do faculty confront students and engage in necessary, meaningful, messy, and, yes, difficult conversations? In this chapter, we outline strategies to help faculty become comfortable in leading discussions around issues of diversity and inclusion, and for students to positively contribute to such conversations.

Why Difficult Conversations in Public Health?

According to the American Public Health Association: "Public health promotes and protects the health of people and the communities where they live, learn, work and play." It goes on further to state: "Public health saves money, improves our quality of life, helps children thrive and reduces human suffering."[1] While all strata of society are included in its purview, at its core, the role of public health is to advocate for the vulnerable, underserved, and marginalized in our society.

Public health is an inherently diverse and multidisciplinary field. It is comprised of individuals trained in a variety of areas, including medicine, nursing, laboratory and basic medical sciences, mathematics, statistics, economics, management, law, anthropology, and the social sciences. Public health is practiced in a variety of settings, including international and domestic federal, state, and local administrative agencies; pharmaceutical companies; clinical research organizations; academic medical centers, local hospitals, and community health centers; community-based organizations, nongovernmental agencies; and civic and faith-based organizations. The underlying structural factors that contribute to societal health are similarly diverse and include race/ethnicity, gender identity, sexuality, socioeconomic status, geography, and ability.[2] Finally, public health practitioners bring varying levels of awareness, understanding, and sensitivity to their work.

From an academic standpoint, students who enter public health classrooms arrive with very different perspectives and life experiences. Structural inequities in society are magnified in academic settings, resulting in a student body of future public health practitioners that often does not reflect the populations they will engage. Conversations that arise in the academic setting include debates over controversial issues in public health such as vaccines, sexuality education, and abortion. They also include discussions about race, class, privilege, white supremacy, and homophobia.

Why Is Navigating Difficult Conversations Important for Students?

The Master of Public Health (MPH) degree is a practice degree based on development of crosscutting competencies.[3,4] Successful graduates must be well equipped to address difficult conversations and topics within the public health workplace. The role of public health is to advocate for the vulnerable, underserved, and marginalized in our society. Students pursuing public health often come from communities outside of those they are training to serve—whether domestic or international. On entering these new environments, students must first be aware of their own biases, fears, and anxieties about race.[5,6] Thus, understanding themselves as racial and cultural beings becomes paramount to developing their professional competencies as public health professionals. In our experience, emphasizing that developing competency in navigating difficult conversations (including those around race and difference) is a professional skill that has allowed students to think of this as an area of growth and learning, not an inherent deficit they can never overcome. Importantly, this development begins prior to orientation for our incoming students.

Why Is Navigating Difficult Conversations Important for Faculty?

As noted for students, faculty must also acknowledge their vulnerability to biases and fears regarding differences in order to effectively lead difficult classroom conversations. A study by Sue et al. sought to identify facilitators and barriers to successful classroom dialogues.[7] Among the strategies deemed "unhelpful" were passivity, or allowing the class to take over the discussion; disengaging, or dismissing the importance of the topic; becoming angry toward the student; simply switching the topic and ignoring the dialogue; and "strategic colorblindness," where faculty claim not to see race for fear that it may indicate that one is racist or biased.[8] Students also report looking to faculty to manage and facilitate these conversations, and paramount to this is faculty self-awareness. This may be particularly critical for students of color in the classroom, who in our experience are not only keenly aware of their fellow students' biases and lack of awareness but are also paying heightened attention to faculty responses.

The Central Goal of Public Health Is to Advocate for the Vulnerable

In order to fully engage in the important work of difficult conversations, it is critical for faculty and administrators to remember that the work of public health is focused on vulnerable populations. Vulnerable populations include the economically disadvantaged, racial and ethnic minorities, the uninsured, low-income children, the elderly, the homeless, those with human immunodeficiency virus (HIV), and those with other chronic health conditions, including severe mental illness.[9] Vulnerable populations may also include rural residents, who often encounter barriers to accessing healthcare services.[10] The vulnerability of these individuals is often enhanced by race, ethnicity, age, sex, insurance coverage (or lack thereof), and absence of a usual source of care.[11,12,13] Their health and healthcare problems also intersect with social factors, including housing, poverty, and inadequate education.[14] As faculty, we must prepare students to be competent in working with these populations, and a first step is for students to begin to recognize their own often invisible advantages and biases.

Recognizing Privilege: "Born on Third Base"

Public health graduate programs are not dissimilar from other graduate programs, wherein there may be an overrepresentation of affluent, majority students and an underrepresentation of minority students.[15] In addition, many majority students in public health are deeply committed to the work of social justice and have a strong desire to work with the underrepresented. This desire does not, however, automatically translate into effective work in diverse communities. Preparation for truly impactful public health work is the "seeing" of privilege. Many people believe that they achieved their status in life solely due to sacrifice and hard work. Privilege is enjoyed by the majority group, but it is often invisible to them. Privilege is deeply problematic for people of color, who try to get people to realize that racial minorities live a different reality than whites. This creates difficulties in dialogue because those in the majority generally believe that they worked hard to achieve what they have, and that if others simply work hard, they also will achieve those same outcomes.[16]

One option to facilitate student recognition of their own privilege is to provide resources including readings, Twitter feeds to follow, movies and music to experience, and websites with interactive exercises such as Project Implicit (https://implicit.harvard.edu/implicit/) prior to the start of class or prior to a planned classroom discussion where issues of privilege and merit will surface. This provides students with an opportunity to delve into their own privileges and biases prior to asking them to reflect on these issues collectively.

Recognizing Microaggressions: "Well-Intentioned Slights"

Microaggressions are defined as "the everyday verbal, nonverbal, and environmental slights, snubs, or insults, whether intentional or unintentional, which communicate hostile, derogatory, or negative messages to target persons based solely upon their marginalized group membership."[17] Generally discussed from the perspective of race and racism, any marginalized group may become a target of microaggressions (e.g., women, LGBTQIA persons, those with disabilities, and religious minorities).[18] Following are four examples of microaggressions from public health classrooms:

1 When discussing a publicly funded insurance program, a student in a class on healthcare management says, "No one in this class is the type of person who would be enrolled in the Mass Health program."

2 A small group of students are randomly assigned to work on a class project. Two students in the group are from China and three of the students, one of whom is Asian American, are from the United States. After class, one of the US students sends the professor an email complaining about having to work with three group members who "don't speak English."

3 After a highly publicized news event involving issues of sexual harassment and gender discrimination, a student makes a joke in a class about how that "could never happen here since everyone here is a girl!"

4 During a discussion about racism and its impact on health, a white student insists on quoting from a popular news source that reinforces the connection between genes and race.

These and other occurrences appear harmless, but research suggests they have a powerful psychological impact on the marginalized.[19] Microaggressions are usually conveyed by well-meaning persons who are unaware of the harm caused by their words.[20] Faculty often fail to recognize microaggressions when they occur.[21,22] Poor handling of these dialogues may result in anger, complaints, and impediments to the learning process as microaggressions accumulate over time and erode individuals' confidence by making them feel unwelcome, devalued, and excluded.

How Difficult Conversations Play Out among the Various Disciplines within Public Health: Examples from Unexpected Places

Nearly all disciplines within public health can and should include difficult conversations about inclusion and diversity. While some fields are explicitly tasked with addressing issues of difference, such as maternal and child health, community health, and social and behavioral sciences, what follows are a few specific examples from disciplines within public health that may not be traditionally expected to include difficult conversations.

Epidemiology and Biostatistics

Race is a frequent source of discomfort and a topic of discussion across all public health disciplines. In the context of quantitative courses, health data (e.g., mortality) are often presented according to race, with emphasis on health disparities. In other instances, race is considered only in the context of multivariable analyses where it is used as a control or adjustment variable. In both situations, little or no discussion is provided to distinguish between the implied biology of race and the well-documented sociology of race in America.[23] Without the contextual lens of sociology, notions of biological superiority/inferiority are tacitly reinforced among majority-, foreign-, and, indeed, some underrepresented minority students. Such perspectives have real-life consequences. A 2015 University of Virginia study found that non-Hispanic white members of the general public, medical students, and medical residents endorsed incorrect views of blacks as related to levels of pain.[24] Fifty-eight percent of whites; 40% and 42% of first- and second-year medical students, respectively; and 25% of medical residents believed that blacks were biologically different (e.g., had "thicker skin") as compared to whites and therefore felt less pain.[25] In STEM fields, unlike the social sciences and humanities, race relations are generally not a focus of study within the discipline. It is therefore even more critical for faculty in epidemiology and biostatistics to begin these difficult conversations and to contextualize the data they discuss, present, and have students analyze.

Environmental Health

The field of environmental health has long addressed environmental racism and disproportionate burdens of environmental hazards experienced by communities of color.[26] Some within the field are, in fact, experts at working closely with communities and modeling the principles of best practices in engaging with the disadvantaged. Environmental health faculty can provide unique opportunities for students to learn from their work and to engage in explicit conversations about bias, privilege, and diversity. While seemingly focused on science and data, environmental health is an expansive field that incorporates issues of power, privilege, autonomy, community status, and policy. Hearing directly from those affected by environmental injustices can be very powerful for students. Environmental justice advocates who are members of impacted communities can be brought into classrooms through TED Talks, Skype lectures, and YouTube videos, offering students the opportunity to discuss and debate critical issues in public health and to engage in difficult conversations.

Health Policy and Management

Within the field of health policy and management there are multiple opportunities to address salient and difficult conversations around privilege and different populations. Some students may be interested in the work of designing health systems that effectively serve vulnerable populations and can learn from faculty who have worked extensively in this field. Rather than assuming healthcare to be "colorblind," explicitly opening conversations about racism, privilege, and diversity allows students in this field the opportunity to better understand work in diverse communities. Interpreting policy through a race-conscious and bias-conscious lens will better prepare students for working in diverse places of employment.

Global Health

Building on a long history of complicated relationships and cultural navigation, global health departments are rich in opportunities for difficult discussions. As beautifully described by Dr. Paul Farmer, recognizing the specific histories of slavery, colonialism, and current global inequity is crucial to the work of global public health.[27] Global health departments often attract a wide range of students who come to the United States eager to learn public health and perhaps are as yet unexposed to the peculiarities of US racial dynamics and history. An important component of teaching global public health involves exposing non-US students to the social determinants of health within the United States. This almost certainly includes discussions of the history of the United States' and other first-world countries' role in colonization. Recent discussions in many global public health classrooms about disrupting the notion of "poverty tourism" and "volun-tourism" are a very good first step. How can faculty navigate difficult conversations between those who live in and are from disadvantaged countries, and those who "spent a summer" in such a place? Recognizing the differences in experiences and then facilitating open and honest conversation about how to recognize privilege in a global context is crucial to developing skilled future professionals who are comfortable navigating challenging situations.

Tips for Engaging in Difficult Conversations

Before Class Begins

We would suggest that the first approach to ensure that we can engage in difficult conversation is in prevention and preparation. Specifically, preparing students for difficult conversations and preparing faculty to facilitate them is crucial to success. To this end, our institution has undertaken a number of strategic initiatives to prepare for and support our community in these conversations. We provide a few examples in the following sections.

Targeted Teachings
Offer programming aimed at building awareness among faculty of the implicit biases that can be introduced into the classroom by both faculty and students. At our institution, formal antibias training was offered over the course of a year and a half for faculty, starting with department chairs. The workshops were specifically designed to develop skills among all members of the school community to be more adept at productively raising and managing difficult topics that arise during class discussions.

New Student Orientation
Include discussions of diversity and inclusion topics during orientation programming for incoming students. These sessions can provide opportunities for students to discuss their fears and concerns about approaching these topics during the academic year, including in class. Programming can include the following: (1) an introduction to the data and framework of why social determinants (e.g., race and class) are critical components of public health; (2) a workshop for students to self-identify their own privileges and biases in a safe and supportive environment; (3) a concrete, guided discussion around how to confront, and be confronted, when inadvertently offending a classmate; and (4) introduce resources for how to learn and develop professional skills around navigating issues of diversity and inclusion while on campus and within the

community. Orientation sessions for new students admittedly do not reach every student, and yet they do provide a starting point for conversations. Further, they offer all faculty the opportunity to refer back to this conversation when difficult conversations do arise during the semester.

Common Language

Include more explicit conversations about race, class, diversity, and social justice throughout the curriculum. In 2016, we launched a new MPH curriculum that included core competencies around diversity and inclusion, as well as expanded examples of frameworks used to consider health outcomes. We further launched a "one school, one book" program aimed at uniting the school community around a single book and examining it from many perspectives. SPH Reads involves assigning a book to all incoming SPH students, faculty, and staff in the summer, with the goal of addressing the topic throughout the semester/academic year in various settings (e.g., classes, nonclass academic events, and social events). This initial exercise of sharing a book focused on diversity allows the entire school community to discuss issues of race, difference, gender, and so forth focused around a single narrative.

Language in Syllabi

Include a specific statement regarding difficult conversations in course syllabi. Language in the syllabus can send a message to all taking the class that difficult conversations will be encountered during the course of the semester, and that faculty are both anticipating and prepared to handle these conversations. The syllabus can also describe the expected standards of behavior for students, such as not making assumptions, giving people the benefit of the doubt, and holding one another (and ourselves) accountable.

Collective Buy-In

Invite the class to collectively brainstorm class ground rules for discussions on diversity. With the inclusion of voices from the entire class, there can be an increased sense of ownership for students. Ground rules can include reminders about confidentiality, not ascribing intent, and not relying on minority students to represent their community. These ground rules can then be referred to throughout the semester when necessary.

Racial microaggressions often trigger difficult conversations in the classroom because they either offend students of color or challenge others to feel accused of being racist.[28] However, if these situations are handled skillfully, they can result in opportunities for growth, improved communication, and learning.[29,30] As classrooms become increasingly diverse, the opportunities for microaggressions and difficult dialogues on race and other topics also increase. Mastering the skill of difficult conversations, as both a speaker and a listener, requires patience, openness, forgiveness, resilience, courage, and time. For faculty feeling overwhelmed at the prospect of facilitating these discussions, there are specific things to do to enter dialogues with compassion and courage. In our own experience as faculty, we have found the following three critical components.

First, allow students to see faculty as vulnerable and open to feedback when we make mistakes or assumptions.[31,32,33] As we have repeatedly emphasized, faculty must acknowledge their vulnerability to biases and fears regarding diversity. By doing so, they can be freed of the constant need to defend against being labeled racist, sexist, or against any other group.[34] Doing so also sets an example for students to follow when seeking open and honest dialogue and participation.

Second, be willing to temporarily suspend one's own beliefs and worldviews in order to entertain, without judgment, others' beliefs and viewpoints.[35] This will require active listening (listening with one's whole heart),[36] followed by rephrasing (restating an individual's concerns using different words). These actions not only help assure student(s) that they have been heard, but they also help to provide clarity to both sides involved in the conversation.[37]

Third, do not rely on students of color, LGBT students, or other disadvantaged groups to speak for their particular identity. While some students are willing to step into this role, it is up to faculty to educate themselves beyond their respective topic(s) of expertise in order to include diverse perspectives in the syllabus in a thoughtful and coherent manner.

Continuing Education

Logically, faculty and administrators who may be feeling overwhelmed at the thought of opening up conversations about race and difference in the classroom may ask how to develop these so-called soft skills. We have found that ongoing opportunities for faculty to talk with one another and to experience facilitating difficult dialogues, particularly on race, are key to developing a culture within the school where these critical conversations, however difficult, are seen as the norm. At our institution, this has included ongoing education and training through faculty development opportunities, including open discussions about classroom experiences, specific anti-bias training, classroom consultations for faculty who are apprehensive about approaching these conversations, and providing faculty with resources for navigating difficult conversations. Carter et al. report that developing a self-understanding is a critical component of faculty development.[38] That is, faculty must begin to see and understand themselves as racial and cultural beings in order to assist others in difficult dialogue.

Experiential Learning

Others have argued that it is critical for educators themselves to have a lived reality outside of classrooms involving interaction and dialogue with people who differ in race, culture, and ethnicity in real-life settings and situations, such as within minority communities or through public forums.[39] Given that many public health faculty members engage in community-based research and work in diverse communities, many in our community already have these lived experiences. Faculty should, however, also be provided with ongoing opportunities to interact with those different from themselves—just as we encourage our students through their practicum placements, public health faculty should also continually engage with diverse communities.

After Class

In the aftermath of a difficult conversation, it is important to take the time to consider the experience (rather than sweep it under the rug) and to glean as many useful lessons as possible from the experience. Faculty often feel constrained by limited time allotted in each semester and, specifically, in each class session. We have lots of material to get through, so the thought of pausing or spending classroom time to reflect on past experiences is initially undesirable. Nevertheless, it can be well worth the time and effort to rearrange lesson plans to accommodate continued discussion and learning.

Reflect

Allow students—and yourself—to debrief through shared journaling. This activity can be facilitated outside of class time through a discussion board or similar feature in online course management systems such as Blackboard. It is important to set ground rules for conduct at the outset. It is also important to focus the feedback by asking students to respond to specific prompts.

Rework and Revisit

Emerging themes from a debrief can be addressed during future class sessions, allowing greater preparation for appropriate response. The time between classes, as well as the feedback from student reflections, can be used to shape the narrative for a future class (or classes). The class schedule should be updated to revisit the discussion, with the appropriate tools, materials, and preparation, so that the original learning objectives are met while addressing the difficult topic.

Conclusion

Difficult conversations are just that—difficult. They are also unavoidable. Most faculty will experience at least one difficult classroom conversation during their career. These conversations often center around race but can involve any number of social statuses, including gender, sexual identity, and class. They are most often triggered not out of malice but through microaggressions or misunderstandings. Whatever the stimulus, these discussions must be, and can be, handled skillfully by faculty. Most importantly, faculty must recognize that they often have all the necessary tools to successfully navigate these conversations. Where this is not the case, our hope is that this chapter has provided the reader with a starting point for developing a road map for pursuing this important work.

REFERENCES

1. American Public Health Association. "What Is Public Health?" https://www .apha.org/what-is-public-health (accessed December 28, 2017).

2. Commission on Social Determinants of Health. "Closing the Gap in a Generation: Health Equity through Action on the Social Determinants of Health. Final Report of the Commission on Social Determinants of Health." Geneva, Switzerland: World Health Organization, 2008. http://www.who.int/social _determinants/final_report/csdh_finalreport_2008.pdf (accessed December 31, 2017).

3. Council on Education for Public Health. "Home." https://ceph.org (accessed December 31, 2017).

4. Associated Schools and Programs of Public Health. "Study." https://www .aspph.org/study (accessed December 31, 2017).

5. Carter S. P., M. Honeyford, D. McKaskie, F. Guthrie, S. Mahoney, and G. D. Carter. "What Do You Mean by Whiteness?" *College Student Affairs Journal* 26 (2007): 152–159.

6. Sue, D. W., A. I. Lin, G. C. Torino, C. M. Capodilupo, and D. P. Rivera. "Racial Microaggressions and Difficult Dialogues on Race in the Classroom." *Cultural Diversity and Ethnic Minority Psychology* 15, no. 2 (2009): 183–190.

7. Sue et al., "Racial Microaggressions and Difficult Dialogues on Race in the Classroom."

8. Trent, S. "We Can Talk about Race without Fighting or Getting Defensive, if We're Willing to Learn How." *Washington Post.* May 18, 2015. https://www .washingtonpost.com/news/inspired-life/wp/2015/03/09/why-americans-fear -talking-about-race-and-how-you-can-lead-the-way/?utm_term=.05cb9e968a49.

9. The Foundation for Accountability and the Robert Wood Johnson Foundation. "A Portrait of the Chronically Ill in America." 2001. http://research.policyarchive .org/95521.pdf (accessed December 31, 2017).

10. Agency for Healthcare Research and Quality. National Healthcare Quality and Disparities Report Chartbook on Rural Health Care. Rockville, MD: October 2017. AHRQ Pub. No. 17(18)-0001-2-EF. www.ahrq.gov/research/findings/nhqrdr/index .html (accessed November 18, 2018).

11. National Center for Health Statistics. "Health, United States, 2016." Washington, DC: US Department of Health and Human Services, 2016. https://www.cdc.gov /nchs/data/hus/hus16.pdf (accessed December 31, 2017).

12. Aday, L. A. "Who Are the Vulnerable?" In *At Risk in America: The Health and Health Care Needs of Vulnerable Populations in the United* States, 2nd Edition. San Francisco: Jossey-Bass, 1991.

13. Healthy People 2020. "Public Health Infrastructure." US Department of Health and Human Services: Office of Disease Prevention and Health Promotion. https://www.healthypeople.gov/2020/topics-objectives/topic/public-health-infra structure (accessed April 7, 2018).

14. The Foundation for Accountability and the Robert Wood Johnson Foundation, "A Portrait of the Chronically Ill in America."

15. Mau, W. C. J. "Characteristics of US Students That Pursued a STEM Major and Factors That Predicted Their Persistence in Degree Completion." *Universal Journal of Educational Research* 4, no. 6 (2016): 1495–1500.

16. MacIntosh, P. *White Privilege and Male Privilege: A Personal Account of Coming to See Correspondences through Work in Women's Studies.* Wellesley, MA: Wellesley College, Center for Research on Women, 1988.

17. Sue, D. W. "MicroAggressions: More Than Just Race." *Psychology Today Blog.* November 17, 2010. https://www.psychologytoday.com/blog/microaggres sions-in-everyday-life/201011/microaggressions-more-just-race.

18. Sue, "MicroAggressions."

19. Sue et al., "Racial Microaggressions and Difficult Dialogues on Race in the Classroom."

20. Sue, "MicroAggressions."

21. Young, G. "Dealing with Difficult Classroom Dialogues." In *Teaching Gender and Multicultural Awareness*, edited by P. Bronstein and K. Quina, 337–360. Washington, DC: American Psychological Association, 2003.

22. Sue et al., "Racial Microaggressions and Difficult Dialogues on Race in the Classroom."

23. Desmond, M., and M. Emirbayer. *Racial Domination, Racial Progress: The Sociology of Race in America.* New York: McGraw-Hill, 2010.

24. Hoffman, K. M., S. Trawalter, J. R. Axt, and N. Oliver. "Racial Bias in Pain Assessment and Treatment Recommendations, and False Beliefs about Biological Differences between Blacks and Whites." *Proceedings of the National Academy of Sciences of the United States of America* 113, no. 16 (2016): 4296–4301.

25. Hoffman et al., "Racial Bias in Pain Assessment and Treatment Recommendations, and False Beliefs about Biological Differences between Blacks and Whites."

26. Cole, L. W., and S. R. Foster. *From the Ground Up: Environmental Racism and the Rise of the Environmental Justice Movement.* New York: New York University Press, 2001.

27. Farmer, P. "An Anthropology of Structural Violence." *Current Anthropology* 45, no. 3 (2004): 305–325.

28. Constantine, M. G., and D. W. Sue. "Perceptions of Racial Microaggressions among Black Supervisees in Cross-Racial Dyads." *Journal of Counseling Psychology* 54, no. 2 (2007): 124–153.

29. Young, "Dealing with Difficult Classroom Dialogues," in Bronstein and Quina, *Teaching Gender and Multicultural Awareness.*

30. Sue et al., "Racial Microaggressions and Difficult Dialogues on Race in the Classroom."

31. Sue et al., "Racial Microaggressions and Difficult Dialogues on Race in the Classroom."

32. Sue, D. W. *Overcoming Our Racism: The Journey to Liberation.* San Francisco: Jossey-Bass, 2003.

33. Young, "Dealing with Difficult Classroom Dialogues," in Bronstein and Quina, *Teaching Gender and Multicultural Awareness.*

34. Sue, *Overcoming Our Racism.*

35. Robbins, S. L. *What If? Short Stories to Spark Diversity Dialogue.* Boston: Davies-Black (Nicholas Brealey Publishing), 2009.

36. Fernandez, C. P. "Managing the Difficult Conversation." *Journal of Public Health Practice* 14, no. 3 (2008): 317–319.

37. Fernandez, "Managing the Difficult Conversation."

38. Carter, "What Do You Mean by Whiteness?"

39. Sue, *Overcoming Our Racism.*

[21]

Public Health Education and Service Learning

DANIEL GERBER AND JEN DOLAN

S ERVICE LEARNING is defined as "a teaching and learning strategy that integrates meaningful community service with instruction and reflection to enrich the learning experience, teach civic responsibility and strengthen communities."[1] Service learning is much more than "just volunteering." It is a teaching tool that helps the instructor facilitate the learning of the course material. Unfortunately, when students say, "I came to college to learn," they often equate learning with lectures or textbooks. And while lectures and textbook learning are still the dominant ways in which we transfer knowledge in higher education, this kind of pedagogy can be deeply enhanced if the professor also uses other teaching tools, such as service learning. For example, students can learn about a current public health problem from a lecture, articles, or a textbook, but the learning is greatly enriched if students are able to observe health problems in a real-world setting, discuss the problem with the people who are actually experiencing it, and, when possible, help with solutions. That is public health service learning.

Why would a public health professor want to include a service learning component in their course? And what does the professor want their students to learn from the service learning project? The overall goal for any public health service learning course is to bring to life the theory and knowledge students are learning in the classroom in order for them to have a deeper understanding and appreciation for today's current health problems, the communities that experience them, and to then pose possible solutions. An important corollary is that students learn about themselves as future public health professionals.

There are different ways of designing and implementing service learning in courses, but Kolb's experiential learning cycle[2] is an excellent model for integrating a service learning project into a course.[3,4] The experiential learning cycle is implemented as follows:

1 Experiencing or concrete experience: the student participates in an experience (e.g., the professor explains what the service learning project is, someone from the community partner visits the class to explain who they are and about the community the students are going to be entering, the students make their first visit to the service learning site)

2 Reflection or reflective observation: the student reflects on this experience (e.g., the student is asked, What is your understanding or experience with the health problem or community and what are your thoughts about the service learning project, guest speakers, or visits to the service learning site?)

3 Thinking or abstract conceptualization: additional information is given to the student to help them understand the service learning project, the community the service learning project is taking place in, or their experience or role with the project (e.g., the student is given readings on the health problem that is to be addressed, the community they are entering, and any programs that already exist that are trying to solve the health problem)

4 Applying or active experimentation: the student is asked to reflect on the readings and how this new knowledge enhances or changes their thinking. This cycle is repeated over and over again as the students become more involved with the service learning project. Having students internalize their thoughts, feelings, and attitudes through reflection of their new experiences and knowledge deepens their learning and assists them in becoming more experienced and competent public health professionals.[5]

How to Begin Developing a Service Learning Component

The biggest issue in developing a service learning component is finding a community partner organization that is engaging in a current health problem that is connected to the course content and is willing to work with students on a service learning project. The good news from a curricular point of view is that there are more health problems to solve than we have solutions. Additionally, partner organizations need not be a "public health institution" such as the local health department. Many nonprofit organizations are working on solving today's health problems. Regardless of the industry or section, the partner organization must be accessible for students and have a role for students to be involved. These two components are vital for success. Finding appropriate organizations and building partnerships up front is the most important aspect of achieving a successful service learning component for the course. To begin to design a service learning course, the professor needs to ask two core questions.

First, what organizations are working on the health problem that is covered in the course and is within, at most, a 30-minute drive from campus? There are times when the organization is farther away, and consequently, the organization sends a representative to the class and the students work on the service learning project remotely. Without additional support such as appropriate technology, these service learning experiences can have limited learning potential.

Second, which organizations have successfully utilized student volunteers in the past? This does not mean that faculty cannot approach organizations that have never worked with student volunteers, but utilizing students well and giving them a worthwhile experience is a skill that some organizations have mastered.

How Do You Build Meaningful Community Partnerships?

Once an appropriate organization is identified, the professor begins a discussion with that organization about using a group of students to assist with a specific project. This discussion has two objectives. The first objective is to identify a project that the students can do where they will have a real-life understanding and appreciation of a current health problem, possible solutions, and the community with whom the partner organization works. The second objective is to ensure that the partner organization benefits by working with the students. In many instances, the community partner's staff feel an additional benefit in the satisfaction of helping students learn. These community partner staff see themselves, and rightly so, as field experts. We call these collaborations "community partnerships" to emphasize the mutual benefits to both parties through the partnership. Examples of potential projects include researching a health problem for the community partner or assisting with organizing or running a specific event.

University and college outreach programs have been around for decades. Outreach refers to situations where faculty or staff of higher education institutions go into communities to offer their expertise in support of a community project or initiative. More recently, the term "engagement" is replacing the term "outreach." Engagement conveys a reciprocal relationship, and this is very important in a service learning course. The community partner must benefit from the students working on something worthwhile while the higher education institution benefits by students receiving a real-world learning experience that deepens their classroom learning. Consequently, labeling service learning projects as engaged programs emphasizes that all partners are giving and receiving something of value.

Starting the Service Learning Project

Once the professor and the community partner decide on a project for the students, the next big challenge is to prepare the students to enter the community. One of the greatest challenges in service learning projects is overcoming students' preconceived perceptions and attitudes about the community they will engage with. Students are usually not from the community they are going into, and these communities are often very different from the students' home communities. At our university, most of the students are white and grew up in suburbia, whereas the communities where we usually implement service learning projects are nearby urban communities comprised of majority black or Latinx residents of lower economic status. These differences make for an incredible learning opportunity for the students, but without proper preparation, the service learning project can be negative for both the students and the community. Students too often enter a different community with ill-conceived perceptions and stereotypes. One criticism of service learning that has emerged in the literature in the past few years is that service learning groups many times fail to recognize the intersectional societal aspects they are dealing with.[6] Preparing students to enter a community different than their own means educating them beforehand about the rich cultural differences of the community and helping them become aware of their own preconceived perceptions and attitudes about the community and the role of an outsider coming in to "help" the community.

One way to begin to address this challenge is by providing the students with readings that describe life in the community they are entering or inviting someone from the community into the classroom to talk about the community. Readings or a guest speaker talking about what they love about their community and about its struggles allows students to see the community as a place where people live their lives with problems but also with the joys of everyday life.

Time management is another challenge that must be addressed before the service learning course begins. Classes are run on a semester or trimester basis, and community projects are not. Implementing a worthwhile service learning project has its own timeline, which may not fit a semester schedule. The importance of up-front planning between the service learning partner and the professor teaching the course is crucial. Even with the best planning, the project is being implemented in the real world, and sometimes things just happen. The professor, the students, and the community partner must work closely together to adjust accordingly.

Developing and Accessing Goals

The overall goal for any public health service learning course is to bring to life the theory and knowledge that is being taught in class to deepen understanding and appreciation for today's current health problems and solutions. A second goal is ensuring that students understand and appreciate the communities they enter and the roles they have to play as future public health professionals. Assessing the overall goal can be accomplished by having students investigate and write papers explaining the current research on the health problem and any solutions that have been posed. The second goal is harder to teach and to assess. One approach to deepen learning and as a means of assessment is through journaling. Weekly or biweekly reflection papers can focus on what students find important about what they are learning in class, what they are learning from their reading assignments, and how their experiences in the service learning project are enhancing their learning. The key is having students reflect on what it all means to them as a future public health professional.

The third goal is successfully achieving a service learning project that the community partner finds worthwhile to their mission. This goal has two parts. The first is in the successful implementation of the project. The second is in the time and energy put into the project. Ideally, the students put more time and energy into the service learning project than do the staff in managing the students. Students must be an asset to the community partner and not a burden to the community partner's staff by requiring too much supervision. Consequently, it is important for the professor to have periodic check-ins with staff at the partner organization to assess progress on project implementation and management. This can be achieved with regular phone calls or emails, but it is important that the professor reaches out and periodically checks in so that adjustments can be made, as needed.

A Case Study of Two Public Health Service Learning Courses

In the previous sections, an overview of how to design and implement a service learning course was offered. In this section, the approach outlined earlier is applied to a case study in which we describe the classes that were taught, how the service learning component was applied, what worked, what challenges emerged, and provide recommendations for improvements.

At a large university in New England, undergraduate students have the opportunity to participate in a university service learning certificate program that consists of a series of four public health courses over the course of two years. The two second-year courses are upper-level health policy and community development public health courses. The start of the second year of the program invariably brings a new community of students to the class, with some knowing one another and some not. Believing that students knowing one another creates a healthier learning environment, the professor makes it a point to engage in various team-building exercises at the start of the fall semester.[7] Once relationships have been established or at least initiated, the learning commences on a deeper level than might have happened otherwise.[8]

Because Kolb's experiential learning cycle in the classroom asks students to share their personal views and experiences, creating a safe classroom environment is important. One way this happens is at the start of each class, everyone has a chance to share how they are feeling, report anything interesting they are doing, or share something they are struggling with. This is an important way for students to bring their whole selves to the class.

As with any class, the goal of the service learning component is to bring to life the theory and knowledge that is being taught in class in order to deepen the understanding of the course content. In both health policy and community development courses, students read many articles and case studies, but they can only learn so much through passive involvement in their education. Having guest speakers speak directly to course topics being covered and offer practical real-world experience and knowledge about these topics is a good start, but it is still a passive learning experience. Active learning begins with the students traveling off campus into a community to learn and implement the service learning project. Ideally, students start working at their service learning site by the first or second week of the semester, and is the beginning of Kolb's cycle—experiencing. The course readings and writing assignments are structured as part of Kolb's experiential learning cycle (reflective and thinking), and meanwhile the students get involved with their community partners as soon as possible (again, the experiencing phase). The professor designed each of the courses to have a final research paper associated with issues the community partners were addressing. Each student and their on-site supervisor worked together to come up with a project that was meaningful and beneficial to the organization and also fit the scope of the class research paper. An example of this coordination was a student who was working at an organization that offers services for those who are struggling financially. This organization offers meals, a secondhand store, food distribution, and, more recently, a free medical clinic. A number of university students volunteer at the facility because there are many different volunteer options in close proximity to the university. One student was particularly interested in the free dental program that was offered. Although the dentist was only on-site twice a month, the student made it a point to get to know her and made her class research paper about dental insurance for the poor. The dentist was very willing to engage with the student and shared the concerns she had with health insurance as it relates to dental care. This student also talked with many of the patients and learned how difficult it is for them to get access to dental care. She heard firsthand that it is nearly impossible for young children to pay attention in school and be successful if they are distracted by the pain of a toothache. At a class-sponsored, daylong visit to the State House, the student was able to meet with state legislators and share the issues that she witnessed at her service site in regard to dental care. The legislators were eager to talk with her and seemed sincere in their desire to change the current policy so that access to dental care, especially for those under 18, would be barrier-free. During the ride home from the State House, the professor could see how proud the student felt knowing that her efforts that day might someday lead to better dental care and better futures for young children.

The university where these two service learning courses are taught does not have a set number of hours that translate to course credits. The courses are four credits and generally involve between 36 and 65 hours per semester for the service learning project. The professor initially decided that 60 hours would be the number of hours to be completed in order for the students to have a good experience and have sufficient time for the community partner to benefit. The challenge was that not all community partners had 60 hours of work. Thus, the hours were subsequently revised to 45 hours, which was more manageable for both student and the community partner. Service learning is not about counting hours, yet students compare experiences so there must be a degree of equity regarding the amount of time worked outside class when credits are awarded.

Benefits for Students and Partner Organizations

Students and partner organizations benefit in numerous ways by actively engaging in their learning. For example, a student who was working in the children's room at a shelter for battered women decided to test the theory she learned in another course. She put a puppet on her hand and started "talking" to a child. Much to her surprise, delight, and fear, the child started discussing some of the abuse he witnessed at home. The supervisor was close by and was able to follow up with the child. Without the hands-on experience, the student would never have known firsthand how effective the written theory actually might be.

College students are in a unique position in that they are generally viewed as adults but are not so old that younger students cannot relate to them. College students are often in a position of being positive role models for their younger clients. Organizations that have young children as their primary clients are able to truly benefit from the involvement of service learning courses such as Big Brothers Big Sisters. Other programs, such as the Boys and Girls Club and Girls Inc., that offer academic tutoring services are able to provide their clients not only with tutors but also service learning students that their clients can relate to (assuming the student mirrors the community they are serving). The young children can look at their tutor and hopefully think, "He looks like me, he is from my community, and he is going to college. Maybe I will be able to go to college, too."

Service learning is a form of engaged learning that can have a high impact on students' learning.[9] It allows information to move from working memory to long-term memory.[10] Students retain information much longer if it is learned through an active experience such as a service learning project. Additionally, public health courses in particular provide students, professors, and community partners the opportunity to address real-life health issues that not only can be incredible learning experiences for the students but an opportunity to afford community partners additional help to address the public health needs of the community.

REFERENCES

1. National Service-Learning Clearing House. https://gsn.nylc.org/clearinghouse (accessed April 10, 2018).

2. Petkus, E. "A Theoretical and Practical Framework for Service-Learning in Marketing: Kolb's Experiential Learning Cycle." *Journal of Marketing Education* 22, no. 1 (2000): 64–70.

3. Eyler, J. "Reflection: Linking Service and Learning—Linking Students and Communities." *Journal of Social Issues* 58, no. 3 (2002): 517–534.

4. Eyler, J., D. Giles, and A. Schmiede. *A Practitioner's Guide to Reflection in Service Learning.* Nashville, TN: Vanderbilt University, 1996.

5. Zull, J. *From Brain to Mind.* Sterling, VA: Stylus Publishing, 2011.

6. Mitchell, T. "Teaching Community On and Off Campus: An Intersectional Approach to Community Engagement." *New Directions for Student Services* 157 (2017): 35–44.

7. Quay, S., and R. Quaglia. "Creating a Classroom Culture That Inspires Student Learning." *Teaching Professor* 18, no. 2 (2004): 1–5.

8. National Service-Learning Clearing House. https://gsn.nylc.org/clearinghouse (accessed April 10, 2018).

9. NSSEville State University. "NSSE 2016 High-Impact Practices." 2016. http://nsse.indiana.edu/2016_Institutional_Report/pdf/NSSE16%20High -Impact%20Practices%20(NSSEville%20State).pdf (accessed April 10, 2018).

10. Zull, *From Brain to Mind*.

22

Technology in Teaching

WAYNE LAMORTE AND KATHLEEN RYAN

EDUCATION HAS BENEFITED from technology for many centuries. At first, formal education consisted primarily of regularly scheduled lectures, during which a professor would transmit information to a group of students who could take notes if they had the means. Paper and writing implements were initially crude and expensive, but other technological advances slowly made them more accessible.

Scribes were the only means for reproducing texts until the invention of the printing press around 1440. Printing presses were abundant throughout Europe by 1500 and greatly facilitated the ability to disseminate information. However, the inability of the instructor to present problems, diagrams, or ideas to the entire class simultaneously was a major limitation until large slabs of slate were introduced to the classroom in about 1801. In the 1960s, green chalkboards were introduced, which had the advantages of being more durable, more pleasing to the eye, and easier to see after erasure. Most recently, we have dry-erase boards, electronic whiteboards, and slide and video presentations.

Lecturing, the taking of notes, and readings from textbooks have been the mainstays of formal education for several centuries, and these continue to have value as learning activities. Lecturing continues to be an effective method for transmitting information, but it is not the most effective method for promoting student thought, changing attitudes, or teaching behavioral skills. Brown and Long concluded: "Over the past two decades, a great deal of research has focused on how people learn. Previously, teaching was most often a kind of 'broadcast' of course content at regularly scheduled intervals, from an expert to student 'receivers.' The learning literature agrees that learning can be enhanced, deepened, and made more meaningful if the curriculum makes the learners active participants through interactivity, multiple roles (such as listener, critic, mentor, presenter), and social engagement (such as group work, discussion boards, wikis)."[1]

Technological innovations have provided us with an ever-increasing array of additional tools that can facilitate learning when they are utilized thoughtfully and appropriately. Technology in teaching is not an end; it is a series of newer tools that can help our students achieve learning goals.[2]

Finding Time to Incorporate Teaching Technology to Foster Active Learning

Effective teaching requires both the transmission of content and thoughtfully designed opportunities for students to actively use information, concepts, and methods to discuss, debate, and solve problems. However, instructors are often reluctant to use classroom time for active learning for fear that it takes up too much time and will prevent them from covering all of the necessary content. Ideally, one must find an appropriate balance between information transmission and active learning. One useful solution proposed by Fink is to thoughtfully design courses with an integration of in-class learning activities and out-of-class activities, as illustrated in figure 22.1.[3,4]

With this approach, the instructor can take advantage of educational technology to provide content and active learning exercises before, during, and after live classroom sessions. When some course content is provided outside of class, through readings, online modules, videos, or podcasts, it creates opportunities to incorporate active learning during class time while still preserving time for minilectures and explanations. Given the broad and multidisciplinary nature of public health, the specific teaching tools that one chooses will vary depending on the subject and the goals of each specific class or learning activity.

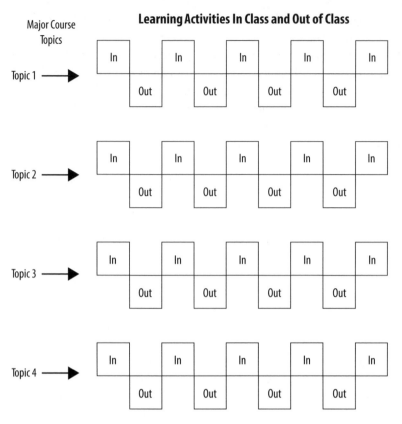

Figure 22.1. Integration of In-Class Learning Activities with Out-of-Class Activities. During a semester, each of the major topics covered in the course should be addressed with an orderly sequence of coordinated learning activities that take place inside and outside the classroom. Adapted from figure 9 in L. Dee Fink, "A Self-Directed Guide to Designing Courses for Significant Learning." https://www.deefinkandassociates.com/GuidetoCourseDesignAug05.pdf.

Key Questions

The key questions to consider for any particular learning activity are:

- What are the learning objectives?
- What are the best teaching methods and teaching tools to employ to achieve those learning objectives?
- How can we, as teachers, achieve clarity and engage and inspire our students?

- How can we best help our students not only to acquire factual knowledge but also to build analytical and critical-thinking skills, the ability to research and weigh alternatives, and the ability to work collaboratively?

Addressing these key questions is best achieved through an appropriate mix of learning activities and teaching methods tailored to the learning objectives for each lesson. In the remainder of this chapter, we discuss some of the available technologies that we have found most useful for teaching students of public health.

Selected Teaching Technologies

Learning Management Systems

Our institution uses Blackboard as its learning management system (LMS), but many other excellent systems exist (e.g., Canvas, Desire2Learn, Sakai, Moodle) and provide similar functions. Several common features, outlined in the following sections, are particularly valuable to almost all courses.

Organization of Course Content
LMSs offer the opportunity to post course content (syllabus, slides, documents, etc.), which often forces the instructor to organize material in a logical fashion.

Communication
LMSs allow the instructor to send announcements to all students, selected groups, or individual students. It is frustrating to students when they are stuck on a difficult concept, and email is a quick, easy way of alleviating this. If one or more students send emails on a difficult concept, the instructor might send a thoughtful response to the entire class. These responses can be saved in a "Discussion Forum" that becomes an archive of frequently asked questions that can be made available in subsequent semesters.

Discussion Boards and Blogs
LMSs provide the option of creating online discussions. For example, the instructor can require students to contribute to a discussion of a

controversial topic and to comment on posts from other students, encouraging them to engage and share their thoughts on complex questions or concepts.

Accessibility and Mobile Learning

The content in LMSs can be accessed any time from any device with an internet connection, which is greatly appreciated by students.

Teams and Groups

LMSs facilitate the creation of student groups or teams and provide them with communication and collaboration tools.

Online Quizzes

LMSs generally provide a means of creating quizzes that can be utilized for formative or summative assessments using a variety of question types. Many systems provide automatic grading and feedback, although open-ended questions need to be graded by the instructor or teaching assistants. A particular favorite of ours is the calculated numeric question type available in Blackboard, which asks the student to solve a problem and submit a numeric answer for which the instructor can set an acceptable range. The instructor also has a number of options for providing brief or detailed feedback.

Another attractive feature available in Blackboard is the ability to create pools of questions on a topic, and then the system creates quizzes or tests that draw a specified number of questions from the pool at random. This provides a way to create formative assessments to promote mastery learning by choosing options that allow students to take a quiz for a given topic multiple times without getting the same questions each time.

Slide Presentations

Slide presentations are not new; increasingly sophisticated methods for projecting text, images, animations, and videos have been used for decades. In a sense, they represent an extension of the chalkboard in that they provide a means of displaying information and images to many students simultaneously.

Many educators deplore the use of PowerPoint because of the tendency for many presenters to write out a talk and then convert it to a series of slides with bullet points that are read to the audience. But it does not need to be this way. When the audience is presented with text on a slide, the natural tendency is to read the text at the expense of listening to the speaker. This practice should be condemned, but PowerPoint or similar systems are well suited to presenting images, diagrams, tables, problems, discussion questions, short embedded videos and podcasts, and animations that can effectively illustrate concepts and present case studies that catalyze in-class discussions. The keys to effective use of slides are to avoid using bullet points as a crutch, to minimize text, and to use images and graphs to convey concepts.

Note-taking has merit for promoting listening, but some instructors post slides before class to diminish the need to take copious notes, allowing students to focus on the discussion and make thoughtful annotations, rather than furiously trying to transcribe.

Videos

A picture can say a thousand words, and well-done videos can say much more. The combination of auditory and visual displays can be engaging, bring concepts to life, and ultimately improve retention. Videos can also present case studies that bring real-world examples into the classroom to stimulate discussion. The key is to find or create brief (three to six minutes is ideal), high-quality videos that effectively explain concepts, ideas, or cases.

Many excellent video clips are available from public health organizations such as the Centers for Disease Control and Prevention and sites such as YouTube, but finding high-quality videos that align with learning objectives can be challenging. Educational videos should be closed-captioned to provide access to hearing-impaired students, although hearing students often also prefer closed-captions. Videos on professional or educational sites generally have accurate captioning, but other sites (e.g., YouTube) generate automated captioning, which often has many errors.

Screen Capture Software

A number of software packages (e.g., Camtasia, QuickTime, Echo360 Personal Capture, Kaltura, Movavi, Adobe Presenter, and Explain Everything) make it possible for instructors to create their own educational videos, which can be shown in class or uploaded to an LMS such as Blackboard, Sakai, or Moodle. With some screen capture packages, it is even possible to embed quiz questions into videos to make them more interactive. There are two general strategies. First, when the goal is to explain a concept or summarize a teaching segment, it is useful to create a sequence of illustrative slides using PowerPoint or Keynote along with a thoughtful script for the narration. The screen is recorded in slide mode, moving from slide to slide while reading the script, which keeps the presentation on track, resulting in a more professional product. The script can also be posted as a text file to improve accessibility. Second, when the goal is to illustrate how to use a software package, such as Excel, again a script can be written and followed as the screen capture software is used to record actions that are taken with the software package.

Recording Classroom Session

There are several methods for recording classroom sessions (e.g., digital camera or Echo360 Lecture Capture), but instructors are divided on the benefit of recording and posting classroom sessions. Some argue that recording and posting recorded lectures may discourage class attendance, although this is less of a problem when classes include active learning exercises. Potential benefits for recording and posting class sessions include: (1) students do not have to transcribe lectures, which is especially useful for nonnative English speakers; (2) students are able to review difficult material and clarify their notes; (3) some students will use them for exam review; and (4) students absent due to illness, religious observance, or inclement weather can review class proceedings.

Before recording classroom sessions, students must be alerted about the recording. It is best practice to capture audio and video of just the instructor and screen to avoid privacy issues. Students need to know if they are being recorded, and some institutions require formal consent. Recording discussions around sensitive topics is particularly problematic. It is also advisable to edit recordings before posting them in order to delete dead space or errors.

Audience Response Systems

Audience response systems consist of a receiver on the instructor's computer and polling devices ("clickers") that the students use to respond to questions that are posed. Software enables the instructor to create polling questions (e.g., multiple-choice, true-false, numeric) before a session, and then to display them at intervals during a classroom session. Most systems enable polling questions to be integrated with PowerPoint for convenient display of the question and the summarized results. Students respond to questions by pressing buttons on the polling device. When the instructor closes polling for a given question, the software summarizes the responses and displays the summary visually.

There are now many options for conducting electronic polling in the classroom or during online classes. Institutions can purchase and license systems with dedicated polling devices, or students can purchase or rent the polling devices. Polling systems enable instructors to register devices to specific students, providing the ability to track responses and attendance; however, many instructors and students prefer anonymous polling because it encourages risk-free participation. Other systems have become available, for which students use their phone as a polling device after installing an app, although many instructors discourage any use of cell phones in the classroom.

Polling systems are popular with students, and they are useful in several ways. They provide breaks in a lecture, during which students can actively participate and gauge their understanding. Students tend to remain more focused if they know that a polling question may be coming. There are several reasons why these systems are appealing. They encourage full participation because students can answer anonymously; they provide the instructor with an immediate way of assessing the extent to which the students are understanding the material; and the results of any questions can be used to generate discussion and clarification. For example, "I see that most of you answered correctly; would one of you be willing to explain why you chose this answer?" or "I see many of you chose a different answer than I did; did you have a different way of thinking about this?" This alerts the instructor to the need to stop and explore misunderstanding and provide clarification.

Online Interactive Learning Modules and Case Studies

There is now widespread acceptance of the importance of incorporating active learning into the classroom, but incorporation of active learning has been impeded largely by the notion that active learning exercises consume a disproportionate amount of classroom time, making it impossible to cover all the material in the syllabus. One solution is to create interactive online learning modules that succinctly present the didactic content for each class. Modules can provide an orchestrated combination of text, images and graphs, embedded videos and podcasts, embedded quiz questions and exercises, hyperlinks to other learning resources, and a wide variety of learning activities. Online modules require the creation of HTML-based web pages, but there are a number of user-friendly software packages that enable an instructor with no programming experience to create very professional learning modules quite easily.

Several instructors at our institution have used SoftChalk software to create interactive web pages that are rigorous in their content, highly interactive, and easy to navigate. Students are required to work through each module before class, and compliance is encouraged by requiring that all students complete a short online preclass quiz with questions that are taken from the module. The modules are engaging and include relevant images, videos, activities, and embedded quiz questions (not for credit) that intermittently test understanding of each section and provide the student immediate feedback.

By requiring students to review each module before class, the instructor can reduce presentation time, allowing more time for discussion of more complex concepts and more time for active learning exercises, questions, and discussion. After each class, students might then complete and submit a more extensive problem set (see section on online quizzes earlier in the chapter).

In addition to allowing more time for active learning and discussion, online learning modules have many benefits. These include that (1) they enable self-paced learning and review at any time; (2) multiple instructors teaching the same course can collaborate in building the modules; (3) using the same modules for multiple sections of a course fosters consistency; (4) learning modules foster integration among courses; (5) corrections, updates, and improvements are easy; (6) learning modules foster student engagement and invite them to explore topics in greater detail through hyperlinks; (7) students come to class better prepared and ask more and better questions; (8) the modules can be accessed any time from any device with an internet connection; (9) modules for introductory courses can be used for review or remediation for higher-level courses; (10) online learning modules can be made accessible to learners across the globe; (11) and online learning modules can provide training for the public health workforce.

In a core epidemiology course, end-of-semester student ratings indicated that 98% of the students strongly agreed (75%) or agreed (23%) that the modules were a significant aid to learning.

Web Conferencing Software

It is beyond the scope of this chapter to discuss distance education (e.g., classes conducted remotely). However, web conferencing software can also enhance face-to-face courses by providing a way to conduct online sessions for office hours or help sessions after hours, to teach a class remotely during inclement weather, to bring guest instructors into the classroom if they are unable to participate in person, or to provide group review sessions.

Active Learning Platforms

Active learning platforms (ALPs), such as Echo360, are comprehensive systems containing elements of many of the technologies described previously. Some of our instructors have begun to use the Echo360 ALP embedded within our LMS. The instructor creates and uploads traditional slides, and from those creates interactive slides within the cloud-based platform to project during class.

During class, students follow along on their own devices (laptop, tablet, smartphone) with the same slide set. In real time, students can take notes and post questions that are linked to specific slides. Short videos and polling questions can be interspersed with the content. After class, the student can view the recording, concurrent with their notes and the questions and responses that are discussed in class.

The platform can stream to allow remote attendance, which is particularly useful during inclement weather. Key advantages of using an ALP include enhanced interaction and communication, real-time analytics on concepts discussed in class, and a convenient method for organizing and archiving content.

ALPs enhance interaction by providing immediate feedback, which allows students to benchmark own performance against peers as a mode of self-assessment. The system also provides analytics showing polling responses and "hot spots" in the class where students were taking notes or marking slides as confusing. We are currently using the analytics to assess student utilization of features and to identify content in need of clarification.

One potential downside of using an ALP is that students need to use an electronic device in class. While it may promote learning, there is also the risk of distraction, although many students are already using devices during class. Engagement with an ALP may actually cut down on recreational device use during class.

Accessibility and Clarity: Universal Design for Learning

The Americans with Disabilities Act (ADA), enacted in 1990, prohibits discrimination against individuals with disabilities in all areas of public life. The purpose of the law is to ensure that people with disabilities have the same rights, access, and opportunities as others, including in education. Vision, hearing, and physical disabilities are the most obvious to consider in education. Audio presentations must be closed-captioned for hearing-impaired learners. Blind learners using screen readers need simple, straightforward navigation and descriptively labeled hyperlinks. Complex images, graphs, and tables should be accompanied by text and audio explanations.

These considerations are important not only for hearing-impaired and blind learners but also for students with less severe limitations that can interfere with learning. For example, students who are not fluent in English and students with dyslexia, color-blindness, or limited ability to use a keyboard or mouse also need to be considered. Universal design for learning embodies a set of principles that go beyond the ADA to try to facilitate access, clarity, and ease of learning for all learners.[5] Learning resources should be designed to meet the learning needs of people with diverse abilities and should ideally accommodate a range of preferences. Learning resources should be clear and intuitive to use. Navigation and interaction should be obvious. Learning activities and assessment questions should be designed to allow the learner to get the wrong answer without a significant penalty, and the learner should be given feedback. Poor color and design choices, difficult navigation, poor organization of information, inadequate size and use of space around headings, text blocks, and interactive elements can all interfere with learning. Resources should be designed responsively, meaning they are optimized to operate in different digital environments (e.g., smartphones, desktops, laptops, tablets) and, when possible, outside of a digital environment (e.g., downloadable and printable hard copies).

Conclusion

There is now an abundance of new technology tools available for teaching—far too many for most of us to master. Instead of trying to master all these tools, the most useful approach is to become adept at using selected methods that are best suited to your courses, your skills, and your teaching style.

Teaching technology is not a panacea, nor an end. Instead, teaching technology should be viewed as an aid to promote learning when used thoughtfully and appropriately.

REFERENCES

1. Brown, M., and P. Long. "Trends in Learning Space Design." In *Learning Spaces*, edited by D. G. Oblinger, 9.1-9.11. Louisville, CO: EDUCASE, 2006.

2. US Department of Education. "Use of Technology in Teaching and Learning." https://www.ed.gov/oii-news/use-technology-teaching-and-learning (accessed April 10, 2018).

3. Fink, L. D. *Creating Significant Learning Experiences—An Integrated Approach to Designing College Courses.* San Francisco: Jossey Bass, 2003.

4. Fink, L. D. "A Self-Directed Guide to Designing Courses for Significant Learning." https://www.deefinkandassociates.com/GuidetoCourseDesignAug05.pdf (accessed April 10, 2018).

5. Faye, E., and W. LaMorte. "Universal Design: Accessible and Inclusive eLearning." Boston University. http://sphweb.bumc.bu.edu/otlt/MPH-Modules/UniversalDesign/ (accessed April 10, 2018).

23

Teaching Support, Training, and Supporting Teaching Assistants

GREG EVANS AND RACHEL SCHWARTZ

W ITH THE GROWTH of programs and schools of public health, especially at the undergraduate level, has come an increased dependence on graduate teaching assistants (GTAs) as members of teaching teams and as instructors of record. GTAs can benefit both graduate and undergraduate students as well as professors in multiple ways, providing additional assistance with everything from basic grading and course preparation to working as instructors of record, tutors, and liaisons between professor and students.[1] They offer new perspectives on content; can develop stronger connections with students, who are closer to them in age; and bring familiarity with technology and cultural references that can be of use to faculty. GTAs also benefit professionally, whether they complete a doctorate and go on to work in academia, continue in field research and application, or work in public health practice. Through their teaching experience, GTAs develop skills such as communication, leadership, and content.[2]

There are, however, challenges in GTA engagement. Research in multiple disciplines indicates that graduate students are often thrown into classroom settings without adequate training, and that they report feeling unprepared for the task. In most cases, these GTAs will simply replicate the teaching styles they experienced as undergraduates, often relying on lectures and standard testing formats. Given that the courses supported or taught by GTAs are often gateway courses that may determine whether undergraduate or graduate students continue in the field, it is crucial that GTAs employ evidence-based, pedagogically sound methods designed to engage students on a variety of levels, to address issues of cultural diversity, and to develop a professional skill set.[3]

In order to respond to the lack of GTA training, some schools of public health have developed tailored training programs for their GTAs, ranging from programs that run for a few weeks and provide basic pedagogical techniques to credit-bearing semester-long or yearlong courses dedicated to developing a broad range of teaching skills, understanding pedagogical theory, and producing a variety of course materials.[4,5,6,7] We recognize that while such training is often preferable, most schools cannot devote the resources or the credit hours they call for and may, in fact, have success in training GTAs using a less costly or time-consuming approach.

We present a GTA training program that is more practical and realistic for many schools, taking into account limitations on time and resources. And while ideally every GTA would be trained beyond the recommended minimums laid out here, the presence of an experienced and dedicated mentor/supervisor can fill in many gaps. We note that depending on class size, funding, and availability of GTAs, some classes might have two or more GTAs, while others have only one. Ideally, in the case of multiple GTAs, senior GTAs could mentor new GTAs and work together as a teaching team.

For such a model to work, it is necessary to invest in support and resources for mentors/supervisors, such as basic mentorship training, access to pedagogical materials, and opportunities to discuss their experiences with other mentors/supervisors. In addition, the school may consider recognition—perhaps in the form of buy-out or credit for service—to accommodate the extra responsibilities of the mentor/supervisor.

The mentor relationship need not be restricted to that between the supervisor and the GTA. In fact, GTA2s (second-semester GTAs) who have been through the process of GTA training can serve as supplemental mentors to peers and undergraduate students and can offer recommendations regarding a variety of teaching issues. Often, GTAs will feel more comfortable bringing certain issues to their peers than to faculty supervisors. Moreover, the experience of serving as a GTA2 mentor is a step toward developing the more senior student's own professionalism.

To further reinforce the success of this GTA training process while lightening the load on mentors/supervisors, a GTA course website should be created. This site provides an open discussion board to complement GTA support group meetings. It also includes links to online training in Family Educational Rights and Privacy Act, Title IX, disability services, and other modules available at most universities. Furthermore, the site serves as a centralized online reference library containing links to materials relevant to GTAs. New information could be added by GTAs and mentors, as well as by a library liaison, if available, designated for the purpose of curating and supplementing materials on the site.

Any GTA training program must be carefully calibrated, using a scaffolding process in which skills introduced in the first semester are reinforced and broadened over the course of the GTA's teaching experience. Such an approach ensures that GTAs retain what they have learned and that their skill set grows alongside their responsibilities. Many of the skills necessary for good teaching are accessible through an entity like a Center for Teaching and Learning (CTL; different schools may use different names for units specializing in faculty development and pedagogy) and, in some cases, technological training offered by the information technology department. Other resources for the GTA might include the dean of students' office, the Title IX officer, faculty handbooks, librarians, writing centers, and Colleges of Graduate Studies (see table 23.1 for listing of specific resources).

In this chapter, we outline a career trajectory of a student's teaching development as a GTA in a school of public health. She begins her teaching experience by developing a strong mentoring relationship with the course professor and learning the most basic course skills. As she gains experience, she takes on more responsibilities, receives additional training and support, and reaches a level of teaching ability and skills that not only allows her to teach her own course but also prepares her to be a new faculty member or health educator.

At the end of the chapter, we include a table that lists teaching skills needed by GTAs and resources to provide them. This table may serve as a guide for a GTA training program and can be tailored to specific needs and resources.

A GTA's Experience

Carla, who holds a Master of Public Health degree in epidemiology, is accepted into a doctoral program in epidemiology at a midsize state university. In addition to taking courses, Carla is selected as a level-one graduate teaching assistant (GTA1) during her first year. Each semester of her three years of doctoral studies, she is trained and mentored in teaching pedagogy and practice. As her skills develop, she takes more responsibility for teaching in the classroom. She begins her teaching in the Epidemiology 101 course for undergraduate students with her mentor/supervisor, and by her fourth semester, she is responsible for developing and teaching an upper-level course on her own, as well as mentoring new GTAs.

Responsibilities and Expectations

The week before classes begin, Carla meets with the professor to whom she has been assigned as a GTA. The professor will serve as more than the professor of record in the undergraduate course; she will also be Carla's supervisor and, ideally, her teaching mentor, modeling teaching and mentoring excellence. The relationship between Carla and her mentor/supervisor will become central to Carla's success as a teacher and professional.

Before turning to the course itself, the professor discusses her own teaching philosophy, how she runs her classroom, whether she favors lectures or active learning or a mixture of both, the types of assignments she gives and why, and how she handles classroom dynamics in a large class. She and Carla will discuss Carla's own experience when she took this class as an undergraduate or graduate and what she found most and least helpful. Throughout the semester, the professor recommends content- and pedagogy-based literature to help in Carla's preparation. In addition, the professor helps Carla begin building a teaching portfolio, which, by the time she completes her degree, will become a valuable resource to be used in her job search.

As part of the GTA training process, Carla keeps a journal in which she reflects on her experience as a GTA—what she has learned, concerns she might have, observations regarding her own teaching style and philosophy, and ideas for her own classroom. This journal serves as the basis for discussions with her mentor/supervisor, who will be able to assess Carla's progress and offer her resources that might assist her.[8]

For Carla to be a successful part of the teaching team, she must understand the professor's goals and objectives for the class, as well as the student learning outcomes (SLOs, or the skills that students should have once they complete the course) she has created. The professor discusses these with Carla, explaining how they align with the assignments and assessments she has chosen. Together, they review the syllabus, noting where major assignments fall and where Carla will be providing special assistance, grading, and tutoring. If Carla is assisting in a graduate-level course, she will have significant input based on her own experience. She and her mentor/supervisor also discuss classroom policies regarding issues including student behavior, plagiarism, diversity training, and so on.

As part of this meeting, the professor clarifies the responsibilities and expectations of her GTA. This conversation is revisited throughout the semester and as long as they work together as new needs arise and as Carla's responsibilities expand. Carla and her supervisor/mentor establish the importance of clear lines of communication between them and lay out a strategy for keeping each other informed about classroom matters.

As a GTA in her first semester, Carla provides basic support to her professor. This includes preparing handouts, posting assignments to the course website, keeping track of student attendance, collecting assignments, and grading multiple-choice question tests. Carla will also observe her professor's teaching methods and is prepared to discuss them. She attends each class, taking notes on what material is covered and what material students find difficult so that she can share it with her mentor/supervisor. She circulates during in-class group work to offer assistance.

Carla also holds weekly office hours, during which she will meet face-to-face with students, explaining concepts and providing general assistance. In preparation, she attends sessions offered by the campus CTL for GTAs and GTA2s on topics ranging from pedagogy and teaching tools to working with groups and creating effective assignments. She also discusses challenges with her peer GTAs in bimonthly meetings and with her mentor/supervisor. She keeps records of student meetings to share with her professor at their regular debriefing sessions.

In addition to her conversations with her mentor/supervisor and her classroom observations, Carla is encouraged to participate in various faculty/graduate student development teaching workshops and seminars. Before the first day of class, she attends a seminar at CTL titled "The First Day of Class," which prepares her for her first experience as part of an instructional team. She follows up with more seminars on a variety of pedagogical techniques, use of learning management systems, collecting and responding to student feedback, and using technology in the classroom. Through mentoring and additional workshops in the CTL, Carla gains skills in writing appropriate emails, Family Educational Rights and Privacy Act and Title IX rules, and professional presentation in the classroom and out.

Second Semester: GTA1

With her first semester experience of Epidemiology 101 behind her, Carla is prepared to take on additional responsibilities in teaching the course during the second semester. She and her mentor/supervisor work more closely on the course-development level, with Carla helping to update the syllabus and taking on a more active role in selecting relevant case studies, developing problem sets and review questions for exams, and writing test questions. To this end, she receives training from CTL and from her mentor/supervisor in what makes a good test question and how to grade essay questions and papers. Carla learns the difference between summative and formative assessments and where it is most appropriate to use each.

As part of her training, Carla assists her mentor/supervisor in writing lesson plans and developing and implementing in-class exercises. Using backward design and a series of SLOs developed with her professor's assistance, Carla prepares and teaches a session on a concept she and her professor select. As part of the session, Carla creates a method of assessment, such as a pretest, a posttest, or a reflective response, and will work with her professor to create an engaging experience using a variety of in-class teaching methods. The mentor/supervisor observes as Carla teaches and afterward provides feedback on everything from content to how Carla handled classroom dynamics. Based on this feedback, Carla revises the course plan and has it available for use during the following semester, when she teaches the course on her own.

TABLE 23.1. A Process Map for Training Teaching Assistants

Teaching Skills for TAs	1st Semester
Understanding of classroom roles and responsibilities	Introduce
Addressing issues of diversity in the classroom	Introduce
Gaining self-awareness as teacher through reflective process	Introduce
Developing a professional persona in and outside the classroom	Introduce
Understanding and addressing a variety of student learning styles	Introduce
Learning and applying course policies and procedures	Introduce
Developing a teaching philosophy	Introduce
Using a learning management system	Introduce
Creating an effective syllabus	Introduce
Developing course learning objectives and methods to measure to what degree they are attained	Introduce
Learning effective teaching methodologies, including active learning, service learning, flipped classroom, backward design	
Learning pedagogical techniques, including problem-based learning, flipped classroom, blended classes, and innovative uses of technology such as i-clickers, smart rooms, and social media	Introduce
Writing review and exam questions	Introduce
Teaching an introductory course	Introduce
Eliciting verbal and written feedback from students	Introduce
Synthesizing and applying lessons learned from student and mentor feedback	Introduce
Applying lessons learned from teaching specialist observer	
Developing tutoring techniques for one-on-one sessions with students	Introduce/ apply
Teaching an upper-level course	
Mentoring other TAs	
Developing teaching portfolio	Introduce/ apply

2nd Semester	3rd and 4th Semesters	Resources
Reinforce	Reinforce	Mentor, faculty and departmental handbooks and bylaws, dean of student, TA course website, CTL, COGS, observing other instructors[3,4,6,7,1,2]
Develop	Reinforce	Mentor, CTL, diversity office, safe place training, Title IX office[3,6,3,4]
Develop	Reinforce	Mentor, reflective journal, TA support group[3,6,11,12]
Reinforce	Reinforce	Mentor, CTL, reflective journal, TA support group, observing other instructors[5,6,8,12,5]
Reinforce	Apply	Mentor, CTL, TA course website[2,3,4,6,6]
Apply	Apply	Mentor, CTL, TA course website, faculty and departmental handbooks and bylaws[3,6,7]
Develop	Complete	Mentor, CTL, TA course website, TA support group, reflective journal[6,8,15]
Apply	Apply	IT, CTL, department online specialist[3,7,10]
Develop	Apply	Mentor, CTL, TA course website[6,9,10]
Develop	Apply	Mentor, CTL, TA course website, University Assessment staff[6,9,10,8]
		CTL, mentor, TA course website, TA support group[4,6,9,10,14,15,16,9]
Reinforce	Apply	Mentor, CTL, IT, TA course website[6,7,9,10,15,16]
Apply	Apply	Mentor, CTL[6,9,16,10]
Reinforce	Apply	Mentor, CTL, TA support group, reflective journal, teaching specialist observations[3,6,7,10,17]
Reinforce	Apply	Mentor, CTL, University Assessment staff[6,9,10]
Apply	Apply	Mentor, CTL[6,7,9,10]
Introduce	Apply	CTL, TA support group[6,7,10]
Apply	Apply	Mentor, CTL, dean of students, TA course website[3,7]
	Apply	Mentor, CTL, TA support group, COGS[3,6,15,17]
	Apply	TA support group, TA online course, CTL[3,6,15]
Apply	Apply	Mentor, CTL, TA mentor, TA support group[3,6,17]

Carla also sits in on at least one other class taught by a GTA as well as another class where she can observe the teaching approach of a different teacher in her department. Reflecting on these observations in her journal helps her come to a better understanding of her own teaching preferences and style.

During the summer, Carla is again encouraged by her department and her mentor/supervisor to attend training workshops and seminars offered by the CTL, and begins reworking the syllabus as needed. Conversations with her mentor/supervisor and the CTL staff are especially helpful in assessing her readiness to teach and addressing weaknesses or concerns.

Third Semester: GTA2

Before the semester begins, Carla submits her course syllabus, SLOs, assignments, and assessments to her mentor/supervisor for review. They meet and discuss any points of concern, and her mentor/supervisor offers resources to address difficulties. Though Carla is now responsible for teaching the course on her own, her mentor/supervisor's oversight and her availability to discuss course matters are crucial to Carla's development and success as an instructor. The professor observes Carla twice during the semester and provides feedback regarding all aspects of the teaching process. Carla is also observed by a teaching specialist (perhaps from the CTL) at midterm and again near the end of the semester. Observations by other professors and peers, while not required, are encouraged, and an appropriate rubric is distributed so that specific feedback is provided. Carla uses midterm comments and the comments of students to revise the second part of the semester, as needed. The teaching specialist returns for another observation and feedback session near the end of the semester.

During the semester, her mentor/supervisor checks in with Carla on issues of work-life balance, helping her meet her goals without undermining her personal life or shortchanging her own coursework.

Also important during this semester is support from peers. Teaching can be an isolating experience, especially for new instructors. Monthly meetings with fellow GTAs to discuss their experiences, share ideas, and even vent about problems will strengthen the teaching skills of all involved, allowing them to learn from one another while creating a community of practice to which they can turn if needed. Such sessions can be facilitated by an experienced GTA2 and might include the sharing of excerpts from the GTAs' reflective teaching journals.

Carla continues to observe others in their classrooms, but her focus is on the upper-level class she will be teaching the following semester on her own.

By this point, Carla has developed a substantial teaching portfolio, including a teaching philosophy that will guide her as she develops future classes. She is ready to discuss her philosophy with incoming GTA1s, and to invite them to observe her class, both to learn from her and to give her feedback.

Fourth Semester: GTA2

In this semester, Carla teaches her first upper-level course. The content is fresh in her mind from her own studies, and she brings to the classroom three semesters of new teaching ideas and experiences. She also faces a unique challenge. In the first three semesters, Carla has been teaching an introductory-level course, which has, for the most part, been predesigned by her mentor/supervisor and others. And though Carla has played a role in developing the intro-level course, she is now in the position of taking on a course she has no experience teaching. She must take the lessons she has learned and adapt them to the new course and to her own teaching style and philosophy, updating it and possibly including new technologies and teaching methods.

At this stage in her development as an instructor, Carla no longer meets regularly with her mentor/supervisor, though an appropriate faculty member reviews her syllabus and assessments. She will have developed a teaching support network made up of fellow GTAs, CTL, IT staff, and other professors whose teaching has influenced her. Carla also plays an important role in mentoring and supervising new GTAs by facilitating discussions, offering suggestions on dealing with teaching issues, and conducting observations and providing feedback.

A bonus to teaching an upper-level course in her specialty will be the opportunity for Carla to integrate elements of her own research and interests into the classroom. This will serve her well as she writes her dissertation and begins planning future research, grant applications, and job opportunities. The lesson plans, syllabi, and other teaching materials she has included in her teaching portfolio provide evidence of her development in communication and leadership skills in addition to her skills as an instructor.

Teaching Skills for GTAs

Table 23.1 is intended to be used as a guide to creating a GTA training process that meets departmental and student needs without overly stretching resources. It lists teaching skills that GTAs should develop as new instructors; notes where each skill is either introduced, reinforced, or applied; and, finally, offers a variety of resources for the training process.

The resource section relies heavily on mentoring but also includes a variety of campus service units that specialize in particular student-related issues. In addition, the resource section provides a listing of additional materials, texts, and websites according to skill. These can be used by GTAs and mentors/supervisors throughout training and beyond to improve teaching at all levels.

Conclusion

The prevailing approach of placing untrained and unsupported GTAs into the classroom has been shown to be harmful to the professors, students, and to GTAs themselves. However, the challenges of running an intensive and often-lengthy GTA training program are beyond the capacity of many programs and schools of public health. The proposed compromise takes into account the fact that GTAs play an important role in marketing public health to potential majors, and that many of them will be future faculty, expected to take on teaching roles. Their experiences in this process help them to market themselves through a robust portfolio, a strong teaching record, and a clear understanding of what goes into creating a successful learning experience.

REFERENCES

1. O'Neal, C., M. Wright, C. Cook, T. Perorazio, and J. Purkiss. "The Impact of Teaching Assistants on Student Retention in the Sciences." *Journal of College Science Teaching* 36, no 5 (2007): 24–29.

2. Austin, A. E. "Preparing the Next Generation of Faculty: Graduate School as Socialization to the Academic Career." *Journal of Higher Education* 73, no. 1 (2002): 94–122.

3. Border, L. L., and L. M. von Hoene. "Graduate and Professional Student Develop Programs." In *A Guide to Faculty Development, 2nd Edition*, edited by J. J. Gillespie and D. L. Robertson, 327–343. San Francisco: Jossey-Bass, 2010.

4. Kobinsky, S. A., K. M. Hrapczynski, and J. E. Clark. "Preparing Future Faculty and Professionals for Public Health Careers." *American Journal of Public Health* 105, no. S1 (2015): S125-S131.

5. Lederer, A. M., C. M. Sherwood-Laughlin, K. D. Kearns, and V. D. O'Loughlin. "Development-Level Public Health Pedagogy Course for Graduate Student Instructors." *College Teaching* 64, no. 1 (2016): 19–27.

6. Ridgway, J. S., I. Y. Ligocki, J. D. Horn, E. Szeyller, and C. A. Breitenberger. "Teaching Assistant and Faculty Perceptions of Ongoing, Personalized TA Professional Development: Initial Lessons and Plans for the Future." *Journal of College Science Teaching* 46, no. 5 (2017): 73–83.

7. Gallardo-Williams, M. T., and L. M. Petrovich. "An Integrated Approach to Training Graduate Teaching Assistants." *Journal of College Science Teaching* 47, no. 1 (2017): 43–47.

8. Stevens, D. D., and J. E. Cooper. *Journal Keeping: How to Use Reflective Writing for Effective Learning, Teaching, Professional Insight, and Positive Change.* Sterling, VA: Stylus Publishing, 2009.

9. Fink, D. L. *Creating Significant Learning Experiences: An Integrated Approach to Designing College Courses.* Hoboken, NJ: John Wiley and Sons, 2013.

10. Huston, T. *Teaching What You Don't Know.* Cambridge, MA: Harvard University Press, 2009.

11. Brown, C. I. "Reaching Resisters in a Teaching Assistant Training Program." *InSight: A Journal of Scholarly Teaching* 11 (2016): 90–101.

12. Luo, J., M. L. Grady, and L. H. Bellows. "Instructional Issues for Teaching Assistants." *Innovative Higher Education* 25, no. 3 (2001): 209–230.

13. Gallego, M. "Professional Development of Graduate Teaching Practices through Reflective Teaching Journals." *Journal of the Scholarship of Teaching and Learning* 14, no. 2 (2014): 96–110.

14. Barkley, E. F. *Student Engagement Techniques: A Handbook for College Faculty.* Hoboken, NJ: John Wiley and Sons, 2009.

15. Major, C. H., M. S. Harris, and T. Zakrajsek. *Teaching for Learning: 101 Intentionally Designed Educational Activities to Put Students on the Path to Success.* London: Routledge, 2015.

16. Howard, J. R. *Discussion in the College Classroom: Getting Your Students Engaged and Participating in Person and Online.* Hoboken, NJ: John Wiley and Sons, 2015.

17. McKeachie, W., and M. Svinicki. *McKeachie's Teaching Tips, 14th Edition.* Boston, MA: Cengage Learning, 2013.

18. Groccia, J. E., and L. Cruz, eds. *To Improve the Academy: Resources for Faculty, Instructional, and Organizational Development*, Volume 32. San Francisco: Jossey-Bass, 2013.

24

Innovations in Evaluating and Valuing Public Health Teaching

The Challenges of Course Evaluations

DELIA L. LANG AND ELIZABETH REISINGER WALKER

THE BODY OF research devoted to examining student ratings of undergraduate or graduate learning environments spans nearly nine
decades and represents the most researched topic in higher education.[1,2,3]
Today, collecting student ratings has become a staple in US institutions
of higher learning.[4,5] Notwithstanding the vast volume of data available on the topic, new investigations into the purpose and utility of student ratings continue to perpetuate conflicting evidence regarding the
validity and utility of such data.

One noteworthy contributing factor to the debate is the varied terminology used in the literature, often interchangeably, to describe student ratings, including student evaluations of teaching, student course
evaluations, student ratings of instruction, or student ratings of teaching.[6] Each term carries a different connotation of what is being measured, which may or may not always reflect the actual assessment instrument. Specifically, the terms "student evaluations of teaching" or
"student course evaluations" can be misleading, as they fail to distinguish between the individuals who provide ratings—students—and
those who review, evaluate, and subsequently make decisions based on
the ratings.[7] The latter could include faculty, who use student ratings
for instructional and course improvement, or department chairs and
other administrators, who may consult these data to inform personnel

decisions based on teaching performance. The terms "student ratings of instruction" and "student ratings of teaching" are restrictive, as many instruments assess teaching, content, and structure. Therefore, throughout this chapter, we use the broad term "student ratings," defined as data obtained from the structured administration of a survey instrument by institutions of higher education to matriculated students during either the midpoint or final weeks of an academic term.[8]

Interestingly, while students, faculty, and administrators alike have continued to fervently question the validity of student ratings, all have simultaneously used them to varying degrees to inform course selection, quality of instruction, and faculty performance reviews and promotions, as well as to demonstrate institutional accountability to external curriculum reviewers.[9,10,11] Schools and programs in public health are no exception. Student ratings have been integral to the development of undergraduate and graduate public health training programs that have increasingly focused on strengthening teaching effectiveness of competency-based curricula.

Within this context, student ratings are insufficient in addressing the needs and interests of the diverse constituents that utilize them (e.g., students, faculty, administrators), yet they represent one necessary tool used to evaluate learning environments and, thus, can contribute to building strong teaching cultures. In this chapter, we highlight key empirical literature describing ways in which student ratings have been traditionally employed across disciplines, including associated benefits and drawbacks. Next, we examine reliability and validity of underlying constructs typically measured by current student rating instruments and review the degree to which these constructs are valid indicators of teaching effectiveness and student learning outcomes. We also examine other strategies for measuring teaching effectiveness, such as external evaluations, self-reflections, and documentation of professional development, that can present a more holistic view. We conclude with considerations specific to public health education.

Uses of Student Ratings

Historically, student ratings were applied primarily as information loops serving both students and faculty. The least disputed use of student ratings was to benefit future student cohorts, who could consult peer ratings from previous academic terms and select courses and instructors accordingly.[12] Evidence suggests that when students utilize ratings for this purpose, they tend to make course selections based on student ratings of faculty alone rather than ratings related to course content or structure.[13]

The information feedback loop for faculty was intended for formative purposes to inform course improvement.[14,15] Not surprisingly, some faculty welcome student feedback regarding their course and teaching methods,[16,17] while others deem such data as uninformative.[18,19] As long as faculty retain the academic freedom to decide how to use students' ratings, if at all, not much controversy surrounds the use of student ratings strictly for formative purposes. It is at the intersection of formative and summative purposes—where utilization of student ratings enters the sphere of performance evaluation—that the discourse garners substantial vigor among faculty.

Over time, the primary use of student ratings has evolved, and student ratings are currently employed primarily for summative purposes. Academic administrative units routinely utilize student ratings as a measure of teaching effectiveness that subsequently informs hiring, annual performance evaluations, faculty retention, promotion and tenure processes, as well as institutional compliance with external oversight (e.g., quality assurance of teaching, meeting required competencies and learning outcomes).[20,21,22,23] The primary rationale among supporters of this practice is that students are best positioned to offer their perceptions of instructors and to evaluate the degree to which they learn as a result of instructors' teaching effectiveness.[24] Others argue that the degree to which student rating instruments measure teaching effectiveness or student learning is debatable.[25,26] It is within this context that the controversy around the validity of student ratings resides and where much of the ongoing research on student ratings as an indicator of teaching effectiveness and learning outcomes persists.

Reliability and Validity of Student Rating Data

Conflicting findings on the reliability and validity of student rating instruments maintain the ongoing debate around their use as indicators of teaching effectiveness and associated learning outcomes, which are subsequently considered for summative purposes. Many researchers caution against conceptualizing student ratings as a marker for teaching effectiveness. Instead, they have advocated for viewing these assessments as student satisfaction surveys that can be heavily influenced by factors unrelated to teaching effectiveness, such as instructors' personality and demographic characteristics such as gender or ethnicity; students' own characteristics, grade expectations, interests, and motivation to learn; and contextual factors such as academic discipline, class level, class size, meeting times, or required versus elective courses.[27,28,29,30,31,32]

Some of the earlier studies on student ratings demonstrate that reliability can be achieved when student rating instruments are well constructed and psychometrically validated. Measures of student satisfaction or perceived educational quality have resulted in consistent and stable scores over time and between raters.[33,34,35] However, with increased focus on assessing competency-based learning and the predominant use of student ratings for summative purposes, many institutions have developed in-house, more student-focused instruments for the specific purpose of assessing teaching effectiveness. Such instruments are typically not subjected to the rigor of psychometric testing, as some of the earlier measures of student satisfaction,[36,37] largely due to lack of consensus on the operational definition of effective teaching.[38]

The question of validity permeates all forms of student rating instruments, including those that may achieve reliable scores. Among many faculty, concerns around the validity of student ratings have persisted and are in part supported by recent research, calling into question previously documented validity of student rating instruments.[39]

Frequently expressed concerns regarding utilization of student ratings highlight the possibility that students are not motivated to complete ratings of courses[40] or, in extreme cases, may even deliberately falsify their ratings.[41] Students' motivation to participate in the rating process is, in part, related to whether or not they perceive that this process is a means by which they can offer meaningful feedback to inform teaching and course content.[42,43] In fact, students often fail to see how course changes, even if they occurred, would affect them, as most student ratings are collected at the end of the semester. Additionally, many students experience this request as a burden at busy times of the semester.[44] Lastly, face validity may be lacking because instruments developed by administrators may not align with students' definitions of teaching effectiveness.[45,46] Such findings call into question not only the motivation of students to give serious consideration to the rating process but also highlight a potential disconnect between instrument developers and users related to their respective definitions of constructs under examination.

Furthermore, challenges related to construct-related validity have also received much attention in the literature. Agreement exists among researchers that student ratings of teaching effectiveness must be multidimensional to comprehensively assess the various factors that encompass effective teaching. However, in the absence of a theoretical foundation to inform both the adequate number and appropriate content of such dimensions, we are left with an overwhelming variety of instruments covering as few as two and as many as twelve dimensions. Consequently, it is difficult to decide what utility such dimensions have, particularly when used for summative purposes. Instead, administrators often rely largely on one global, unidimensional score to assess teaching effectiveness.[47] Marsh suggested that multidimensional scores can be used for formative purposes, while a unidimensional score may offer sufficient evidence for summative purposes.[48]

A sizeable body of literature published between 1975 and 1995, including several notable literature reviews and meta-analyses,[49,50] reported small-to-moderate correlations between student ratings of teaching effectiveness and student learning, measured by final exam scores. Results from these studies were accepted as evidence supporting the convergent validity of student ratings, which persisted even until recently.[51] Most of these early conclusions were derived from multisection study designs that involved random assignment of students to equivalent course sections, each one taught by a different professor.[52,53] However, random assignment to multiple course sections is often impossible; therefore, other variables such as prior student learning may confound the association between student ratings and learning. In a recent meta-analysis, Uttl et al. reanalyzed studies used in previous meta-analyses, accounting for sample size and previous learning. They demonstrated that student ratings of teaching effectiveness and student learning are not associated as previously thought, concluding that students do not necessarily learn better from higher-rated instructors.[54]

Ultimately, at the root of faculty discontent with student ratings is the concern over validity and that student rating scores may be misused or misinterpreted by administrators.[55,56,57] A comprehensive evaluation of teaching effectiveness can include student ratings but should also encompass other methods of assessment.

Assessing Teaching Effectiveness and Student Learning

The idea that student ratings should be considered in concert with other indicators to evaluate teaching and performance is not new.[58] Such indicators can include external evaluations, instructor reflections, and documentation of professional development.

One component of evaluating teaching effectiveness includes external evaluations, such as student ratings derived from psychometrically validated instruments and peer/expert teaching reviews. In one of the few studies of teaching evaluation in public health, Vian and Ashigbie describe implementing peer review of teaching among faculty teaching in a Master of Public Health program. A main purpose of the peer-review program was to review, share, reflect on, and discuss teaching practices. The peer review provided feedback for formative purposes and was not used for formal performance assessment.[59] Faculty find peer reviews to be valuable and report making changes to their courses based on constructive feedback.[60,61] Considerations with peer review of teaching mirror the issues with student ratings to some degree. Key decisions about peer ratings include whether they will be used for formative or summative purposes, whether reviews will be conducted by peers or experts, and what mechanism for delivering potentially sensitive feedback will be used. Additionally, one critique of peer reviews is that the process of being reviewed may alter the instructor's preparation and teaching in such ways that the observed session is not representative of their overall instruction.[62]

Alternative ways of soliciting student feedback on teaching include qualitative or mixed-methods data collection either at midterm or at the end of the semester. The Small Group Instructional Diagnosis is an example of a structured procedure to provide instructors with constructive feedback. A faculty member not associated with the course facilitates a discussion with the students about the course's strengths and weaknesses, and then provides the instructor with a summary of the feedback and recommendations.[63] Focus groups at the end of the semester provide in-depth information to supplement formal student ratings.[64] Additionally, conducting qualitative interviews or focus groups with alumni can provide insight into longer-term impacts of teaching and learning.[65]

A second component of assessing teaching effectiveness is based on instructor reflections on their own teaching. Documentation of instructor reflections can include teaching philosophy statements, descriptions and examples of innovative and inclusive teaching, descriptions of pedagogical strategies used in various learning environments, and associated course materials (e.g., syllabi, examples of assignments and assessments). Additionally, descriptions of and reflections on professional development, such as completion of workshops related to teaching, mentorship, and scholarship of teaching and learning (SoTL) projects can also be considered.[66]

Teaching portfolios have emerged as a way to present evidence of teaching effectiveness from a multidimensional perspective.[67] A comprehensive teaching portfolio provides a breadth of data sources from diverse perspectives that could subsequently be used for formative or summative purposes. Student ratings would be one factor that, depending on how the instrument was constructed, would serve to assess student satisfaction with a course and instructor. For formative purposes, these could inform next action steps. However, for purposes of promotion and tenure, a faculty member's teaching philosophy, engagement in professional development opportunities, peer reviews, and teaching consultations could be viewed in concert with student ratings toward a more holistic approach to evaluate teaching.

Conclusion

To date, limited research has emerged from within public health on student ratings, teaching effectiveness, and learning outcomes. There is great potential and a need to focus on such discipline-specific research in an effort to develop a much-needed evidence base guiding effective teaching practices in public health.[68] While we can apply many of the core lessons from the vast literature on these topics to public health, considerations unique to our field are worth noting. As a discipline, public health draws students from a broad array of academic and professional backgrounds and is tasked with equipping them to thrive in an equally diverse and dynamic workforce. The public health educational curriculum expects students at undergraduate, master's, and doctoral levels to achieve foundational public health competencies irrespective of subdiscipline.[69] These competencies must be assessed and documented through multiple data sources drawn from various institutional domains and stakeholders, including students (e.g., student satisfaction, student ratings) and faculty (e.g., instructor reflections, peer observations, documentation of professional development). The resulting wealth of data could contribute to the growing SoTL in public health, mirroring similar extensive research that has informed the education of other health science professionals for decades.[70] Recently, schools of public health began establishing centers and offices dedicated to faculty development around teaching and pedagogical scholarship. Continued development and support of such academic support units is important for fostering student learning within a rigorous academic culture that values innovative, inclusive, and evidence-based public health pedagogies.

Public health is uniquely positioned to apply its theoretical and methodological expertise to SoTL, thereby identifying, implementing, and evaluating existing and new teaching strategies. Research addressing the valid assessment of multidimensional student ratings and other methods of evaluating teaching effectiveness remains integral to this process. Consequently, holistic approaches to examining teaching effectiveness, student learning, and learning environments are needed to promote strong teaching cultures in public health education.

REFERENCES

1. Annan, S. L., S. Tratnack, C. Rubenstein, E. Metzler-Sawin, and L. Hulton. "An Integrative Review of Student Evaluations of Teaching: Implications for Evaluation of Nursing Faculty." *Journal of Professional Nursing* 29 (2013): e10-e24.

2. Linse, A. R. "Interpreting and Using Student Ratings Data: Guidance for Faculty Serving as Administrators and on Evaluation Committees." *Studies in Educational Evaluation* 54 (2017): 94–106.

3. Ory, J. C. "Faculty Thoughts and Concerns about Student Ratings." *New Directions for Teaching and Learning* 87 (2001): 3–15.

4. Murray, H. G. "Student Evaluation of Teaching: Has It Made a Difference?" Paper presented at the Annual Meeting of the Society for Teaching and Learning in Higher Education. Charlottetown, Prince Edward Island, 2005.

5. Zabaleta, F. "The Use and Misuse of Student Evaluations of Teaching." *Teaching in Higher Education* 12 (2007): 55–76.

6. Gravestock, P., and E. Gregor-Greenleaf. *Student Course Evaluations: Research, Models and Trends.* Toronto: Higher Education Quality Council of Ontario, 2008.

7. Linse, "Interpreting and Using Student Ratings Data."

8. Linse, "Interpreting and Using Student Ratings Data."

9. Kogan, L. R., R. Schoenfeld-Tacher, and P. W. Hellyer. "Student Evaluations of Teaching: Perceptions of Faculty Based on Gender, Position, and Rank." *Teaching in Higher Education* 15 (2010): 623–636.

10. Kozub, R. M. "Student Evaluations of Faculty: Concerns and Possible Solutions." *Journal of College Teaching and Learning* 5 (2008): 35–40.

11. Spooren, P., B. Brockx, and D. Mortelmans. "On the Validity of Student Evaluation of Teaching: The State of the Art." *Review of Educational Research* 83 (2013): 598–642.

12. Beran, T. N., and J. L. Rokosh. "Instructors' Perspectives on the Utility of Student Ratings of Instruction." *Instructional Science* 37 (2009): 171–184.

13. Beran, T. N., C. Violato, D. Kline, and J. Frideres. "The Utility of Student Ratings of Instruction for Students, Faculty, and Administrators: A 'Consequential Validity' Study." *Canadian Journal of Higher Education* 35 (2005): 49–70.

14. Beran and Rokosh, "Instructors' Perspectives on the Utility of Student Ratings of Instruction."

15. Goldschmid, M. L. "The Evaluation and Improvement of Teaching in Higher Education." *Higher Education* 7 (1978): 221–245.

16. Balam, E. M., and D. M. Shannon. "Student Ratings of College Teaching: A Comparison of Faculty and Their Students." *Assessment and Evaluation in Higher Education* 35 (2010): 209–221.

17. Kulik, J. A. "Student Ratings: Validity, Utility, and Controversy." *New Directions for Institutional Research* 109 (2001): 9–25.

18. Beran and Rokosh, "Instructors' Perspectives on the Utility of Student Ratings of Instruction."

19. Nasser, F., and B. Fresko. "Faculty Views of Student Evaluation of College Teaching." *Assessment and Evaluation in Higher Education* 227 (2002): 187–198.

20. Arthur, L. "From Performativity to Professionalism: Lecturers' Responses to Student Feedback." *Teaching in Higher Education* 14 (2009): 441–454.

21. Beran, T. N., and D. Kline. "What's the 'Use' of Student Ratings of Instruction for Administrators? One University's Experience." *Canadian Journal of Higher Education* 37 (2007): 26–43.

22. Edström, K. "Doing Course Evaluation as if Learning Matters Most." *Higher Education Research and Development* 27 (2008): 95–106.

23. Spooren, Brockx, and Mortelmans, "On the Validity of Student Evaluation of Teaching."

24. Murray, "Student Evaluation of Teaching."

25. Spooren, Brockx, and Mortelmans, "On the Validity of Student Evaluation of Teaching."

26. Uttl, B., C. A. White, and D. W. Gonzalez. "Meta-Analysis of Faculty's Teaching Effectiveness: Student Evaluation of Teaching Ratings and Student Learning Are Not Related." *Studies in Educational Evaluation* 54 (2017): 22–42.

27. Beran and Rokosh, "Instructors' Perspectives on the Utility of Student Ratings of Instruction."

28. Denson, N., T. Loveday, and H. Dalton. "Student Evaluation of Courses: What Predicts Satisfaction?" *Higher Education Research and Development* 29 (2010): 339–356.

29. Donnon, T., H. Delver, and T. Beran. "Student and Teaching Characteristics Related to Ratings of Instruction in Medical Sciences Graduate Programs." *Medical Teacher* 32 (2010): 327–332.

30. Linse, "Interpreting and Using Student Ratings Data."

31. Spooren, Brockx, and Mortelmans, "On the Validity of Student Evaluation of Teaching."

32. Uttl, White, and Gonzalez, "Meta-Analysis of Faculty's Teaching Effectiveness."

33. Annan et al., "An Integrative Review of Student Evaluations of Teaching."

34. Marsh, H. W. "SEEQ: A Reliable, Valid, and Useful Instrument for Collecting Students' Evaluations of University Teaching." *British Journal of Educational Psychology* 52 (1982): 77–95.

35. Ramsden, P. "A Performance Indicator of Teaching Quality in Higher Education: The Course Experience Questionnaire." *Studies in Higher Education* 16 (1991): 129–150.

36. Annan et al., "An Integrative Review of Student Evaluations of Teaching."

37. Richardson, J. T. E. "Instruments for Obtaining Student Feedback: A Review of the Literature." *Assessment and Evaluation in Higher Education* 30 (2005): 387–415.

38. Spooren, Brockx, and Mortelmans, "On the Validity of Student Evaluation of Teaching."

39. Uttl, White, and Gonzalez, "Meta-Analysis of Faculty's Teaching Effectiveness."

40. Chen, Y., and L. B. Hoshower. "Student Evaluation of Teaching Effectiveness: An Assessment of Student Perception and Motivation." *Assessment and Evaluation in Higher Education* 28, no. 1 (2003): 71–88.

41. Clayson, D. E., and D. A. Haley. "Are Students Telling Us the Truth? A Critical Look at the Student Evaluation of Teaching." *Marketing Education Review* 21 (2011): 101–112.

42. Chen and Hoshower, "Student Evaluation of Teaching Effectiveness."

43. Sojka, J., A. K. Gupta, and D. R. Deeter-Schmelz. "Student and Faculty Perceptions of Student Evaluations of Teaching: A Study of Similarities and Differences." *College Teaching* 50 (2002): 44–49.

44. Powell, N. J., C. Rubenstein, E. M. Sawin, and S. Annan. "Student Evaluations of Teaching Tools." *Nurse Educator* 39 (2014): 274–279.

45. Pan, D., G. S. H. Tan, K. Ragupathi, K. Booluck, R. Roop, and Y. K. Ip. "Profiling Teacher/Teaching Using Descriptors Derived from Qualitative Feedback: Formative and Summative Applications." *Research in Higher Education* 50 (2009): 73–100.

46. Spooren, Brockx, and Mortelmans, "On the Validity of Student Evaluation of Teaching."

47. Spooren, Brockx, and Mortelmans, "On the Validity of Student Evaluation of Teaching."

48. Marsh, H. W. "Students' Evaluations of University Teaching: Dimensionality, Reliability, Validity, Potential Biases and Usefulness." In *The Scholarship of Teaching and Learning in Higher Education: An Evidence-Based Perspective*, edited by R. P. Perry and J. C. Smart, 319–383. Dordrecht, Netherlands: Springer Netherlands, 2007.

49. Abrami, P. C., S. d'Apollonia, and P. A. Cohen. "Validity of Student Ratings of Instruction: What We Know and What We Do Not." *Journal of Educational Psychology* 82 (1990): 219–231.

50. Cohen, Peter A. "Student Ratings of Instruction and Student Achievement: A Meta-analysis of Multisection Validity Studies." *Review of Educational Research* 51 (1981): 281–309.

51. Marsh, "Students' Evaluations of University Teaching," in Perry and Smart, *The Scholarship of Teaching and Learning in Higher Education*.

52. Abrami, d'Apollonia, and Cohen, "Validity of Student Ratings of Instruction."

53. Uttl, White, and Gonzalez, "Meta-Analysis of Faculty's Teaching Effectiveness."

54. Uttl, White, and Gonzalez, "Meta-Analysis of Faculty's Teaching Effectiveness."

55. Boysen, G. A. "Significant Interpretation of Small Mean Differences in Student Evaluations of Teaching Despite Explicit Warning to Avoid Overinterpretation." *Scholarship of Teaching and Learning in Psychology* 1 (2015): 150–162.

56. Boysen, G. A., T. J. Kelly, H. N. Raesly, and R. W. Casner. "The (Mis)Interpretation of Teaching Evaluations by College Faculty and Administrators." *Assessment and Evaluation in Higher Education* 39 (2014): 641–656.

57. Spooren, Brockx, and Mortelmans, "On the Validity of Student Evaluation of Teaching."

58. Kulik, J. A., and W. J. McKeachie. "The Evaluation of Teachers in Higher Education." *Review of Research in Education* 3 (1975): 210–240.

59. Vian, T., and P. G Ashigbie. "Accelerating Educational Innovation in the MPH Degree Program: What Is the Role of Peer Review of Teaching?" *Journal of Health Education Teaching* 6 (2015): 43–56.

60. Brickman, P., C. Gormally, and A. M. Martella. "Making the Grade: Using Instructional Feedback and Evaluation to Inspire Evidence-Based Teaching." *CBE Life Sciences Education* 15 (2016): 1–14.

61. Vian and Ashigbie, "Accelerating Educational Innovation in the MPH Degree Program."

62. Thomas, S., Q. T. Chie, M. Abraham, S. J. Raj, and L. Beh. "A Qualitative Review of Literature on Peer Review of Teaching in Higher Education: An

Application of the SWOT Framework." *Review of Educational Research* 84 (2014): 112–159.

63. Coffman, S. J. "Improving Your Teaching through Small-Group Diagnosis." *College Teaching* 39 (1991): 80–82.

64. Lang, D. L., E. R. Walker, R. J. Steiner, and R. C. Woodruff. "Implementation and Mixed-Methods Evaluation of Team-Based Learning in a Graduate Public Health Research Methods Course." *Pedagogy in Health Promotion* 4, no. 2 (2018): 140–150.

65. Lattuca, L. R., and J. M. Domagal-Goldman. "Using Qualitative Methods to Assess Teaching Effectiveness." *New Directions for Institutional Research* 136 (2007): 81–93.

66. Gravestock and Gregor-Greenleaf, *Student Course Evaluations.*

67. Appling, S. E., P. L. Naumann, and R. A. Berk. "Using a Faculty Evaluation Triad to Achieve Evidence-Based Teaching." *Nursing and Health Care Perspectives* 22 (2001): 247–251.

68. Merzel, C., P. Halkitis, and C. Healton. "Pedagogical Scholarship in Public Health: A Call for Cultivating Learning Communities to Support Evidence-Based Education." *Public Health Reports* 132 (2017): 679–683.

69. Council on Education for Public Health. "Accreditation Criteria: Schools and Programs of Public Health." Silver Spring, MD: CEPH, 2016. https://ceph.org/assets/2016.Criteria.pdf (accessed March 25, 2018).

70. Richardson, "Instruments for Obtaining Student Feedback."

PART IV THE PRESENT AND THE FUTURE

[25]

Responding Interprofessionally to a Complex World

The Impact on Public Health Education and Workforce

LAURA MAGAÑA VALLADARES, JULIAN FISHER, NELLY SALGADO
DE SNYDER, AND SILVIA E. RABIONET

THE WORLD IS becoming increasingly complex, dynamic, and inter-connected. Natural and created systems constantly need to adapt. The patterns of global interaction and emerging technologies pose threats and opportunities to achieve large-scale, sustainable economic development. Health is one of the major resources linked to sustainable development; however, the burden of diseases is a major source of global inequalities.[1] The complexities of current events and social conditions make health elusive for many and too costly for others. Despite decades of substantial investments to boost prosperity, reduce poverty, and improve health, substantial inequalities persist worldwide.[2] Health is a basic human right and a cornerstone for sustainable global economic growth and social justice; therefore, examining the drivers of these inequalities is imperative. We should also stay abreast of current movements, scientific developments, and technological capacities that can transform and enhance the leadership role of the public health workforce. The healthcare workforce, broadly defined, needs to understand and have the competencies to address the internal inequalities created by the healthcare system while addressing external forces and social determinants of health.

Poverty, lack of education, imbalances of power, use of violence, and irresponsible utilization of environmental resources leading to natural disasters create pathways to poor health. These pathways can trigger social fractures, the spread of infectious diseases, and inadequate access to care that could ease the burden and progression of communicable diseases. To illustrate these pathways, we have evidence that low-income children and women have unequal opportunities to thrive. For example, in developing countries, children from low-income households are four times less likely than children from high-income households to be enrolled in primary education. Most of the approximately 780 million illiterate adults worldwide are women. Moreover, low-income people face higher risks of malnutrition and death in childhood and lower odds of receiving primary or key healthcare intervention at any age.[3]

Active conflict zones, including civil wars, criminal violence, sectarian battles, territorial disputes, transnational tensions, and interstate conflicts, affect all continents.[4] A major outcome of war and violence is the displacement of people and an increase in the refugee population distributed worldwide. By the end of 2017, nearly 68.8 million people were expected to be displaced, as compared with 35.4 million in 2011. Every region of the world is affected by the influx of refugees.[5] From a humanitarian and healthcare perspective, refugees' needs should be addressed with intention and understanding to avoid public health crises, prevent the spread of disease, and integrate them into society.

The interdependency of the environment, well-being, and health can be further illustrated by considering the effect of natural disasters on the most vulnerable and poorest regions of the world. According to the World Health Organization (WHO), natural disasters kill nearly 90,000 people and affect 160 million people worldwide. Furthermore, natural disasters add substantially to the number of displaced people worldwide. Disasters have an immediate impact on the physical, biological, and social resources of the affected people, and have a long-term impact on their health, well-being, and survival. During and in the aftermath of a disaster, a disruption of health services, food insecurity, stress, unemployment, and powerlessness occurs, especially among those in the lower socioeconomic strata. Evidence indicates a long-lasting effect on individuals and their ecosystems. Many health and emergency aid workers who are deployed to disaster areas in their country or internationally without adequate training in disaster response experience danger and frustration.[6]

Historically, events such as wars, natural disasters, migration, and urbanization have challenged public health and marked defining moments in the evolution of the field. During the past decade, the WHO's Health Promotion and Social Determinants of Health initiatives have spearheaded the realization and documentation that health is fundamentally a social and political choice rather than a personal choice.[7] In 2015, the United Nations General Assembly agreed on a bold agenda by enumerating 17 sustainable development goals (SDGs) to achieve by 2030. Although most of the goals relate to health and well-being, SDG 3 (ensure healthy lives and promote well-being for all at all ages) directly targets health.[8] Central to this goal is a realization of the importance of health as a resource and underscores the intersection of health with other sectors, issues, and goals. The SDGs call for comprehensive action on the social determinants of health and intersectoral action by emphasizing their interrelatedness and equity across all goals.

We live in an era of important scientific and technological developments that redefine how we treat and even eradicate diseases. Information technology has made data accessible. Digital technologies can accelerate and broaden the transfer of information and enhance interactions among patients, communities, and health workers. Exchanges of ideas and evidence have been enhanced by social media and internet-based communications. A proliferation of models of grassroots mobilization and patient-centered care are being implemented, evaluated, and documented. Health in All Policies (HiAP) has become a standard for countries to achieve and is defined in the following paragraph.[9] The next cadre of health professionals should be competent not only in the use of new knowledge but also in the translation of emerging technologies to eliminate the pathways that trigger poor health and social inequalities.

Embracing HiAP—a collaborative approach that integrates and articulates health considerations into policy-making across sectors—and equipping the public health workforce with new competencies to work interprofessionally to address the social determinants of health (which reflect the societal policy drivers of all determinants of health: physical, social, cultural, behavioral) is critical to facilitate the intersectoral work. The health professions need to embrace transdisciplinary learning and acquire the skills to respond to and negotiate intersectoral responses in a complex world. Health systems need to embrace the value of intersectoral work, flexibility, internal and external synergies, and innovation to address their core undertakings—maintaining health, preventing disease, and avoiding or delaying unnecessary deaths in the population.

Public Health Education for a Complex and Multifaceted World

Public health has undergone major changes since it was first conceptualized by C. E. A. Winslow a century ago.[10] In recent decades, global forces have had a major impact on the way in which we think about health. Now it is widely accepted that health issues are no longer strictly a health ministry's national concern but have important multisectoral and international dimensions.[11] Despite these changes, public health education has not transformed itself with the same speed.

The literature shows that globalization is intimately related to public health, but the linkages between globalization and health are complex.[12] Globalization has led to a constant, dynamic exchange of goods and services, along with increased movement of people, cultures, and lifestyles across borders, which may result in an increased spreading of health-related problems worldwide. Global health focuses on the international transfer of health risks and factors, which are parallel to economic interdependence.[13]

Public health has taken a prominent place on national and international agendas. Public health issues can have a negative impact on a nation's economic growth and development and on national and international security. In the past, health issues were considered to be linked to development concerns. In recent times, however, health issues have become part of political agendas associated with national and global security themes. Pandemics, infectious disease threats, fears about bioterrorism, and issues related to trade and health have provided an incentive for foreign policy decision makers to devote more attention to health matters.[14]

The links between global health policy and governance gave rise to global health diplomacy that calls for professionals with strong and multilayered negotiating skills among all the other cross-cutting competencies to work in an interconnected and complex world.

Today, public health goes beyond preventing disease, prolonging life, and promoting health. The demographic, epidemiologic, and democratic transitions occurring worldwide, influenced by globalization, have transformed the way in which we view population health. Public health education must include an awareness of the health risk interdependence that exists among all sectors and all nations. As such, public health training must transcend sectors and borders, and a new generation of public health professionals must understand that economic transformations have created a complex mosaic of living conditions that influence population health. Health is the meeting ground between the social sciences and the health sciences.[15] Interdisciplinary and intersectoral collaboration, particularly the inclusion of disciplines such as political geography, international economy and law, and demography, is necessary to respond to national and global health problems.[16]

Given the complexity of local and global health and the need for intersectoral approaches, public health graduate students need to develop competencies in policy, negotiation, diplomacy, dialogue, and collaboration.[17] The multifaceted nature of public health calls for professionals who are proficient in an array of cross-cutting competencies to respond to current complex challenges, including the following:

- Ability to work in multidisciplinary, multisectoral, and multinational teams
- Negotiation skills to address and participate in discussions of trade, investment, commerce, security, migration, housing, and foreign relations
- Advocacy, communication, and diplomatic competencies to successfully work in multicultural, multisector settings that may involve private and public interests but remain loyal to principles of social justice and health for all
- Skills in data analysis and knowledge building, knowledge sharing, and knowledge translation to foster evidence-based collaborations with other sectors and disciplines.

Public health is dynamic and multifaceted; therefore, it calls for training imaginative and creative professionals with a strong understanding of the political and economic processes worldwide.[18] They may come from various disciplines and sectors, but public health professionals must be able to negotiate, create synergies, and think strategically and tactically to provide answers and solutions to the many challenges they will face. In its 2016 meeting, the Advisory Committee on Health Research of the Pan American Health Organization recommended prioritizing the training of new generations of public health profession-als with a wide variety of skills and emphasizing "long-range planning, problem-solving under pressure, visionary thinking, negotiating with people from outside the health sector, learning to identify areas of op-portunity, and the ability to use institutional, social, and financial re-sources to maximum effect."[19]

It will take profound change and innovation for public health edu-cation to overcome these challenges. Schools and programs of public health need to evolve from informative lectures to formative environ-ments and transformative learning.[20] Public health education should be viewed as a lifelong process. Rather than adding more content to exist-ing graduate curriculum, competency-based education allows for some competencies to be mastered over time, through professional practice, rather than within a limited time frame.

Rethinking In-Service Training: Lifelong Learning Systems to Retain a Competent Workforce

The public health workforce has an important contribution to make to the United Nations 2030 Agenda for Sustainable Development as a whole and has an important leadership role in the implementation of SDG 3, which includes achievement of universal health coverage by 2030.[21] Public health workforce education and training within a life-long learning framework is a strategic priority for the profession to pre-pare for and respond effectively to the health and development chal-lenges of the twenty-first century.

This approach will require that training the public health workforce in the desired range of competencies is viewed as a lifelong learning pro-cess and is aligned with the health needs and changes in health labor market demands, health services, and local communities, including those resulting from protracted and acute public health emergencies and hu-manitarian crises.[22] Such a transformative and socially accountable ap-proach could catalyze and drive new thinking and enhance collabora-tion and cooperation among ministries of education, health, labor, and finance, as well as other ministries, professional organizations, and stakeholders.

This reorienting of the public health workforce has been given added impetus through a report of the United Nations High-Level Commission on Health Employment and Economic Growth, its ten recommendations, and the accompanying five-year action plan.[23] Strikingly, the commission's report calls for the health workforce to be geared toward the social determinants of health, health promotion, disease prevention, primary care, and people-centered, community-based services.

The social determinants of health and universal health coverage must be addressed in an integrated and systematic manner, which will, in turn, support the implementation of the United Nations 2030 Agenda as a whole. This framework creates an enabling environment for the public health workforce to address the many cross-cutting issues that do not fit neatly into health program areas covered in the 13 health targets in SDG 3.[24]

A HiAP approach can enable public health professionals working in various sites, levels, and sectors to consider the health implications of decisions, seek synergies, and avoid harmful health impacts to improve population health and health equity.[25] Interprofessional and intersectoral workforce training within a lifelong learning framework can support a HiAP approach and help define intersectoral action in a coordinated, convergent, and mutually reinforcing manner.

National public health institutes, universities, schools and programs of public health, and collaborating centers need to work together with health systems to find innovative educational models, strategies, and environments to support workforce development and update changing competencies. In this regard, regulation and accreditation are key instruments that could catalyze transformative public health workforce education and training and facilitate the necessary institutional and instructional reforms.

The WHO published the National Health Workforce Accounts to facilitate the standardization of health workforce information systems for interoperability (e.g., the ability to exchange health workforce data within broader subnational or national health information systems, as well as within international information systems).[26] The National Health Workforce Accounts includes the indicator—standards for the social determinants of health in accreditation mechanisms—and draws on a HiAP approach in the module for governance and health workforce policies.

Innovation and transformation of public health teaching will require strengthening lifelong learning systems to achieve integrated, people-centered prevention and care;[27] ensuring community-based and distributed public health education and training;[28] engaging and empowering communities in public health curriculum development;[29] transforming what, where, and how students learn to better address needs;[30] and transforming faculty development and leadership.

Lifelong learning systems can profoundly expand and transform the public health workforce. The conventional pipeline model cannot readily adapt the competencies and skills of public health professionals to the evolving health needs of communities and populations or ask them to acquire the competencies and skills necessary for effective cross-sectoral collaboration and teamwork. The emphasis and orientation that public health competencies are only developed in academic programs and settings—at the expense of continuing professional development—must be challenged.

A shift toward intersectoral planning for public health workforce education and training is needed. Schools, colleges, universities, and other tertiary educational institutions, community-based learning facilities, and health workplaces could gradually become integrated learning centers, which would form mutually reinforcing learning networks. It would be useful to establish diverse learning pathways with multiple entry and exit points that support continuous learning and career progression. Learning pathways could enable public health professionals to navigate between sites or levels and gain recognized competencies and qualifications throughout the life course. Together, such learning networks and learning pathways could form flexible, responsive lifelong learning systems. Such systems would help engage and empower communities in public health workforce curriculum development and foster people-centered, community-based, engaged, and distributed learning (learning that can occur independent of time and place in noncentralized locations).

To promote lifelong learning, many countries have developed a national qualifications framework to enable effective education, training, and employment policies, as well as a strategy for strengthening the governance of labor market and qualification systems. Information and data at all levels will be important to support evidence-based intersectoral planning and to monitor and evaluate public health workforce education, training, and opportunities for lifelong learning. Public health professional graduate tracking will provide valuable data on education and employment outcomes. WHO National Health Workforce Accounts and health workforce registries are first steps toward standardizing the health workforce information architecture.

A final point for public health workforce lifelong education is to expand and broaden the use of innovative information communications technology and social media. For example, professionals would benefit from opportunities for intersectoral communication to promote understanding of all perspectives, encourage the exchange of experiences, address complex intersectoral policy development, and foster policy implementation dialogue with stakeholders. The expanded use of information communications technology and social media could help public health professionals deliver effective, rapid, and evidence-based multisectoral responses during public health emergencies, natural disasters, and humanitarian crises.

There is a pressing need for socially accountable, transformative public health workforce education and training as part of a wider reorientation of the health system. Diverse and innovative learning pathways are necessary to evolve and expand effective learning opportunities linked to health employment. These learning pathways should include flexible and innovative models that could include hybrid and social media approaches for developing technical and applied experiential knowledge, skills, and attitudes that are relevant to practice.

Conclusion

Health education systems are obsolete, fragmented, and heavy on content and memorization. The education of those in the health professions has not kept pace with worldwide needs, evolving challenges, lifestyle changes, and technological and cognitive advances. Public health education, as part of the health education system, requires radical transformation to meet current and future population health challenges. World economic growth and development depends on a healthy population.[31] The need for a more competent health workforce requires a transformative approach to education and lifelong learning.

Our complex world requires reinventing the health education system to be more holistic, interprofessional, and ongoing. Health education must be viewed as a lifelong learning endeavor that requires the development of fundamental competencies within the formal system of education and diversification and mastery of them through practice and experience. Viewing education as lifelong requires a shift from the traditional time-based silos of formal educational programs to a continuum of formal, informal, practice-based, and team-based learning experiences. Competencies, assessment, learning experiences, and interprofessional approaches need to be continuously revisited and redefined. The time is ripe for change, but we must all work together to make it happen.

REFERENCES

1. World Health Organization. *WHO eBook on Integrating a Social Determinants of Health Approach into Health Workforce Education and Training.* Geneva: World Health Organization, 2015. http://www.who.int/hrh/resources/ebook _integrating_social_determinants/en.

2. World Bank. *Poverty and Shared Prosperity 2018: Taking on Inequality.* Washington, DC: World Bank Group, 2018.

3. World Bank. *Poverty and Shared Prosperity 2018.*

4. Council on Foreign Relations. "Global Conflict Tracker." https://www.cfr.org /interactives/global-conflict-tracker#! (accessed April 10, 2018).

5. United Nations. "United Nations High Commission for Refugees Global Report 2016." 2016. http://reporting.unhcr.org/sites/default/files/gr2016/pdf/Book _GR_2016_ENGLISH_complete.pdf (accessed April 10, 2018).

6. World Health Organization. *Working for Health and Growth: Investing in the Health Workforce.* Geneva: World Health Organization, 2016. http://www.who .int/hrh/com-heeg/reports/en.

7. World Health Organization. *Promoting Health in the SDGs.* Geneva: World Health Organization, 2017. http://www.who.int/healthpromotion/conferences /9gchp/shanghai-conference-report/en.

8. United Nations. "Transforming Our World: The 2030 Agenda for Sustainable Development." 2015. https://sustainabledevelopment.un.org/post2015 /transformingourworld/publication (accessed April 10, 2018).

9. Government of South Australia and the World Health Organization. *Progressing the Sustainable Development Goals through Health in All Policies: Case Studies from around the World.* Adelaide: Government of South Australia, 2017.

10. Winslow, C. E. A. "The Untilled Field of Public Health." *Modern Medicine* 2 (1920): 183–191.

11. Frenk, J., and S. Moon. "Governance Challenges in Global Health." *New England Journal of Medicine* 368 (2013): 936–942.

12. Woodward, D., N. Drager, R. Beaglehole, and D. Lipson. "Globalization and Health: A Framework for Analysis and Action." *Bulletin of the World Health Organization* 79 (2001): 875–881.

13. Frenk, J., O. Gomez-Dantes, and F. Chacón. "Global Health in Transition." In *Routledge Handbook in Global Public health*, edited by R. Parker and M. Sommer, 11–17. London: Routledge, 2011.

14. Fidler, D. P. "Health as Foreign Policy: Between Principle and Power." *Articles by Maurer Faculty* (2005): https://www.repository.law.indiana.edu/facpub /525.

15. Kickbusch, I., T. E. Novotny, N. Drager, G. Silberschmidt, and S. Alcazar. "Global Health Diplomacy: Training across Disciplines." *Bulletin of the World Health Organization* 85 (2007): 901–980.

16. Giovannini, M. J., and A. T. Brownlee. "The Contribution of Social Science to International Health Training." *Social Science and Medicine* 16 (1982): 957–964.

17. Fernandez, C. S., and D. Roberts. "Strengthening Negotiation Skills, Part I: How to Use Facets of Knowledge to Create Influence for Public Health Leaders." *Journal of Public Health Management and Practice* 21 (2015): 214–216.

18. Rayner, G. "Multidisciplinary Public Health: Leading from the Front?" *Public Health* 121 (2007): 449–454.

19. Pan American Health Organization. *46th Session of the Advisory Committee on Health Research*. (2017). http://iris.paho.org/xmlui/bitstream/handle /123456789/34305/PAHOKBR17019-eng.pdf?sequence=1&isAllowed=y (accessed December 15, 2017).

20. Frenk, J., L. Chen, Z. A. Bhutta, et al. "Health Professionals for a New Century: Transforming Education to Strengthen Health Systems in an Interdependent World." *Lancet* 376 (2010): 1923–1958.

21. United Nations, "Transforming Our World."

22. World Health Organization. *Global Strategy on Human Resources for Health: Workforce 2030*. Geneva, Switzerland: World Health Organization, 2016. http://www.who.int/hrh/resources/globstrathrh-2030/en.

23. International Labour Organization, Organisation for Economic Co-operation and Development, and World Health Organization. *Health Employment and Economic Growth: A Five-Year Action Plan (2017–21)*. Geneva: World Health Organization, 2016. http://www.who.int/hrh/com-heeg/com-heeg_actionplan2016 .pdf?ua=1.

24. United Nations, "Transforming Our World."

25. World Health Organization. *Health in All Policies: Training Manual*. Geneva: World Health Organization, 2015. http://apps.who.int/iris/bitstream /10665/151788/1/9789241507981_eng.pdf?ua=1&ua=1.

26. World Health Organization. *National Health Workforce Accounts: A Handbook*. Geneva: World Health Organization, 2016. http://www.who.int/hrh /documents/handbook_health_workforce_14a.pdf?ua=1.

27. Fisher J., K. Holmes, and B. Chakroun. "Transforming the Health Workforce: Unleashing the Potential of Technical and Vocational Education and Training." In *Health Employment and Economic Growth: An Evidence Base*, edited by J. Buchan, I. S. Dhillon, and J. Campbell, 281–306. Geneva: World Health Organization, 2017.

28. Transformative Education for Health Professionals. "Route 90 Collaborative." http://whoeducationguidelines.org/content/multimedia/video/route-90 -collaborative (accessed April 10, 2018).

29. World Health Organization. *Transforming and Scaling Up Health Professionals' Education and Training: Recommendations at a Glance*. Geneva, Switzerland: World Health Organization, 2013. http://whoeducationguidelines.org/content /recommendations-glance (accessed April 10, 2018).

30. Pálsdóttir, B., N. Cobb, J. Fisher, et al. "Enabling Universal Coverage and Empowering Communities through Socially Accountable Health Workforce Education." In *Health Employment and Economic Growth: An Evidence Base*, edited by J. Buchan, I. S. Dhillon, and J. Campbell, 307–340. Geneva: World Health Organization, 2017.

31. Pálsdóttir et al. "Enabling Universal Coverage and Empowering Communities through Socially Accountable Health Workforce Education." In Buchan, Dhillon, and Campbell, *Health Employment and Economic Growth*.

Envisioning a Future for Public Health Education across the Life Course

SANDRO GALEA AND LISA M. SULLIVAN

PUBLIC HEALTH ASPIRES to create a healthier world, one where we elevate the social, economic, and cultural forces that produce health.[1] This is a dynamic vision for public health, and one that requires that we work across sectors and are responsive to the emerging needs of populations, locally and globally. It requires a bold imaginative scope to grapple with the structures of health systems in West Africa, without which we may have outbreaks of Ebola in North America; federal pricing subsidies, which are in part responsible for widely available corn and encourage the production of calorie-dense, nutrient-poor foods that fuel the obesity epidemic; and issues around drug availability and the proliferation of prescription drugs that gave rise to the opioid epidemic that currently ravages the United States. Those of us who are entrusted with the responsibility to teach public health are faced with a challenge: how do we best train our profoundly passionate students to serve the mission of public health when they graduate while equipping them to deal with public health challenges 20 and 40 years hence, when they will be in positions of leadership in the field?

This book is an effort to help map out the universe of options that can provide an answer to that question. To do so, we aim to provide an overview of the core issues relevant to teaching public health today, but with an eye toward the future. Part I of the book grounded us in history and led to the present, as a survey of where public health teaching sits today. It also provided a conceptual orientation to public health teaching, touching on the key components that we need to consider in structuring our pedagogic approach to public health.

Part II discussed opportunities for public health teaching across the life course continuum. We started with bringing public health to high school students, then moved to undergraduate education, community colleges, and then to the currently modal teaching approaches in graduate schools of public health, at the master's and doctoral level. Part II concluded with an extension of the scope of public health teaching beyond formal programs into lifelong learning and asked readers to consider how we may best teach public health across professions, preparing our students to think beyond the public health sector.

Part III includes chapters on a range of innovative approaches to public health teaching that show promise both in their present incarnations and with an eye toward the future. We discuss course design and how innovative course design can transform the traditional "sage on a stage" approach to education. This can well be enhanced by efforts to maximize student engagement. We are alert to the rapidly changing demographics of the public health workforce and student body, as well as the need for public health to prepare students to serve whole populations. Therefore, we included chapters that discuss cultural competence and ways to teach in more diverse classrooms. As pedagogic scholarship evolves, it is becoming increasingly clear that active, engaged learners retain what we teach, and are also better equipped for learning, long after they complete formal degree programs. Chapters on active learning, practice-based teaching, teaching by the case method, group projects, and team-based learning presented the reader with primers on how to adopt these approaches in their classrooms toward the end of creating the best possible learning experience, one that stays with students and prepares them for a lifetime of learning. Part III also includes chapters on some of the—perhaps chronic—challenges that we teachers have faced, including how best to manage difficult conversations, how best to evaluate our teaching, and how to determine best practices around engaging teaching assistants. A chapter on service learning offered ways we can embed teaching in the community and how students can learn well by providing a service—doing well for themselves by doing good in the community.

Part IV looks toward the future, with the preceding chapter outlining the promise and potential of public health teaching. As we conclude the book, rereading it in its entirety and taking a 30,000-foot view, three observations strike us that we wish to share with the reader in hopes of sharpening our collective thinking and perhaps pointing a way forward toward ever-more effective teaching in public health.

First, academic public health has responded well, admirably so, to the evolving challenges of teaching and preparing our students to become the next generation of doers, teachers, and researchers in public health. The range of approaches that are covered in the book represents an extraordinary show of innovation that aims to find ways to better convey the core material of public health, engaging students and preparing them well for a future that shall, undoubtedly, look quite different than the present. Some of the material presented here represents a quantum leap in the field's thinking about our pedagogy. The embrace of student-centric teaching approaches such as case-based, practice-based, and active learning represents, to our minds, an effort by the field to be responsive to changing student learning styles, to the literature that teaches us how we learn best, and to anticipate what the future might hold and how we might best prepare students for successful careers and for the learning they will be doing over the course of their lives. This suggests a dynamic field, one that has not simply accepted a way of teaching that has lived on for decades but one that is making an effort to prepare itself for the pedagogic requirements of its second century. Our learning outcomes and pedagogy will appropriately continue to evolve. Measuring and critically reviewing markers of what we care about rather than concerning ourselves with what we can measure will strengthen all members of our learning communities. Adoption of these approaches makes public health teaching relevant, authentic, and practical, perhaps exactly as it should be as we prepare students for an uncertain world with the bold aspirations of public health powering their ambitions.

Second, public health education is inclusive, not only of a diversity of students and populations that we aim to serve but also of perspectives and ideas that shape the contours of our educational programs and initiatives. Chapters about teaching to diverse student bodies are, in some ways, the self-evident manifestation of this development. But chapters such as the one on handling difficult conversations offer guidance to the reader about how we may draw out and handle diversity of opinion in the classroom. Certainly, in our experience, we have no shortage of diversity of perspectives in the classroom, and recognizing this is a step in the right direction. Public health should be diverse, and it is part of our responsibility to ensure that we prepare our students for an ever-more diverse world. A student body that can embrace difficult issues, engage in respectful conversations with no simple answer, and work with diverse populations across (oftentimes competing) sectors is exactly the type of workforce that we collectively should want in our public health workforce. That public health teaching, as suggested by the chapters in this book, is indeed taking this approach is heartening.

Third, gone are the days when public health education meant only attaining a Master of Public Health (MPH) degree. The MPH remains a cornerstone of our educational programs, but we were struck, on reading the book, that the MPH is the subject of just one of twenty-six chapters. That does not, of course, diminish the importance of the MPH. It remains the foundational degree of nearly all public health programs as well as the de facto credential of the public health professional throughout the country and, increasingly, throughout the world. However, public health education has moved well beyond the MPH. Recognizing that our goal as a profession is to create a world whose social, economic, and cultural structures produce health, it is clear that we must engage in teaching across the life course, starting with high school and continuing all the way through to the end of our students' lifetime. That we have chapters showing examples of how we do just that is a testament to the field's responsiveness to this challenge, providing ongoing education that both creates the next generation of professionals dedicated to public health and works to educate the world about the forces that create health in populations, toward making those populations healthier.

Therefore, the book well suggests that public health education is relevant, authentic, and practical; that public health education is inclusive; and that public health education is ongoing. We have previously[2] suggested these as principles that can guide public health education and that can serve us well as we look ahead to public health gaining more prominence in our collective efforts to build a healthier world. We look forward to a world where these principles further shape our educational efforts, where our students remain engaged in learning throughout their lifetime, and where we embrace our responsibility to engage all sectors in the task of creating a healthier world. We hope that the book provides a useful primer to all its readers, allowing us to get ever better at our teaching toward this end.

REFERENCES

1. Galea, S., and G. J. Annas. "Aspirations and Strategies for Public Health." *Journal of the American Medical Association* 315, no. 7 (2016): 655–656.

2. Sullivan, L., and S. Galea. "A Vision for Graduate Public Health Education." *Journal of Public Health Management and Practice* 23, no. 6 (2017): 553–555.

cooperative learning, 46–49, 134–35, 210–11

core competencies: bachelor's degree programs, 56; cultural competency, 163; DrPH programs, 92–94; establishment, 209; in interprofessional education, 115–17, 120; MPH programs, 76–77; new/revised, 76–77, 139; traditional, 76, 139

core curriculum: changes, 139; clinical training-oriented, 16; for diverse student body, 172–78; innovative approach, 19–21; integrated, 80–81

Cornell Center for Teaching Innovation, 134

corporate university model, 105

Council on Education for Public Health (CEPH), 8, 16, 209

Council on Education for Public Health accreditation criteria, 31, 55, 75, 108; Applied Practice Experience, 232, 234; competency basis, 129–30; cultural competency training, 163; curriculum changes, 139; DrPH programs, 92, 93–94; Integrative Learning Experience, 232, 234; MPH programs, 75, 77; professional development, 57; revised, 18–19, 22; undergraduate programs, 55, 56–57, 61

Council on Linkages between Academia and Public Health Practice, 18

course design, 127–46; competencies, 129–31; content, 131–32; evaluation and response, 136–38; general principles, 128–32; in group-based service learning, 223–24; learning objectives, 128, 129–31, 132, 133–34, 140–41; in practice-based teaching, 200–206; special considerations, 138–41; structure, 133–35; syllabus, 135–36; Understanding by Design (UbD) framework, 130–32

course evaluations. See student ratings

Coursera, 83, 104, 107

critical analysis, 93

"Critical Component Elements" (ASPPH), 31

cross-cutting skills, 28, 30, 32, 34, 56, 76, 81, 93, 315

culminating projects. See capstone projects

cultural competency, 93, 164–66, 324

cultural competency training, 158–67; in service learning, 265–66. See also difficult conversation navigation; diverse classroom teaching

cultural exchange activities, 162

culture, 161

curriculum, 5, 9, 28–30, 34–36, 55–56, 57, 139. See also core curriculum; course design

data analysis skills, 84, 93–94, 315

De Beaumont Foundation, 31

Delphi process, 53, 76

dental care, 268–69

Dental Science (DDS)/MPH programs, 78

Des Moines University, 121–22

Dialogue Initiative, 175

difficult conversation navigation, 169, 246–60, 278–79; about microaggressions, 250–51, 256, 258; about race, 248, 249, 251–53, 256–57; in specific academic disciplines, 251–54

digital badges, 20, 103, 107

digital technology, 149

diplomacy skills, 314, 315

disabled individuals, technology for, 282–83

discussions, 184–85, 210–11, 236–37, 275–76. See also difficult conversation navigation

disequilibrium theory, 44–45, 170

displaced persons, 312

dissertations, 96–97

distance learning, 189

diverse classroom teaching, student-centered approach, 168–81, 324, 325–26; case study, 172–78; classroom behavior and environment, 176–77

diversity: difficult conversation navigation about, 246–61; faculty, 169; in interprofessional practice, 115–16; as MPH core competency, 76; of public health field, 246, 247; of public health workforce, 324; of US population, 168; in workplace, 27. See also cultural competency

syllabi, 132, 135–36, 255, 256
systems thinking, 76, 77

teaching assistants, 13, 188, 216–17
teaching assistant training programs, 284–95; mentor/supervisor relationship, 285–91
teaching effcctiveness evaluation, 300–302. *See also* student ratings
teaching portfolios, 302
team-based learning, 12, 20, 80, 153–54, 236, 237–38, 239; in interprofessional education, 121–22; with learning management systems, 276; in service learning, 267–68
teamwork, 117, 140, 203, 213, 221–22, 229
technology, in teaching, 23, 101–2, 272–83; in global public health, 81, 82; for individuals with disabilities, 282–83; in practice-based teaching, 201–2; types, 275–82
tell-help-share activities, 135
thinking: collaborative, 151–52; independent, 42–43; strategic, 153, 315
think-pair-share activity, 135, 150–51
360-degree evaluation, 229
Title IX, 286, 289
"Toss the Ball" learning activity, 46
TRAIN Learning Network, 102–3, 104, 108
transformational learning, 316
transparencies, 189–91
Trello, 202
Triple Aim, 114, 115, 118
Tulane University School of Public Health, 82

undergraduate education, public health, 19, 41–63; approach and strategies, 42–48; Critical Component Elements, 55–56. *See also* associate degree; bachelor's degree
Undergraduate Public Health and Global Health network, 67

underrepresented minorities, 168–69, 170–71, 249–50
Understanding by Design (UbD) framework, 130–32
United Nations (UN), 313, 316–17
universal design for learning, 155, 282–83
universal health coverage, 316, 317
University of Alabama at Birmingham School of Public Health, 80
University of Florida, 121
University of Memphis School of Public Health, 123
University of Minnesota, 122, 123
University of South Carolina, 122
University of Virginia, 252
University of Washington School of Public Health, 82
US Department of Education, 16, 19
US Department of Health and Human Services, 109
US Public Health Training Center, 109

values and ethics, 76, 93, 122
Vanderbilt University School of Public Health, 16
Veterans Health Administration, 102–3
veterinarians, 79, 105
Vygotsky, Lev, 47

web conferencing software, 281
Welch, William, 7, 8, 16
Welch-Rose report, 7, 16, 17–18
Who Will Keep the Public Healthy? (IOM), 110
Winslow, C.E.A., 89, 98, 314
workforce, in public health, 34–36, 107–8, 324; National Health Workforce Accounts, 317, 318–19; readiness, 31, 32, 69
World Health Organization (WHO), 113–14, 176, 312, 313, 317, 318–19

YouTube, 190, 277

zone of proximal development, 47